KT-423-810

Youth Policy and Social Inclusion

Critical debates with young people

Edited by
Monica Barry

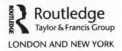
Routledge
Taylor & Francis Group

LONDON AND NEW YORK

First published in 2005 by Routledge
2 Park Square, Milton Park, Abingdon,
Oxon, OX14 4RN

Simultaneously published in the USA and Canada
by Routledge
270 Madison Ave, New York, NY 10016

Transferred to Digital Printing 2007

Routledge is an imprint of the Taylor & Francis Group, an informa business

© 2005 Monica Barry

Typeset in Sabon MT by J&L Composition, Filey, North Yorkshire
Printed and bound in Great Britain by TJI Digital,
Padstow, Cornwall

All rights reserved. No part of this book may be reprinted or
reproduced or utilised in any form or by any electronic,
mechanical, or other means, now known or hereafter
invented, including photocopying and recording, or in any
information storage or retrieval system, without permission in
writing from the publishers.

Every effort has been made to ensure that the advice and information in this book are true and accurate at the time of going to
press. However, neither the publisher nor the authors can accept
any legal responsibility or liability for any errors or omissions
that may be made. In the case of drug administration, any medical
procedure or the use of technical equipment mentioned within
this book, you are strongly advised to consult the manufacturer's
guidelines.

British Library Cataloguing in Publication Data
A catalogue record for this book is available from the British
Library

Library of Congress Cataloging in Publication Data
A catalogue record has been requested

ISBN 10: 0-415-31903-X (hbk)
ISBN 10: 0-415-31904-8 (pbk)
ISBN 13: 978-0-415-31903-4 (hbk)
ISBN 13: 978-0-415-31904-1 (pbk)

CN 362.7
AN 77076

Youth Policy and Social Inclusion

Critical debates with young people

Northern College
Library

NC01764

CANCELLED
N COLLEGE LIBRARY
BARNSLEY S75 3ET

Are socially excluded young people becoming an 'underclass', expecting everything but doing nothing to help themselves? Or are adults the problem – ignoring and exacerbating the real issues facing young people today?

Many young people lack status, rights and power because they fall between the two stools of protection and dependence as children and autonomy and self-determination as adults. They are also often considered by their elders to be rebellious and troublesome, and labelled with phrases such as 'underclass youth' and 'dangerous youth'.

This book critically examines these discriminatory attitudes and looks at the 'problem' of adults rather than the 'problem' of young people. Rather than focusing on the problems that young people *present to others* in society, this book emphasises the problems that young people *face from others*.

The authors ask searching questions about society's capacity and willingness to be more socially inclusive of young people in terms of policy and practice, and explore the extent to which young people have access to status, rights and responsibilities as young adults. The book takes an holistic and multi-disciplinary approach to identifying and analysing the factors which promote and exacerbate the social inclusion of young people, with contributors examining important themes and issues such as:

- citizenship;
- drug use;
- education;
- homelessness;
- rights;
- teenage pregnancy;
- unemployment;
- youth offending; and
- youth transitions.

The book is unique in that young people have also contributed their views on the issues and on the chapters in this book. Each young contributor describes their direct experiences and draws out the key issues from the academic contributions, suggesting ways forward for a more inclusive society in the future.

Youth Policy and Social Inclusion will appeal to a wide audience, including students, practitioners, policy makers and academics in the fields of social policy, social work, sociology, youth and community work, criminology, economics, education, housing and politics.

Monica Barry is a Research Fellow at the University of Stirling, working on youth offending, theories of desistance, youth transitions and social inclusion. She has a PhD in Criminology, is the Criminal Justice Research Adviser to the Association of Directors of Social Work and jointly edited the recent publication *Social Exclusion and Social Work: Issues of Theory, Policy and Practice* (Russell House).

Contents

Contributors

Monica Barry is a research fellow at the University of Stirling, working on youth offending, theories of desistance, youth transitions and social inclusion. She is the Criminal Justice Research Advisor to the Association of Directors of Social Work and is joint editor of *Social Exclusion and Social Work: Issues of theory, policy and practice* (1998) and author of *Challenging Transitions: Young people's views and experiences of growing up* (2001).

Saul Becker is Professor of Social Care and Health in the Institute of Applied Social Studies at the University of Birmingham. Prior to that he was Professor of Social Policy and Social Care, and Director of the Young Carers Research Group, at Loughborough University. He has researched and published extensively on informal care (particularly young carers), child welfare, poverty and social care issues.

Lynne Cox is a research assistant with the Centre for Research in Social Policy at Loughborough University. She has contributed to a range of projects, from service evaluations to a longitudinal qualitative study of youth, and has undertaken research on disabilities, including investigating the additional needs and costs of disabled people.

Chris Dearden is a Research Fellow in the Young Carers Research Group, which is located in the Department of Social Sciences at Loughborough University. Her research interests are children's issues, youth and transition to adulthood and issues around social care and informal care giving, especially young carers. She has also evaluated several support schemes and services for young people and is co-author, with Saul Becker, of *Growing Up Caring* (2000).

Michael Freeman is Professor of English Law at University College London. He is the author of *The Rights and Wrongs of Children* (1983), *The Moral Status of Children* (1997) and numerous other books and articles, many dealing with children's rights, child law and children's policy.

Peter Kemp is professor of social policy and director of the Social Policy Research Unit at the University of York. Between 1996 and 2002 he was professor of housing and social policy at the University of Glasgow. From 1990 to 1995 he was the Joseph Rowntree professor of housing policy and founding director of the Centre for Housing Policy at the University of York. His current research interests are housing benefit, social security and welfare to work.

Ruth Lister is Professor of Social Policy in the Department of Social Sciences, Loughborough University. She is a former Director of the Child Poverty Action Group and has published widely around poverty, income maintenance and citizenship. Her latest books are *Citizenship: feminist perspectives* (2nd edn., 2003) and *Poverty* (2004).

Greg Mannion is a lecturer within the Institute of Education, University of Stirling, teaching mainly on the Teaching Qualification in Further Education (TQFE) programme. His research interests include the socio-logical and spatial dimensions of schooling, lifelong learning and the emergence of learners' identities. Recent publications address issues such as school–college transition, social inclusion and adult–child relations.

Sue Middleton is Director of the Centre for Research in Social Policy, Loughborough University. She specialises in the study of poverty and social exclusion, particularly among children and young people, leading programmes of national and international research, much of which focuses on transitions to adulthood.

Ken Roberts is Professor of Sociology at the University of Liverpool. His main research areas are young people's transitions into the labour market, and the sociology of leisure. His books include *Youth and Leisure* (1983), *Youth and Employment in Modern Britain* (1995), *Leisure in Contemporary Society* (1999) and *The Leisure Industries* (2004).

Alison Rolfe is a Research Fellow in the School of Psychology at the University of Birmingham, currently conducting qualitative research on a longitudinal study of untreated heavy drinking. Her previous experience includes research on teenage motherhood, which was conducted in collaboration with NCH and formed the basis of her PhD. She has also completed research on young people and self-harm for NCH.

David Smith is a former probation officer who has taught at Lancaster University since 1976. He became Professor of Social Work in 1993 and Professor of Criminology in 2002. He has researched and published extensively on probation and youth justice. His most recent research has been on racist violence, witness support and Black, Asian and Irish experiences of probation and criminal justice.

Joan Smith has been the Director of the Centre for Housing and Community Research since 1989, which is now housed at London Metropolitan University. She has a particular interest in youth homelessness and social inclusion and her research publications include *The Family Background of Young Homeless People* (1998), *Taking Risks: An analysis of the risks of homelessness for young people in London* (1999), *Moving On, Moving Out* (2001) and *Dispersed Foyers* (2004).

Noel Smith is a Research Associate with the Centre for Research in Social Policy, Loughborough University. He has substantial experience of researching young people, including homeless youth, young Travellers, substance users and the longitudinal study of young people's transitions. His research interests include transitions, agency and social exclusion, and qualitative methodologies.

Kate Stanley is Senior Research Fellow and Head of Social Policy at the Institute for Public Policy Research (IPPR), Britain's leading progressive think tank. Her research covers welfare rights and responsibilities, equalities issues and carers, parents and children. Prior to joining the IPPR, she worked in the Policy and Research Unit of Save the Children UK where she specialised in asylum and refugee issues, children's rights and child poverty and published *Cold Comfort: young separated refugees in England* (2001).

Howard Williamson works in the School of Social Sciences at Cardiff University (Wales, UK) and is also a practising youth worker. Since 1992, he has been Vice-Chair of the Wales Youth Agency. He has conducted research and published extensively on a variety of 'youth issues', most notably the 'status zer0' research of the mid-1990s which led to wide-ranging policy interest in the exclusion of young people from learning. His current research includes a follow-up study (25 years on) of a group of young offenders he studied in the mid-1970s. In 2002 he was awarded a CBE for services to young people.

Rowdy Yates is Senior Research Fellow and facilitator of the Scottish Addiction Studies group in the Department of Applied Social Science, University of Stirling. He has worked in the drugs field for more than 30 years and, prior to this appointment, he was the Director and co-founder of the Lifeline Project, one of the longest established drug specialist services in the UK. He is the current president of the European Working Group on Drugs Oriented Research and vice-president of the European Federation of Therapeutic Communities and in 1994 received an MBE for services to the prevention of drug misuse.

Preface

Young people rarely see themselves as an integral, valued and recognised part of our society. Many young people argue that they need to have a greater 'voice', but my belief is that it is not young people's lack of a voice that is the problem but adults' lack of a willingness or capacity to listen and understand. Likewise many professionals working with young people say that they have too few rights to participation and integration, but I would argue that it is not a lack of legislation that is the problem but adults' lack of a willingness to implement it. In effect, it is suggested in this book that there is institutionalised 'ageism' against young people, perhaps based on a fear of change or a loss of power.

A fuller rationale for involving young people in this book is given in the introductory chapter. Suffice to say at this point that 'giving young people a voice' requires both gentle persuasion and cajoling – not of young people themselves, but of certain 'gatekeepers' whose responsibility to protect young people may at times clash with their desire to empower them. Fortunately, this task was made easier in this instance by the fact that the book was seen as worthwhile and young people's involvement as innovative within academic publishing.

Because of limited financial resources that resulted in academic authors receiving £50.00 per chapter and each young person £30.00 gift vouchers plus a copy of the book, it was not possible to comply with the insistence of one organisation – the National Youth Agency (NYA) – that young people should not contribute their views for anything less than £7.76 per hour. In my view, young people should be able to choose whether or not to contribute their views for less. Indeed, all the young people who wrote postscripts said that payment was not a prime motivation compared to the recognition and self-esteem they gained from contributing to an academic book and this was evidenced by their strong commitment to formulating and sharing their views about youth and youth policy. The NYA experience was fortunately an isolated incident and all the other organisations contacted were fully supportive of the exercise and more than happy to put me in touch with interested young people.

The enormous contribution of both the academic authors and the young people who wrote the postscripts is self-evident from the following chapters of this book, but I would nevertheless like to thank them again sincerely for their belief in the book and their commitment to the task of writing the chapters and postscripts.

The organisations that I would also like to thank include not only Save the Children (which gave both generous financial support to the project and provided access to young people in England, Scotland and Wales) and the publishers but also the following, whose help and encouragement are gratefully acknowledged:

- Article 12 Scotland
- Bethany Christian Trust
- Cardiff Youth Network
- Children in Wales
- Communities that Care
- Lothians Equal Access Programme for Schools
- Salford Foyer
- Sheffield Young Carers Project
- Who Cares? Scotland
- Wales Youth Agency
- Young Women's Christian Association (YWCA)
- Youth Justice Board
- Youthlink Wales.

Monica Barry,
May 2004

Chapter 1

Introduction

Monica Barry

Youth policy and social inclusion

Young people have few legitimate means to having their voice heard. This book offers them that voice. It also offers a major opportunity to turn the problem of 'youth' on its head and to question the extent to which 'adults' – their attitudes, policies and practices – ignore and exacerbate, rather than acknowledge and resolve, the problem of young people's social exclusion. The chapters in this volume ask searching questions about society's capacity and willingness to be more socially inclusive of young people. Whereas much of the academic focus in recent years has been on the problems that young people *present to others*, this book emphasises the problems that young people *face from others*. It addresses the fact that those who are older and more powerful than young people have rights and responsibilities which are not only denied to young people but are also used to further marginalise them.

Many young people lack status, rights and power in our society, not only by dint of their perceived vulnerability because of age but also because they fall between the two stools of protection and dependence as children and autonomy and self-determination as adults. They are also often labelled by their elders as rebellious and troublesome, and phrases such as 'underclass youth' and 'dangerous youth' abound within the overall context of 'a nation at war with its young' (Jeffs 1997). Brown (1998), for example, suggests that there is 'a recurring and ongoing preoccupation with the perceived threat to social stability posed by unregulated, undisciplined and disorderly youth'. And yet there is increasing qualitative research evidence to suggest that young people are largely conformist and conventional in their behaviour and aspirations (see, for example, Jeffs and Smith 1998, Williamson 1997). However, they are set apart from mainstream society by the often limited understanding and increasing pessimism of adults, and many young people are doubly constrained by poverty, their extended dependence on the family and state in the transition to adulthood, and by limited opportunities available to them for higher education, employment, housing and citizenship.

Youth policy is one of the key vehicles for ensuring that young people's social inclusion becomes more of a reality; another is a move towards non-discriminatory practices and attitudes of society, particularly towards young people. The combination of significant changes in attitudes and practices, and an innovative and genuinely inclusive youth policy could well pave the way for young people to begin to experience greater recognition and respect within our society. This book highlights the current and potential obstacles in the way of achieving that aim.

Several major government policy initiatives in recent years have focused on attempting to combat social exclusion (although not necessarily, by implication, to promote social inclusion) and on improving services and opportunities for children and young people. Starting with the early years, Sure Start focuses on poverty and disadvantage amongst pre-school children. Quality Protects is another Department of Health initiative aimed at transforming children's social services. The Connexions Service, developed by the Department for Education and Skills, is a multi-agency approach to tackling social exclusion amongst adolescents and school-leavers. These and other similar initiatives stress the need to give all young people, but in particular those from disadvantaged communities, the best start in life, through improved provision, advice and guidance and opportunities for personal and social development. However, there are still major deficiencies in the provision for, opportunities available to, and participation of, children and young people in the UK which question the effectiveness of such initiatives in promoting social inclusion.

Young (1999) talks of the relative deprivation of both rich and poor alike, with the former anxious to hold onto increasingly diminishing assets and the latter deprived of the rewards of affluence:

> Relative deprivation is conventionally thought of as a gaze upwards: it is the frustration of those denied equality in the market place to those of equal merit and application. But deprivation is also a gaze downwards: it is dismay at the relative well-being of those who although below one on the social hierarchy are perceived as unfairly advantaged.
> (Young 1999: 9)

Young people experience relative deprivation – the 'gaze upwards' – because of their age and, hence, status in the social hierarchy. Likewise, many adults may perceive young people as 'unfairly advantaged' – the 'gaze downwards' – thus creating an impasse that youth policy has yet to overcome. Young people are seen as newcomers to the adult world of potential power and influence. They are the perceived threat to an already precarious status quo and are therefore often scapegoated as a result. Much of the theoretical and policy-oriented literature on young people in the last decade has been predominantly about 'problem youth'; how to manage them and how to incorporate them into the status quo. Ironically, their separateness from 'adults' is merely exacerbated by the perceived need to integrate them into society. There seems to be a dearth of literature which (a) *challenges* existing theory, policy and practice in relation to social exclusion and (b) *questions* not only current inclusive approaches but also the current status of young people in society. This book is unusual in its acknowledgement of young people's potential for social *inclusion* as opposed to their propensity for social *exclusion*. It focuses on policies and practice that may affect opportunities for social inclusion of more disadvantaged young people in the age range 15–25. Topics have been identified which are the key areas of concern to young people and professionals alike.

Critical debates with young people

This book is particularly unusual in including contributions from young people who have direct experience of issues that affect them. It acknowledges that they are 'expert witnesses' in such matters and has provided them with the opportunity to comment and expand on the views of academics and policy makers. The postscripts are intended to supplement and elaborate, rather than to contradict or constrain, the contributions made by the chapter authors. The postscripts make it possible for young people with experience of the topics being addressed to explore their views further. The ultimate aim is to give specific groups of young people a platform from which to voice any concerns they may have about current academic and political thinking on particular issues of relevance to young people.

The majority of young people writing the postscripts suggested that they themselves came from disadvantaged backgrounds, but all the postscript contributors were asked to consider the specific problems that disadvantaged young people may have in terms of youth policy and social inclusion. It was originally felt that only those young people from disadvantaged backgrounds would be suitable commentators on matters relating to social exclusion. However, I have revised this opinion on the basis of the responses I received. It is not so much 'class' or 'poverty' per se but, more specifically, age that is most likely to differentiate young people as a minority group. Significantly, the young people from more affluent backgrounds experienced similar forms of discrimination as those from more disadvantaged backgrounds. Their lack of power, empowerment and rights as 'young people' classifies them as an homogeneous group and separates them from the status of 'adulthood', suggesting that age is possibly more of an inhibiting factor to social inclusion than class per se. Thus, 'disadvantage' comes as much from age as from one's socio-economic background.

Young people were approached by the editor of the book, via the auspices of chapter authors, statutory agencies and voluntary organisations working in the field. Those young people who expressed an interest in contributing to the debate about youth policy and social inclusion were asked to read either a 'user-friendly' summary of the relevant chapter provided by individual authors or the full chapter. They were then asked to comment on the strengths and weaknesses of the ideas contained in the chapter, to offer additional commentary based on their own experiences and to make further policy recommendations where appropriate. Each young person was given a gift voucher in lieu of payment and a complimentary copy of the book.

Seldom have theoretical, empirical or policy-oriented books on this subject ever encouraged written contributions from young people themselves. These postscripts are intended to help stimulate critical debate on topics relating to young people and social inclusion. All the postscripts have been written by young people with direct experience or knowledge of the topic on which they are commenting, and their biographical details at the start of each postscript highlight this fact. Often these biographical details say as much as the postscripts themselves about the premature and misjudged discrimination of adults towards young people.

Engaging with young people in this way has been for me a lesson in humility. They did not need cajoling, as many gatekeepers suggested they might, nor were they incapable of commenting on technical, academic prose. They understood the problem, they engaged wholeheartedly with the subject matter, they were enthusiastic about participating in the exercise and they did so within the tight timescale and budget allowed.

The postscripts are based very much on the contents of the chapter to which they are responding and are the main focus of the concluding chapter to this volume. The final section of this chapter therefore outlines the main thrust of the arguments of the academic contributions contained within the book.

Layout of the book

This volume is split into two parts: Part I contains the chapters relating to the wider issues of youth policy and social inclusion for young people – depicting more the political rhetoric of youth policy rather than the actuality for young people. This section contains six chapters on youth policy, citizenship, young people's rights, education, transitions and leisure (Chapters 2–7, respectively).

Chapter 2 sets the scene for a more in-depth analysis of youth policy initiatives in recent years. Howard Williamson highlights New Labour's commitment to social inclusion, notably in relation to 'status zer0' youth and its focus on opportunities for education, training and employment as a means of reducing the likelihood of further exclusion from, for example, drug use, teenage pregnancy and offending behaviour. However, as with several chapters in this volume, Howard Williamson suggests that the government continues to take a punitive approach to the behaviour of young people, thus labelling young people as the root cause of the problem rather than wider social structures.

Chapter 3 argues that renewed attempts at promoting citizenship amongst young people only serve to reinforce their exclusion by highlighting them as 'deficient' in terms of their potential for political and social apathy and disengagement. Ruth Lister and her colleagues instead suggest that young people themselves see citizenship in more proactive terms – based on their sense of identity, active participation in society and employment opportunities. The authors draw on the findings from their recent longitudinal study of 16–23 year olds' perceptions of citizenship to refute the notion of young people as disengaged or apathetic. On the contrary, these young people demonstrated a high level of commitment and responsibility to the wider society, irrespective of their 'rights'.

In Chapter 4, Michael Freeman stresses the importance of rights in discourses on social inclusion and exclusion. Rights are seen by many policy makers as a 'militant concept' and, as such, while seemingly supported in principle by the state, they are rarely enacted in practice through legislation. Michael Freeman points out that although children's rights are increasingly addressed by governments, there is no similar move to address the rights of young people, but he draws out the main reasons why the UN Convention on the Rights of the Child (up to the age of 18) can as easily apply to young people beyond the age of 18 in terms of participation, education, employment and a respect for autonomy.

Chapter 5 suggests that tackling social exclusion does not necessarily enhance young people's social inclusion, not least in relation to the important sphere of education. Greg Mannion argues that the government's focus on social exclusion is informed by often misleading assumptions – that reducing exclusion requires employment; that social inclusion is a future goal rather than a current need for young people; and that only those young people 'at risk' of social exclusion should be targeted. Drawing on actor network theory (ANT) and concepts of habitus and capital, Greg Mannion explores how learning takes place during the transition from childhood to adulthood and illustrates the significance of young people's preferred sources of information, their support networks and their decision-making processes.

Chapter 6 compares models of youth transition with the reality for many young people. It cites the work of anthropologists who have identified a 'liminal' period in the 'rites of passage' for young people. Within this liminal phase of marginalisation from mainstream society, young people have neither the status nor the attributes of either protected children or autonomous adults and they tend to turn towards their peers for support. Monica Barry draws on the views and experiences of particular groups of disadvantaged young people to illustrate the potentially discriminatory attitudes and structures towards them because of their age and status. She concludes that their lack of opportunities, encouragement and trust merely serve to exacerbate young people's socio-legal exclusion from the wider society.

In Chapter 7, Ken Roberts compares and contrasts the meaning of leisure for young people with that of governments, which tend to view youth leisure in terms of regulating potential trouble. The author is critical of government policy that prioritises leisure as a vehicle towards integration and conformity. For young people themselves, leisure and youth culture are more a vehicle towards self- and social-identity and individuality, a vehicle through which they can gain the freedom to express themselves without undue surveillance and control by their elders. Ken Roberts argues that whilst the unemployed are the most marginalised when it comes to accessing leisure facilities, incorporating leisure on the social inclusion agenda will not in the longer term resolve the low socio-economic status of young people.

Part II of the book examines the reality for certain populations of young people. It contains chapters on both specific issues (youth unemployment, youth homelessness, youth justice and drug misuse amongst young people – Chapters 8, 9, 11 and 14, respectively) and specific groups (young asylum seekers, young mothers and young carers – Chapters 10, 12 and 13, respectively).

Chapter 8 highlights the changes in the youth labour market over the last 30 years which has left the school-to-work transition an extended and fragmented experience for many young people, notably those with multiple disadvantages. Peter Kemp argues that New Labour's focus on employability rather than the availability of appropriate jobs prolongs the 'deficit model'. While he suggests that New Labour's commitment to tackling the issues surrounding young people's social exclusion is evident through its New Deal initiative, he concludes that those young people most at risk of social exclusion are still discriminated against in this and other employment policy initiatives.

Chapter 9 suggests that social exclusion for young homeless people arises not only as a result of changes in family stability and formation but also as a result of government policy relating to employment, state benefits and affordable housing. Joan Smith notes that homelessness is more likely for young people who experienced other forms of disadvantage as children, such as poverty, school exclusion, physical abuse and family instability. She highlights the work of the Foyer Federation, which aims to alleviate social exclusion amongst young homeless people by providing supported accommodation, advice, education and training opportunities.

Having been dependent on people smugglers and traffickers to escape persecution and insecurity in their own countries, many young asylum seekers experience yet further uncertainty and marginalisation on arrival in the UK. In Chapter 10, Kate Stanley highlights the problems facing such young people as a result of government policies that deny them access to certain services and rights based on age, immigration status and country of origin. The chapter concludes that there is an urgent need for a more inclusive approach to young asylum seekers and refugees in the UK to ensure that their needs and aspirations are met, their skills invested in and their lives normalised as quickly and as fully as possible.

Chapter 11 gives an overview of youth justice policy in recent years, drawing similarities between previous Conservative law and order policies and those of the current New Labour administration. David Smith tempers much of the criticism aimed at the present government's approach to youth justice by citing positive research evidence of effective, welfare-oriented policies both north and south of the border. However, he suggests that there is an increasing emphasis on crime and punishment at the expense of wider issues for young people such as unemployment and poverty. He highlights the need for a greater public awareness and understanding of the difficulties facing young offenders and for more constructive programmes to address offending, such as restorative justice.

Chapter 12 compares the government line on teenage pregnancy with the views of young mothers themselves and questions the extent to which policy and practice actually help or hinder the social inclusion of young people with children. Societal reactions towards teenage pregnancy are also misguided, given that rates of teenage pregnancy in England and Wales have been falling since the 1970s, especially amongst under 18 year olds. Alison Rolfe highlights young mothers' feelings of discrimination and marginalisation and concludes that the effect of policies for this group of young people tends to exacerbate rather than alleviate their increasing social exclusion.

In Chapter 13, Chris Dearden and Saul Becker describe the situation for young carers, highlighting the fact that many families do not have access to good quality and affordable community-based services, that community care is under-resourced and that government policy tends to assume the availability of family carers to fill the gaps in service provision. Some four per cent of young people aged 18–24 in the UK will have been regular carers of ill or disabled relatives as children, often on a full-time basis, and such caring work can often have severe repercussions for them both as children and young adults, exacerbating feelings of social exclusion.

In Chapter 14, Rowdy Yates gives an overview of research on drugs and alcohol over the last half century, highlighting the shift from a medical to a social model of substance misuse. The author suggests that there are few services which have adequate resources or staff with specialist training to work with young people experiencing drugs problems, and yet the UK has one of the highest rates of experimentation and problem drug use in Europe. The chapter concludes that policy and practice are perhaps 'out of touch' with the reality for many young people – notably those with other manifestations of social exclusion, such as depression, loneliness and inadequate access to support services.

Finally, Chapter 15, Conclusions, draws together the common threads from the chapters, concentrating in particular on the young people's postscripts to highlight the need to adopt a more holistic approach to the problems facing young people in the UK today. The common themes emerging from policy and practice that impinge on young people's social inclusion are highlighted, as is the need for a change in professional and public attitudes towards young people along the lines envisaged by young people themselves.

References

Brown, S. (1998) *Understanding Youth and Crime: Listening to youth?* Buckingham: Open University Press.

Jeffs, T. (1997) 'Changing their ways: Youth work and "underclass" theory', in R. MacDonald (ed.), *Youth, the 'Underclass' and Social Exclusion*, London: Routledge.

Jeffs, T. and Smith, M. (1998) 'The Problem of "Youth" for Youth Work', *Youth and Policy*, No. 62: 45–66.

Williamson, H. (1997) 'Status Zer0 youth and the "underclass": Some considerations,' in R. MacDonald (ed.), *Youth, the 'Underclass' and Social Exclusion*, London: Routledge.

Young, J. (1999) *The Exclusive Society*, London: Sage.

Part I

Overarching themes

Chapter 2

Young people and social inclusion – an overview of policy and practice

Howard Williamson

A few years ago, I invented a mythical androgenous character called Tommy (or Tammy) Butler and mapped his life chances in each decade since the Second World War (Williamson 2001a). He (for it was more likely to be 'he' – four out of five 'socially excluded' young people are young men (House of Commons Education Committee 1998)) epitomised that classic disadvantaged young person who, as youth transitions became more complex (Furlong and Cartmel 1997), became increasingly at risk of social exclusion. The fact that Tommy's initials are the same as Tony Blair's is no coincidence. In 1999, when the Prime Minister launched *Bridging the Gap* (Social Exclusion Unit 1999a) he made an implicit promise to the likes of Tommy: social *inclusion* was a top priority for the new Labour government. New measures would be put in place to maximise young people's participation in education and training (the best protective factor against social exclusion) and to minimise their risks of dropping out. There would be both *generalised* initiatives to support and involve all young people and more *targeted* measures directed at particular groups of young people (such as young offenders) or at particular issues (such as teenage pregnancy and young motherhood). Prior to this commitment by the government, at least until the mid–1990s, Tommy and Tammy Butler and their contemporaries across different generations had steadily slipped off the policy radar map.

That 'map' has, however, been redrawn quite dramatically in the past few years. When New Labour was elected in 1997, I was asked to depict the framework of policy and practice directed at young people. On a single sheet of paper I portrayed the 'top down' government departments and the various soundbites reflecting Labour's aspirations ('education, education, education', 'rights *and* responsibilities', 'a hand up not a hand out', 'tough on crime, tough on the causes of crime'). I sought to connect these to the issues and needs of young people, both in general terms (education, training and employment; leisure time opportunities) and in relation to groups of young people with specific needs (such as looked after children), in specific circumstances (such as homeless young people) and presenting specific challenging behaviours (such as young offenders). In the middle, I portrayed the policy measures in place at the time: schooling and youth training, the youth service, social services, and the 'correctional' services of police, probation and prisons. That map would be almost unrecognisable today, for it would be overlaid with the raft of new measures with which this chapter is concerned. First, however, the basis for the re-thinking and re-casting of policy and practice needs to be considered.

Youth research tells us many different stories about young people. At times it perhaps tells us more about the theoretical (and political) persuasions of the researchers than about young people themselves. More 'disadvantaged' young people have certainly been a primary focus of youth research, but qualitative studies – through pointing up their strategies of resistance and avoidance (see, for example, Hall and Jefferson 1976) – have, in some ways, romanticised their position at the margins. Such research is engaging and persuasive, but it can conceal the evidence provided by more pedestrian surveys of young people, which indicate forcefully that the vast majority of young people – including those at the margins – aspire to modest and mainstream futures. And what we do know, from both qualitative and quantitative studies, is that an increasing minority of young people, as a result of changing patterns of youth transitions (Johnston *et al* 2000, Barry 2001), are at risk of being unable to fulfil such aspirations – for a job, a home, a family and a car. More vulnerable young people are more at risk (Coles 1997) and public policy during the years of Conservative government often compounded young people's pathways to exclusion (Williamson 1993). Young people may have been perceived as *causing* problems, eliciting punitive policy responses on this front. But in equal, though less acknowledged, measure, they were *experiencing* problems: they had become trapped in a 'chronic crisis of young adulthood' (Williamson 1985). They were, de facto, 'trapped as teenagers' (Williamson 1990). During the 1960s and early 1970s it had been argued that policies of 'non-intervention' (Schur 1973) served young people best. By the 1980s and 1990s, however, such apparent 'benign neglect' was tantamount to 'malign indifference' (Drakeford and Williamson 1998): it was clear that more vulnerable young people required more robust levels of positive intervention and support. In fact, policy towards young people had been working in the reverse direction. Social security (income support) entitlements had been withdrawn from 16 and 17 year olds in 1988 in return for a youth training 'guarantee', but this had been significantly unfulfilled (Maclagan 1992). In 1988, the Prime Minister, Margaret Thatcher, rejected the idea that there should be any public policy response to the burgeoning numbers of homeless young people (*Hansard*, 7th June 1988). These are but two examples. The cumulative outcome of these and similar policies in education (where school exclusions rose at least threefold during the 1990s) and in youth justice (where the mantra advanced by Prime Minister John Major was that we should 'understand a little less, and condemn a little more') was the steady emergence of a population of 'socially excluded' young people. These have variously been depicted as 'status zer0' or 'NEET' young people, although these terms refer specifically to those young people who are not in education, training or employment. This is, however, a crude proxy by which wider forms of 'social exclusion' may be defined, for early drop-out from mainstream pathways in education, training and employment is closely linked to greater probabilities of, for example, substance misuse, offending behaviour and teenage pregnancy (Social Exclusion Unit 1998, 1999a, 1999b, 2000). Non-participation in education, training and employment has therefore become the 'lever' for policy development and implementation across much broader territory. 'Status zer0', although originally devised (as 'status A', then 'status 0' and then 'status zer0') as a technical term to portray those outside of mainstream learning pathways (Istance *et al* 1994, Williamson 1997), has become a metaphor for young people who apparently counted for nothing and were apparently going nowhere. It was to these young people that New Labour's 'youth policy' turned its attention.

From a position of political denial in the early 1990s, there had been a gradual, and often grudging, political acknowledgement of the *scale* of the challenge of young people's social exclusion. Indeed, the Conservative government, shortly before its defeat, had established Relaunch (subsequently re-branded by Labour as New Start in England, and, throughout, called the Youth Access Initiative in Wales). This was a strategy for maintaining the engagement of young people with mainstream schooling and for re-integrating those who had already been excluded. It was hastily conceived, but at least it paid lip service to the issue. More tellingly, an early inquiry under New Labour by the House of Commons Education Committee (1998) asserted that disengagement from learning was 'not a residual policy problem, but a significant policy challenge'. This upped the ante for a government which had at its heart, at least rhetorically, social policy aspirations around social inclusion, active citizenship, lifelong learning and community safety. This suggested the need for a clear focus on 'youth policy' and a more robust and integrated policy response to the needs of more vulnerable and socially excluded young people.

The raft of measures which have been talked up (and sometimes put in place) since 1997 is legion. Even though the *practice* may continue to be subject to criticism, for many reasons, the Labour government (in London) has not only conceded the scale of the 'problems' to be addressed but also has sought – commendably – to distinguish and differentiate between different groups of 'socially excluded' young people. The predicaments facing young people may appear to be much the same (for example, unemployment or homelessness) but the reasons for those predicaments may be diverse – and, in turn, demand a calibrated policy response. Where responsibility for producing that policy response has been devolved to national administrations in Wales, Scotland and Northern Ireland, similar calibration in policy responses has also been attempted. From a policy perspective, such differentiation is a daunting challenge. The Blairite mantra of 'joined-up solutions to joined-up problems' may command an immediate appeal (and makes complete sense) but it rests uncomfortably with the parallel need to deconstruct the analysis of what needs to be done across policy domains (education, housing, health), between social groups of young people (by gender, race, 'class' and geography), and at different levels of administration (UK, devolved government and regional levels). There are, further, initiatives on the 'youth policy' question at supra-national level which, although they are required to take notice of rules of 'subsidiarity', add to the complexity of the challenge. Joining-up is necessary in a variety of both horizontal and vertical directions.

On this account, it is virtually impossible to present the full catalogue of measures which have now been established within and around the challenge of social inclusion. Indeed, specific initiatives directed towards socially excluded young people dovetail with wider measures concerned with the promotion of active citizenship, lifelong learning and community safety. To separate one from the others would produce a false picture, for they all rest within the same grid or along the same continuum, yet to embrace everything risks producing an impenetrable maze. With these points in mind, the remainder of this chapter will highlight some of the most prominent initiatives, endeavour to tease out the extent to which they have contributed to the 'social inclusion' agenda and identify the issues that have emerged during the process of their development and implementation.

The two most immediate, and expensive, developments were concerned with the labour market and the youth justice system. Both had a high political priority, for they enshrined two of the five 'pledges' made by New Labour on taking office: the movement of 250,000 long-term unemployed young adults from welfare to work, and the cutting by half of the time it took for persistent young offenders to come to court (from 142 to 71 days). These were the headline targets to allay populist concerns about idle youth and youth crime. The more detailed policies and practice around the New Deal and the Youth Justice Board were clearly related to analyses which addressed the 'risk' factors to do with social exclusion and the 'protective' factors which might prevent it. The New Deal denied young people receiving benefit for more than 6 months the option of remaining unemployed. It was heralded as radically different from previous government youth training schemes: it was a programme which could be tailored to the needs and aspirations of the individual. It was a national programme, but with local flexibility determined by local labour market information. The New Deal was 'rolled out' nationally in April 1998 – a massive achievement. Within two years, it had met its 'pledge'. Like most recent government initiatives, it has been subjected to academic criticism (see Jeffs and Spence 2000; Chapter 8 this volume), but it should be credited not only for investing some £3 billion in young people but also for some of its innovations, not least the concept of the 'Gateway'. This is a period of up to four months during which delivery partners must seek to address those factors in unemployed young people's lives (such as literacy and numeracy problems, or drug dependency) which constitute 'barriers to employment'. In launching the New Deal, Chancellor Gordon Brown had proclaimed: 'The era of social exclusion is over and the era of economic prosperity has begun'. The extent to which the New Deal has in fact promoted social inclusion, especially of the most disadvantaged, is debatable and can be probed at many levels. Critics will point to the fact that a key indicator of success – 'sustainable employment' – is defined as job retention for more than a meagre 13 weeks. The New Deal kicked off in buoyant economic times, giving it a strong chance of 'success'. For the purposes of this chapter, attention will be drawn to two concerns. First, the New Deal has clearly failed to engage effectively with the *most* disadvantaged people, despite attention being paid to this issue, and alternative strategies proposed, after early indications of significant numbers leaving the New Deal for 'unknown destinations' (see Adebowale 1999). Secondly, the punitive sanctions regime was in fact strengthened, with no consultation, by the Secretary of State, early in 2000 as a result of evidence of the number of young people (around 8%) refusing to participate in the New Deal. These two factors – insufficient flexibility and over-coercion – are common features across policy domains that preclude the possibility of effective practice when it comes to young people facing multiple disadvantage – those who are *most* socially excluded.

The youth justice reforms instituted since 1998 have also come under the academic hammer as manifestations of a 'new authoritarianism' (Pitts 2003) and expressions of the 'criminalisation of social welfare' (Goldson 2002, Chapter 11 this volume). Yet they can be viewed from quite another perspective. Discredited approaches from the past, whether purportedly concerned with 'treatment' or 'punishment', were abandoned in favour of one single objective: the prevention of offending by young people. Since its inception in 1998, the Youth Justice Board has recognised that the best chance of preventing offending, or further offending, by young people is through ensuring swift attention to their family circumstances, their health and their education needs. In this respect, approaches developed within the youth justice system, although also concerned with young people taking responsibility for their offending behaviour, can be viewed as a strategy for social inclusion. Such approaches are not, of course, primarily concerned with social inclusion per se, but the evidence points clearly to the fact that offending behaviour is linked to other indicators of exclusion and that offending histories make the possibility of social inclusion even more remote. Hence, the recently established prevention strategy of the Youth Justice Board, which was foreshadowed by the summer SPLASH programmes that have now been converted, and taken over by the Department for Education and Skills, to more integrated delivery under the banner of Positive Activities for Young People. Few in educational and youth services would deny that such practice is urgently needed as a mechanism for social inclusion, even if they were previously cautious when it was solely within the remit of crime prevention objectives. Further down the offending track, efforts to ensure the proper provision of education for young people in custody and to develop appropriate support and throughcare when offenders return to the community should also be viewed as inherently a social inclusion agenda. The recent PRISE (Planned Resettlement into Secure Employment) initiative, being developed by a partnership of some half a dozen interested organisations, will endeavour to provide better prospects for young offenders than they had before. The Youth Justice Board has also sought to divert young people from custody through its ISSP (Intensive Supervision and Support Programme) initiative, which requires young people to be supervised for a minimum of 25 hours a week. This is designed not only to win public confidence for non-custodial penalties, and the support of the courts, but also, arguably, to provide structure, purpose and direction in the lives of young people whose previous existence was disorganised and chaotic. There are, inevitably, different ways of evaluating such measures, but to dismiss them out of hand is tantamount to colluding with the marginalisation of those who are most at risk in contemporary society. Even the Children's Rights Alliance for England asserted recently that the Youth Justice Board had effected a 'miraculous transformation' in the conditions of young people within the juvenile secure estate, albeit, admittedly, from a very low base (Hodgkin 2002).

The New Deal is a UK-wide programme, though with some significant adaptations within the devolved administrations. The youth justice system referred to above applies only to England and Wales, though Wales is in the process of establishing, in conjunction and consultation with the Youth Justice Board, its own All-Wales Youth Offending Strategy. This is to be closely connected to Extending Entitlement, the youth support service in Wales, which is parallel and equivalent to Connexions in England. Extending Entitlement, in theory at least, encapsulates a broader vision than Connexions and is premised upon a rather different philosophy. In its analysis of the social exclusion of young people, it asserts that for young people to develop the skills and competencies for both 'employability' and full civic participation in society, they need to be exposed to a 'package' of opportunities and experiences. Many young people avail themselves of such a 'package of entitlement' through private means and initiative, and through family support. The 'package' includes, at its heart, retention and achievement in formal education (reflecting firmly the Connexions agenda), but it also includes, inter alia, non-formal learning opportunities, away from home experiences, access to new technologies and the chance to be involved in sports, music and the arts. Socially excluded young people get very little exposure to such a 'package': Extending Entitlement, through the work of Young People's Partnerships at the local authority level, seeks to ensure that they do. Extending Entitlement is, therefore, forcefully premised upon a social inclusion agenda. It attempts to reach those young people who will not, or cannot, gain access to the 'package of entitlement' by other means.

The related Connexions Service in England was the direct outcome of two government documents published in 1999: *Bridging the Gap* (Social Exclusion Unit 1999a) and *Learning to Succeed* (DfEE 1999). Both flagged up the imminent establishment of 'a new support service' for young people, which would bring together the Careers Service and 'some parts' of the Youth Service. The marriage of the two partners has been a stormy one, with suspicion on both sides. Nonetheless, an often uneasy relationship has been sustained and, after a couple of years of pilot development, Connexions throughout England was finally launched in May 2003. Connexions is designed to provide 'the best start in life for every young person'. It has been cleverly marketed as a 'universal service differentiated according to need'. Thus, while all young people between the ages of 13 and 19 will, at least notionally, have a 'personal adviser', those requiring more intensive support and intervention, or who need referral to more specialist provision, will secure a disproportionately greater amount of personal advisory contact time. Early indications are that Connexions has, in some of the pilot areas, made a significant difference to the retention of young people in learning, and early inspection reports by OFSTED have largely (though by no means always) been favourable. A national evaluation by the Youth Studies Unit at De Montfort University will illuminate the matter further and draw firmer conclusions about the extent to which Connexions has ensured appropriate support for more disadvantaged young people, and not simply forestalled their predicted pathways towards a future of unemployment.

In Wales, the youth service was always considered to be a key partner in the vision of Extending Entitlement. This was far from the case in England, where youth services felt that their historical skills in reaching out to, and working with, more marginalised young people, had been overlooked (or noted but ridiculed) in policy development. Indeed, one Minister described the youth service as the 'can't do, won't do service', which some felt was tantamount to its death knell and supplanting by Connexions. This has not, however, materialised. There is, indeed, a new sense of hope and purpose for the youth service since the publication of *Transforming Youth Work* (DfEE 2001) and especially since the publication of *Resourcing Excellent Youth Services* (DfES 2002b). These have, for the first time, placed youth work on a more secure financial footing but, in return, demanded more demonstrable evidence of its efficacy and impact. Youth work would argue, of course, that had it been properly resourced in the past, there would have been little need for new initiatives such as Connexions. Although fundamentally a universal service, youth work had always 'differentiated according to need' and focused much of its attention on the social inclusion (and participation) agenda. Once again, the impact of youth work awaits a national evaluation, which is also to be carried out by the Youth Affairs Unit at De Montfort University. But Tom Wylie, chief executive of the National Youth Agency, maintains that the 'architecture' is now in place for youth work to make a proper and professional difference on a range of policy objectives concerning young people – including social inclusion.

Connexions was also a by-product of the work of the Social Exclusion Unit which, in 2000, as part of its work on a national strategy for neighbourhood renewal (which involved deliberation on key challenges by 16 Policy Action Teams (PATs)), produced a seminal report on the circumstances of more disadvantaged and excluded young people – *PAT 12* (Social Exclusion Unit 2000). This identified both the risk factors at play and the longer-term consequences of social exclusion. It argued for more integrated services and a greater emphasis on prevention. The direct outcome of PAT 12 was the setting up of the Children and Young People's Unit (CYPU), in November 2000, overseen by a high-level inter-departmental Ministerial committee, and the appointment of the first Minister responsible for children and young people. The CYPU drove forward a set of principles upon which practice with children and young people should be developed. At its core were principles of participation and consultation, and a Children's Fund of some £450 million over three years was put at the disposal of the CYPU for the development of community-based preventative initiatives. A dedicated budget for youth participation was also made available, which in some respects may be seen as contributing to the mainstreaming of work that has been pioneered by Save the Children (Treseder 1997) and the Carnegie Young People Initiative (see, for example, Cutler 2002) in the UK. It has also more recently been advocated at the level of the European Union (European Commission 2001), although it has always been central to the thinking within the youth work of the Council of Europe (see Williamson 2002b). The burning issue, however, is whether or not such approaches to engaging with young people, and developing policy from their agendas, ever really reaches more marginalised and 'disorganised' young people (see Kirby and Bryson 2002). It has, however, impacted upon some of the most vulnerable groups of young people, notably looked after children (young people in public care) for whom advocacy and consultation processes have produced renewed policy commitment to their welfare and their futures. *Quality Protects* (DoH 1999), in England, and parallel initiatives elsewhere, have sought to ensure – after a wave of child abuse scandals in children's homes, particularly in Wales – proper support for looked after children, whose record in education has been abysmal (some 75 per cent leaving school with no qualifications whatsoever) and who disproportionately experience unemployment and homelessness on leaving care.

In mainstream schooling more generally, the provision for 'disapplication' of young people in key stage 4 (15 and 16 year olds) has allowed for the development of alternative curricula for young people at risk of exclusion or alienated from the national curriculum. These developments, in the late 1990s, have provided a platform for the restructuring of 14–19 learning, through *Choice and Excellence* in England (DfES 2002a) and *Learning Pathways 14–19* in Wales (Welsh Assembly Government 2002b). Both seek to provide young people with greater flexibility in the pathways they take, which will hopefully instil greater motivation to learning, and lifelong learning, and reduce the likelihood of drop out, alienation and exclusion. In this way, education policy is seeking to address the entrenched problem of significant numbers of young people dropping out of learning at or before the minimum age, never to return, when evidence suggests quite unequivocally that the acquisition of formal educational qualifications remains the best protective factor against social exclusion (House of Commons Education Committee 1999; see also Chapter 5 this volume).

Coupled to the greater flexibility being developed in academic and vocational learning is the emergence of 'citizenship' education. This may be viewed as the mirror image to initiatives specifically designed to combat social exclusion. The promotion of active citizenship has been strengthened not only through the establishment of citizenship education in schools (since September 2002) but also through a range of extra-curricular 'volunteering' measures such as Millennium Volunteers (MV). MV – which requires young people to complete 100 or 200 hours of regular voluntary service in order to achieve national accreditation – was originally envisioned to be part of the social inclusion agenda, just as the European Voluntary Service programme was at the European level (European Commission 1995). The indications are, however, that such opportunities have largely been taken up by more included young people, as value-added elements to their CV, rather than by more excluded young people – although those responsible for these initiatives would challenge this assertion. The same argument is also often levelled at personal development programmes such as the Duke of Edinburgh Award and the ASDAN Youth Achievement Award, though, in the former case, there is evidence of it operating effectively with young people in custody, for whom it may provide a spur to shifting the direction of their lives. In the round, however, there are concerns that such measures, even if they are purportedly directed at socially excluded young people, tend to be seized by less excluded groups, sometimes thereby marginalising the more marginalised even further (see Chapter 3 this volume).

Beyond the formal and non-formal learning sectors, there have been other policy developments which might contribute to the social inclusion of young people. In health, the UK-wide drugs strategy, *Tackling Drugs to Build a Better Britain* (HM Government 1998), has recognised the prevalence of a diversity of illegal drug use by young people (see also Chapter 14 this volume). As a result, it made young people – through education and prevention – one of its key strategic priorities (although these have recently been revised). Yet more critical commentators have alleged that practice rarely reaches those with whom it needs to engage (see Parker *et al* 2001). Moreover, young substance misusers (and it should be noted that the Welsh strategy is concerned with substance misuse, rather than illegal drugs per se) often have a range of mental health problems, as indeed do young offenders. Child and Adolescent Mental Health Services (CAMHS) remain thin on the ground, despite some recent political focus in England and an already launched strategy document in Wales (Welsh Assembly Government 2002a). The picture is almost equally gloomy in relation to sexual health, where sexually transmitted infections are increasingly in prevalence amongst young people and levels of teenage pregnancy remain high. In terms of general health, it is more socially excluded young people whose diet is likely to be least healthy and who are least likely to be engaged in constructive physical activity. Indeed, it is the more socially excluded who are involved in a greater level of health-risk behaviour. Yet, educational messages are least likely to get through to them, and services are often insufficiently available when they are required.

Housing and homelessness is complex policy territory in its own right. What we know is that successful transitions to independent living are invariably supported, usually invisibly, by strong family support (see Ainley 1991, Seavors and Hutton 2003). More socially excluded young people are likely to need even greater support, yet they are less likely to be able to access it; even when parents might be willing to provide it, they are often unable to do so. More 'at risk' young people are often propelled, precipitously, to independent living and are more vulnerable to homelessness. Improved concern and provision for young people leaving care, who in the past have been most vulnerable to such processes, has not yet extended to vulnerable young people more generally, despite the modest, though important, contribution of the Foyer movement (see Ward, 1997; Chapter 9 this volume) and the sterling work undertaken by youth homelessness projects within the voluntary sector.

I have endeavoured to provide a whistlestop journey past some of the main signposts of New Labour's 'youth policy' directed at cementing the social inclusion of young people. Has it worked? Is it working? Not surprisingly, it is hard to say. It is, undoubtedly, a step-change in political approaches to young people – and especially towards more socially excluded young people – but one has to temper such commendation with some caveats, both 'top-down' and 'bottom-up'. Top-down, the political commitment to an 'opportunity focused' and inclusive youth policy must remain in question. The 'problem-oriented' approach to young people has certainly not been submerged, as evidenced in 2002 by the street crime initiative and in 2003 by the anti-social behaviour White Paper (Home Office 2003a). Neither could be condemned out of hand, for they reflected some deep anxieties in the public psyche. But, equally, neither was likely to assist a 'youth inclusion' agenda. And the fact that the portfolio of 'Minister for Young People' changed hands four times within 6 weeks around May 2003 was hardly a testament to the political sustainability of that responsibility. Soon afterwards, however, in the ministerial reshuffle of June 2003, the 'children's' portfolio was consolidated within the Department for Education and Skills, under Minister of State Margaret Hodge. Initially designated Minister for Children (but subsequently, after some heavy lobbying, re-designated as Minister for Children and Young People), this post inherited responsibilities from within the DfES and from the Home Office and Lord Chancellor's Department. The promise it held was immediately undermined by media revelations about Hodge's activities around child support and protection when she was a council leader a decade earlier and this led to considerable delay in the publication of an 'overarching' Green Paper on Prevention (DfES 2003). This itself was triggered by the latest child protection tragedy concerning Victoria Climbié. Much hope is vested in the Green Paper but critics would argue that it may prove to be just the latest in a line of well-intentioned policy aspirations which, once more, will not have sufficient financial and professional resources to make a real difference on the ground. Meanwhile, more structural change and strategic reorganisation in services for young people is proposed.[1]

Bottom-up, as I have written elsewhere (Williamson 2002a), one must differentiate carefully within the group depicted as 'socially excluded' youth, if responses are to be tailored appropriately. My own crude typology has been concerned with the 'essentially confused' (for whom many of the policy measures outlined are likely to pay fairly immediate dividends) and with the 'temporarily sidetracked' (for whom a somewhat more patient approach will also yield a relatively 'quick win'). For what I call the 'deeply alienated', however, who divide into the 'purposeful' and the 'purposeless', the challenge is far more profound and wide-ranging. These socially excluded young people are already cynical of the possibilities being presented to them. Some have already found 'alternative ways of living'. They are skilled in strategies of avoidance. Programmes of intervention lack credibility with them. There is, therefore, a policy question concerning 'reach and relevance': do the policies described really reach the most disengaged and, even if they do, are they considered relevant and meaningful to the young people concerned? Do those agencies responsible for delivery engage in 'perverse behaviour', claiming that that they are working with the most disadvantaged when in fact they are working with less marginal, and more motivated, groups? (This is an understandable position to take, given the targets that are often imposed: it can lead to what a colleague of mine once described as 'hitting the target, but missing the point'!) Moreover, it is one thing having 'push' factors at play but these need to be accompanied and complemented by 'pull' factors. It is one thing to come off drugs, quite another to stay off drugs unless there is a reason and purpose for doing so (Pearson 1987). Such considerations have remained insufficiently thought through in the drive towards more positive 'joined-up' policy.

Yet 'youth policy' is at least firmly positioned on the public policy map, across the UK, within the expanding European Union and, indeed, throughout the 48 countries of the Council of Europe. Social inclusion is one of its paramount agendas. Many of the initiatives portrayed have been designed to that end, in recognition of the growing evidence concerning the 'youth divide' (Jones 2002). They are often in their early stages of development and implementation and it is hardly a surprise that they are routinely subjected to academic critique. There are legitimate concerns that, when Ministers wave the latest strategy document, they give the impression that the job is done. Resource questions (both human and financial) are a recurrent criticism. Further limitations to policy effectiveness are already apparent: making contact, tracking and keeping in touch (see Green *et al* 2001); the lack of sufficient flexibility; the question of eligibility and sanctions; the levels of choice and participation; the age range(s) that they serve. There is an absurd sense of urgency in demonstrating 'success' when it is clear that more socially excluded young people require both time and patience if their needs are to be assessed, an appropriate response identified and their motivation secured (Williamson 2001b). The evidence base demonstrates clearly that more robust support services are needed if socially excluded young people are to be coaxed back into the mainstream, which is where the majority of them would like to be. But their return will not be unconditional: they will have to be persuaded that there is something in it for them, something rather better than they have at present, which may not always seem much to *us*, but appears to be meaningful to them. Even homeless young people have *something*, and therefore something to lose, if the support proffered does not lead to some other meaningful and lasting destination (Blackman 1997). Local cultural pressures and the constrained or 'bounded' choices within them (Evans *et al* 2003) remain an important counterpoint to the aspirations of youth policy and the social inclusion agenda within them. Recognition of this fact will be critical, if the 'Tommy Butler' born in 1990 is to become 'included' as he becomes a teenager in 2003:

> When Tommy goes to secondary school, he will be doing 'citizenship' education and will be supported by a Personal Adviser from the

Connexions Service. If he starts going off the rails, that person will be there to provide both direct and indirect support, putting him in touch with those who can help him best. Tommy may, of course, not be persuaded that he needs their 'help'. He may well encounter the new Youth Offending Panel, which, if he gets into trouble, will frame a 'programme of activities' to divert him from crime. There will be a greater focus on preventative intervention, following the public resources allocated for work with children and young people as a result of the powerful analysis of the reasons for 'social exclusion' by a governmental Policy Action Team on Young People. In school, he may access an 'alternative curriculum offer' instead of being thrown out. Young people are a key strategic priority for a new drugs strategy; substance misuse education will be part of his PHSE (Personal, Health and Social Education) curriculum and treatment services will be more readily available if he moves beyond experimental and recreational drug use into more dependent routines. Tommy will have the possibility of a variety of routes to achievement in learning; work is currently being developed around the concept of 'graduation', first mooted in *Bridging the Gap*, which will enshrine not only academic and vocational qualifications but also attention to key skills, community involvement and personal development. He will be encouraged to engage with extra-curricular activities and volunteering.

How will Tommy respond to all this? Much depends, of course, on his character and circumstance. Certainly this framework of public policy carries the prospect of far fewer young people slipping to the edge, but it fails to acknowledge that motivation to participate (to stay on board) is secured largely by the strength of certainty about the destinations that are likely to be reached. Today's globalised world carries little certainty, and the research evidence tells us that retention in learning and the acquisition of qualifications is the best protective factor against all the indicators of exclusion (teenage pregnancy, criminality, drug misuse, psycho-social disorders). But Tommy is not interested in the research evidence. He will try to make sense of these 'opportunities' in the context of his subjective realities. The power in the messages from his local culture and community (however misguided and misinformed) – about what's the point of education, the exploitative nature of government training schemes, the need for a 'live for today' mentality (for the maintenance of psychological well-being), the suspicion of professionals, that volunteering is a cunning ploy to get you to work for nothing, the fact that there are other ways to 'get by', and so on – must not be overlooked. It is how Tommy Butler weighs such information against that provided by the battalions involved in public policy initiatives which will determine the extent to

which he connects with the inclusion, achievement and citizenship
agenda or opts for something else.

(Williamson 2001a: 3–4).[2]

Endnotes

1 The Green Paper on Prevention (DfES) was published in October 2003. A com-
panion document proposing reforms to the youth justice system was published at
the same time by the Home Office (Home Office 2003b). Soon after the publication of the Green Paper, the departmental structure within the portfolio of the
Minister for Children and Young People was itself reorganised, one consequence
of which was the demise of the Children and Young People's Unit.
2 Quotation reproduced with kind permission of Liza Catan, Director of ESRC's
research programme, 'Youth, Citizenship and Social Change'.

References

Adebowale, V. (1999) *Meeting the Needs of Disadvantaged Young People: a Report
to the New Deal Task Force*, London: Department for Education and
Employment.
Ainley, P. (1991) *Young People Leaving Home*, London: Cassell.
Barry, M. (2001) *Challenging Transitions: Young people's views and experiences of
growing up*, London: Save the Children.
Blackman, S. (1997) 'Destructing a Giro: a critical and ethnographic study of the
youth "underclass"', in R. MacDonald (ed.), *Youth, the 'Underclass' and Social
Exclusion*, London: Routledge.
Coles, B. (1997) 'Vulnerable youth and processes of social exclusion: a theoretical
framework – a review of recent research and suggestions for future research agen-
das', in J. Bynner, L. Chisholm and A. Furlong (eds), *Youth, Citizenship and
Social Change in a European Context*, Aldershot: Ashgate.
Cutler, D. (2002) *Taking the Initiative: Promoting young people's involvement in
decision making in the UK: Update*, London: Carnegie Young People Initiative.
DfEE (1999) *Learning to Succeed: A new framework for post-16 learning*, London:
The Stationery Office.
DfEE (2001) *Transforming Youth Work*, London: The Stationery Office.
DfES (2002a) *Choice and Excellence*, London: The Stationery Office.
DfES (2002b) *Resourcing Excellent Youth Services*, London: The Stationery Office.
DfES (2003) *Every Child Matters*, London: The Stationery Office.
DoH (1999) *Quality Protects*, London: The Stationery Office.
Drakeford, M. and Williamson, H. (1998)'From benign neglect to malign indiffer-
ence? Housing and young people', in I. Shaw, S. Lambert and D. Clapham, (eds),
Social Care and Housing, Research Highlights in Social Work 32, London: Jessica
Kingsley.
European Commission (1995) *Teaching and Learning White Paper*, Brussels:
European Commission.

European Commission (2001) *A NewImpetus for European Youth: White Paper*, Brussels: European Commission.

Evans, K., Rudd, P., Behrens, M., *et al.* (2003) *Taking Control: Young adults talking about the future in education, training and work*, Leicester: National Youth Agency.

Furlong, A. and Cartmel, F. (1997) *Young People and Social Change*, Buckingham: Open University Press.

Goldson, B. (2002) *Vulnerable Inside*, London: The Children's Society.

Green, A., Maguire, M. and Canny, A. (2001) *Keeping Track: Mapping and tracking vulnerable young people*, Bristol: The Policy Press and Joseph Rowntree Foundation.

HM Government (1998) *Tackling Drugs to Build a Better Britain*, London: The Stationery Office.

Hall, S. and Jefferson, T. (eds) (1976) *Resistance through Rituals*, London: Hutchinson.

Hodgkin, R. (2002) *Rethinking Child Imprisonment: A report on young offender institutions*, London: The Children's Rights Alliance for England.

Home Office (2003a) *Respect and Responsibility: Taking a stand against anti-social behaviour*, London: The Stationery Office.

Home Office (2003b) *Youth Justice: The next steps*, London: The Home Office.

House of Commons Education Committee (1998) *Disaffected Children*, London: The Stationery Office.

House of Commons Education Committee (1999) *Access for All? A Survey of Post-16 Participation*, London: The Stationery Office.

Istance, D., Rees, G. and Williamson, H. (1994) *Young People not in Education, Training and Employment in South Glamorgan*, Cardiff: South Glamorgan Training and Enterprise Council.

Jeffs, T. and Spence, J. (2000) 'New deal for young people: Good deal or poor deal?', *Youth and Policy*, 66: 34–61.

Johnston, L., MacDonald, R., Mason, P., *et al.* (2000) *Snakes and Ladders: Young people, transitions and social exclusion*, Bristol: Policy Press.

Jones, G. (2002) *The Youth Divide: Diverging paths to adulthood*, York: Joseph Rowntree Foundation.

Kirby, P. and Bryson, S. (2002) *Measuring the Magic? Evaluating and researching young people's participation in public decision making*, London: Carnegie Young People Initiative.

Maclagan, I. (1992) *A Broken Promise: The failure of youth training policy*, London: Youthaid.

Parker, H., Aldridge, J. and Eggington, R. (2001) *UK Drugs Unlimited*, London: Palgrave.

Pearson, G. (1987) *The New Heroin Users*, Oxford: Blackwell.

Pitts, J. (2003) *The New Politics of Youth Crime: Discipline or solidarity?*, Lyme Regis: Russell House Publishing [revised edition; first published by Palgrave 2001].

Schur, E. (1973) *Radical Non-Intervention: Rethinking the delinquency problem*, New Jersey: Prentice-Hall.

Seavers, J. and Hutton, S. (2003) *With a Little Help from. . . Their Parents?*, Leicester: National Youth Agency.

Social Exclusion Unit (1998) *School Exclusion*, London: The Stationery Office.

Social Exclusion Unit (1999a) *Bridging the Gap: New opportunities for 16–18 year olds not in education, employment or training*, London: The Stationery Office.

Social Exclusion Unit (1999b) *Teenage Pregnancy*, London: The Stationery Office.

Social Exclusion Unit (2000) *National Strategy for Neighbourhood Renewal – Report of Policy Action Team 12: Young people*, London: The Stationery Office.

Treseder, P. (1997) *Empowering Children and Young People*, London: Save the Children.

Ward, C. (1997) *Havens and Springboards: The Foyer movement in context*, London: Gulbenkian.

Welsh Assembly Government (2002a) *Everybody's Business*, Cardiff: Welsh Assembly Government.

Welsh Assembly Government (2002b) *Learning Pathways 14–19: A consultation document*, Cardiff: Welsh Assembly Government.

Williamson, H. (1985) 'Struggling beyond youth', *Youth in Society*, February.

Williamson, H. (1990) 'Trapped as teenagers', *Planet: The Welsh Internationalist*, 80: 14–22.

Williamson, H. (1993) 'Youth policy in the United Kingdom and the marginalisation of young people', *Youth and Policy*, 40: 33–48.

Williamson, H. (1997) 'Culture, politics and social exclusion: a comparison of 'status zer0' young people in two localities', in H. Williamson (ed.), *Youth and Policy: Contexts and consequences*, Aldershot: Ashgate.

Williamson, H. (2001a) 'From 'Tommy Butler' to Tony Blair: a story of marginalised youth and public policy', *ESRC Youth, Citizenship and Social Change Newsletter*, Issue 3 Winter 2000/Spring 2001: 6–8.

Williamson, H. (2001b) *Learning the Art of Patience: Dealing with the Disengaged*, British Youth Council Youth Agenda No.17, London: British Youth Council.

Williamson, H. (2002a) 'Developing diverse responses to disaffection' in Institute for Career Guidance, *Career Guidance – Constructing the Future 2002: Social inclusion – policy and practice*, Stourbridge: Institute of Career Guidance.

Williamson, H. (2002b) *Supporting young people in Europe: Principles, policy and practice*, Strasbourg: Council of Europe.

Postscript on policy and practice

Steven Kidd and Kieran Marshall

Steven Kidd

I am Steven Kidd, a 22-year-old Communications student from Lanarkshire in Scotland. I have recently completed a two year term as Chair of the Scottish Youth Parliament, an organisation run by and for young people, and I am also a trustee of the United Kingdom Youth Parliament. My major passion is the involvement of all young people in decisions which affect their lives, and quite often this 'voluntary' commitment leaves very little room for a social life, though when I can, I enjoy going out with friends, reading, writing and travel.

Throughout my involvement in the youth sector I have come across many Tommy or Tammy Butlers, young people for whom life is never clearly mapped out. Successive initiatives have always promised much in bringing these excluded young people into the mainstream, but have, until recently, delivered little. As Howard Williamson points out, though, there has been a seed change in the way in which young people and their associated issues are viewed by policy makers at the highest level – government has perhaps realised that there are no benefits to being a marginalised group of society and therefore there must be circumstances which keep these people out in the cold, for it cannot be by choice.

Since 1997, the initiatives introduced have clearly reduced the holes in the net, but have not removed them and it is still those from the most excluded backgrounds who seem to fall through. The 'joining-up' of the various initiatives of which Howard Williamson speaks has been the major factor in ensuring that the numbers are increasingly smaller, but, as is the nature of any net, some will escape. While young people now have greater choice than ever before, it is important that they are properly informed and advised on the path which is most appropriate to them, a concept which appears to have been embraced by both the Connexions and Extending Entitlements programmes in England and Wales. These, and other similar initiatives, will be far more useful to young people if they retain the 'best interests of the young person' as the prime consideration – a young person is not a statistic, but a complex collection of skills, abilities, needs and desires, and services directed towards young people would do well to take this on board.

So what of Tommy Butler? Does he perceive himself to be socially excluded? There are undoubtedly many ways for academics and government departments to determine whether, statistically, Tommy is amongst the socially excluded, but Tommy's own perceptions are equally important – I think that what many people may overlook are the beliefs and attitudes which young people have towards a value system. While many young people are aware that certain behaviours and lifestyles are the 'wrong' choice, it does not always preclude them from being the 'accepted' choice. No-one would argue that to start smoking, for example, was the 'wrong' choice, yet how many people have done and continue to do this. The same can be said for truancy, drinking to excess, the misuse of drugs and almost every situation which impinges on what is seen as a young person's social inclusion. This creation of a series of acceptable 'wrong' behaviours is something which is built up by the immediate society surrounding young people, particularly family and friends, and can be evidenced by 'hot spots' of similar 'social exclusion' behaviours in families, in groups of friends and in certain communities. Effectively, an extension of peer pressure is created, as these young people become part of a perpetuating cycle.

What is encouraging, though, is that the government is recognising this and moving away from the 'problem-orientated' approach, though not entirely, as can be seen from the various anti-social behaviour bills. What is needed is an attitudinal shift towards the modification of acceptable behaviours and lifestyles to that which is on a par with society as a whole. The introduction of citizenship classes is a positive move in this direction, though I would argue that this should be a cross-cutting subject, which must also include the modification and standardisation of personal and social education across the curriculum. At a time when it appears that young people, and in particular those from socially excluded backgrounds, are not being given adequate support at home, there is a clear need for education to perform this function, teaching young people to live healthily and happily in the world around them.

I think there is also a need for the media in this country to act more responsibly – if the only stories about young people in a newspaper are sensationalist pieces about youth crime, there is a great difficulty in persuading young people that they are valued as members of society. While I don't expect such stories to be excluded altogether, I would like to see the media giving a more balanced coverage of this nation's young people. The government, too, could benefit from such a stance, increasing the publicity of their policies and initiatives to enable young people to become independently aware of the opportunities available to them.

What appears obvious is that without changing society's opinion of young people in general, and the opinion of young people themselves, the problem of social exclusion will remain. The process has been started with the range of policy moves described by Howard Williamson, but what will be needed to make them work is change in the attitudes of the people they will affect. Howard Williamson has hit the nail on the head with a telling insight into the lives of socially excluded young people, but unfortunately it is, I fear, one of many more nails needed to close the coffin on social exclusion.

Kieran Marshall

My name is Kieran Marshall, I'm 17 years old and live in South Wales. I am currently working as a Youth Peer Educator (Mental Health) for a national charity called Youthlink Wales which is owned and run by young people. Although I like socialising with friends, reading and sport, a lot of my interests are work-related, as I have a deep interest in social science – in particular youth work, community education, social medicine and mental health.

At the start of this chapter, I was quite amused by the author's creation of a 'mythical androgynous character' – Tommy or Tammy – spelling for me the current concern of writers and professionals with gender correctness but also highlighting the current state of concern and practice towards social inclusion and the broader issues of rights, equal opportunities, etc. The first few pages of the chapter mapped for me the 'promise' from government of this character's 'social inclusion' in a very sorry way. Systems are becoming more complex as adult transitions are extended, but there is still an expectation on young people to 'fit' the criteria set by government at every stage of that transition. The angle from which the government were shooting, or the tree under which they were barking, displayed to me their wrong turn in the journey to hit the inclusion button. Calling it a 'social inclusion crisis' years after it happened seemed inevitable. I liked the way Howard Williamson told me this honestly and constructively – buttering the bread evenly – even though there were parts of the chapter with which I disagreed or felt differently about, but who wouldn't when you're not reading your own work!

I think a lot of the causes of the problems faced by young people are a result of the government's interest in 'boxes being ticked' and 'number crunching'. I think the real true focus of many of the issues for young people in the UK have been lost. It is all too easy to say that disability access is putting a ramp and lift to the stairs of a building and thinking it is complete. It's not, and many practitioners and young people know it is not. What about the actual service young people receive? Are the deliverers trained, can they speak their language: even if they can and the young people take in what is said, do they really understand it? And how is that measured?

I think major moves need to be taken to ensure that we, as a country, secure good foundations for social inclusion work, otherwise there will be growing problems because we started building on bad foundations. As a service recipient myself of education and training services on post-16 programmes, I have experienced the system enough to know only too well about the problems the government has in implementing strategies, which I think are only fuelled as a result of the 'number crunching' and 'boxes being ticked' approach. Just because a tick is against what was in the plan, doesn't mean that it is done. It is all too easy to say something is being done because someone has said that it is! Many services are just interested in getting you through the door and being a tick in the box, having too much of a focus on quantitative outcomes rather than an equal balance of quantitative and qualitative outcomes.

Publicity for policies and services is another issue: how the government and devolved administrations communicate and publicise these programmes. If you ask a young person in England 'what is Connexions?', it is highly likely that their response will be they have heard of it in some shape or form. Ask a young person in Wales what they think or feel about Extending Entitlements and the response is likely to be 'what is that?'. I think the ultimate question is not about the programme itself, not just yet anyway, but whether the communication and publicity highlight the right things to the right young people in the right language? Young people may say why waste time on rubbish policy stuff when they could be engaging in their own familiar and clear (in comparison to what policy could do) way of life – crime, drugs, unprotected sex, skipping school and/or training, etc. Not all young people necessarily see the choices as 'exclusion and the bad ways in life' or 'inclusion and the good ways in life'. If vital changes aren't made to offer young people better choices, everything will hang on the luck of the draw.

Policies and programmes need to be accessible (language, etc.), understandable (clear, etc.) and useable (designed for young people to change things or take action, etc.). Why is what appears be the answer turning into a problem? The solution could possibly be the building of forward-thinking programmes, integrating positive, evidenced approaches, with new plans and ideas that have received proper and clear consultancy with young people.

In this chapter it would have been good to see a greater focus on the need for more resources in the youth sector, and the need for better publicity and wider consultation with young people. For example, Extending Entitlements (in Wales) is a strong and valid response to the Education and Learning Bill; it addresses many social inclusion issues and is geared towards a unique and inclusive Welsh approach to better services and entitlements for young people. A cracking idea! But, the programme from a service level is severely under-resourced and implementation has gone 'head first, back to front'. I feel that Howard Williamson's chapter could have paid a little more attention to these issues and explored other routes to the problems and what the possible solutions are. This would have also offered an opportunity to government, business, the public and commissioners to become more aware of the issues being faced and to ensure that more resources are secured, or that alternative economical ways of working are developed. However, the chapter offers a stimulating account of issues around social inclusion and exclusion, and makes a valid contribution to the agendas aimed at tackling social exclusion.

77076

Chapter 3

Young people and citizenship

Ruth Lister with Noel Smith, Sue Middleton and Lynne Cox

Introduction

Citizenship has re-emerged as a central political and academic concept in recent years. Although traditionally understood as a force for inclusion, contemporary citizenship theory tends to emphasise its exclusionary tendencies (Lister 2003). In the UK, the New Labour government has attempted to re-articulate and to promote public debate on its meaning. It is particularly concerned about young people's relationship to citizenship in the face of perceived apathy and disengagement (Advisory Group on Citizenship 1998, Pearce and Hallgarten 2000). Young people are thus typically represented as deficient citizens. This chapter challenges such representations in favour of an understanding of young people as 'citizens in the making' (Marshall 1950: 25, Arnot and Dillabough 2000). More than at other points of the life-course, youth is a time when the relationship to citizenship is in a state of flux.

The chapter reports findings from a 3-year qualitative, longitudinal study of how young people negotiate the transitions to citizenship, which was part of the ESRC Youth, Citizenship and Social Change Programme. A total of 110 young people in the East Midlands town of Leicester, aged 16/17, 18/19 and 22/23 in 1999, were interviewed.[1] There was a gender balance and about one in eight was Asian, predominately of Indian-Hindu background (to reflect Leicester's main minority ethnic community). Given the salience of paid work to contemporary characterisations of citizenship, the group was stratified according to 'insider' and 'outsider' status as a proxy for social class. 'Insiders' conformed with a stereotypical model of the 'successful' young person as on the route through 'A' levels and university and into graduate-type employment; 'outsiders' fell well outside it, with few or no qualifications and a record of unemployment for most of the time since leaving school. By the third and final interview in 2001, 64 of the original group remained.[2]

Both the study and other relevant empirical research are used to throw light on young people's understandings of citizenship and the extent to which they identify themselves as citizens. More specifically, this chapter looks at notions of 'first class' and 'second class' and 'good' and 'bad' citizenship and at perceptions of rights and responsibilities. It concludes by arguing for an inclusive notion of citizenship, which takes on board young people's perspectives.

The meaning(s) of citizenship

Until recently, citizenship has not been a salient idea in the British political tradition. Few people, therefore, have a clear idea as to what it means to be a citizen (Speaker's Commission 1990, Dean with Melrose 1999, Miller 2000). Not surprisingly, citizenship was not part of the everyday language of the young people in our study. Nevertheless, the idea resonated with their own attempts to make sense of their position in society. Five models of citizenship emerged: universal status, respectable economic independence, constructive social participation, social-contractual and right to a voice. Moving from the most articulated (universal status) to the least articulated (right to a voice). These are discussed below.

Universal status

At its most inclusive, everyone is understood to be a citizen by virtue of membership of the community or nation. In a 'thin' version, this reflected a view that 'citizen' means 'person'. This was the response given by a number of 'outsiders' in particular. For one, a 19 year-old white male, citizenship didn't 'mean owt', but he added that 'it's just a person at the end of the day – a citizen'. For another, a 19 year-old 'outsider' white female, 'it doesn't matter what they do, everybody's a citizen'.

A 'thicker' understanding drew on notions of 'belonging' – to either the local or national community. Two participants summed it up: 'Belonging. I think being part of something ... a sense of belonging' (16 year-old 'insider' white female); 'citizenship is about being somewhere, belonging somewhere' (16 year-old 'outsider' Asian female). Overall, there were no obvious gender differences but 'insiders' were more likely to subscribe to the universal status model and young Asians did so more consistently over the three years. However, in another study in the ESRC programme African-Caribbean and Pakistani young people rejected the notion of citizenship as a universal status. Instead, 'many were convinced that citizenship was hierarchised and unequal' (Harris *et al* 2001: 50).

Respectable economic independence

This model is embodied by a person who is in waged employment, pays taxes and has a family and their own house: 'the respectable economically independent citizen', associated with the economic and social status quo. As a 16 year-old 'outsider' white male put it: 'I think as soon as you're living in your own house, out working, paying your bills. That's when you're a citizen'. A 16 year-old 'insider' white male defined a citizen as being 'a working part of the country', which would mean 'when I've got a house, wife, kids, job going on'. The model underpinned understandings of 'first class' and 'second class' citizenship, discussed below. It effectively excludes many of the young people themselves, in the short term, because of age or dependence on their parents and, in the longer term, some 'outsiders' because of anticipated unemployment and their generally disadvantaged labour market position. The young men were more likely to invoke this model; otherwise, there were no clear patterns.

Constructive social participation

Here, citizenship denotes a constructive stance towards the community. This ranged from the more passive abiding by the law to the more active citizenship as a responsible practice – helping people and having a positive impact. A 22 year-old 'outsider' white female summed it up: 'A citizen is where you're helping in the community . . . . You're helping people and you're trying to do your best. Trying to support where you are'. On this basis she considered that people 'who can't be assed to get off their beer bellies and help are not a citizen or anything. They don't care what happens around them'. A 16 year-old Asian male was one of a number of 'insiders' who talked about being responsible and contributing as part of a reciprocal relationship with the community or society: 'Being responsible; being mature about everything and again, not just taking, giving back . . . . It's helping out in as many ways as you can'. This 'constructive social participation' model underpinned notions of 'good' citizenship discussed below. 'Outsiders' were rather more likely to subscribe to it than 'insiders', but there were no clear gender or ethnic differences. The model was also prominent in a recent national survey of school students (Kerr et al 2003).

Social-contractual

A small number, particularly females, referred spontaneously to rights and/or responsibilities. An 'insider' white female, for instance, stated that citizenship means 'being a part of society and having rights and requirements of living within the law'. This represents one element of what Dean with Melrose (1999) identified as a 'social contractual' citizenship discourse. An earlier American–British study of adults found that, in both countries, the majority subscribed to the social-contractual model (Conover et al 1991).

Right to a voice

The right and genuine opportunity to have a say and be heard is at the heart of this model, which emerged from the responses of a small number of participants. As one 22 year-old 'outsider' white male explained: 'To feel a citizen, I'd say I should have a right to say what goes on'. A 16 year-old 'insider' Asian female talked about 'being able to help in decision-making . . . just having your say in what's gonna happen'. A 16 year-old 'insider' white female thought she'd feel like a full citizen 'when people do respect you for your views and they listen to you'.

The five models were not mutually exclusive in that some young people subscribed to more than one, sometimes drawing on different models simultaneously. Overall, the 'universal' model dominated. However, over the three years it diminished in importance and the 'respectable economic independence' and 'constructive social participation' models, with their invocation of economic and civic responsibility, were articulated with increasing frequency.

To be a citizen?

The importance of identity to citizenship is increasingly being recognised in the citizenship literature (Jones 1994, Turner 1997, Isin and Wood 1999, Stevenson 2001, Jones and Gaventa 2002). Hall *et al* observe that 'in the contemporary political and policy arena, much of the rhetoric of citizenship is about citizenship as an identity – encouraging young people in particular to think of themselves *as* citizens' (Hall *et al* 1998: 309, emphasis in original). Like other identities, citizenship identity is constructed and evolves and it is possible to identify processes of differential citizenship identity formation (Hobson and Lindholm 1997). John Shotter underlines the difficulties involved:

> . . . to be a citizen is not a simple matter of first as a child growing up to be a socially competent adult, and then simply walking out into the everyday world to take up one's rights and duties as a citizen. This is impossible. For . . . it is a status which one must struggle to attain in the face of competing versions of what [it] is proper to struggle for . . .
> (Shotter 1993: 115–16).

National identity

One of the difficulties is the tendency to conflate citizenship and national identities (Fulbrook and Cesarani 1996). Alongside citizenship, national identity is a current preoccupation of British politicians, concerned to stimulate debate on what it means to be British – and also English – in a changing world and a devolved United Kingdom. In the study, participants, who had engaged readily with questions about citizenship, struggled when asked about nationality and national identity and showed little enthusiasm for the topic. This echoed the difficulties Conover *et al* (1991) reported among their British respondents.

White participants frequently used the terms British and English interchangeably but, for the most part, found it difficult to articulate what they meant other than in comparison with other nationalities or in the context of British multi-culturalism. The most common response was to associate nationality with country of birth, parental heritage and long-term residence. Culture (articulated in such terms as language, food, customs, history, humour, monarchy, the pound) tended to be a secondary theme. In terms of their own identification, responses ranged from a sense of significance and pride (sometimes expressed in relation to sport) through indifference to negativity.

In the case of a small number of white 'outsiders', discussion of nationality was tinged with hostility to Asian residents and asylum seekers, who were perceived as receiving more help from the state than white people whose families had paid tax through the generations. Some also talked about cultural, religious and language differences. The majority was, however, more accepting. They thought it only understandable that those of Asian background would want to be in touch with and have pride in their roots and culture and one noted the ways in which people's roots are in any case 'all getting very global and mixed up'. The Asian participants themselves found it easier to talk about nationality, for it opened up discussion about the balance between, or compound of, British and Asian identities. Some described themselves simply as British, some as equally British and Indian and others emphasised that they were as British as anyone else, referring to their Indian origin as 'just background'. The study by Harris *et al* (2001) of African-Caribbean and Pakistani young people found more of a sense of 'not belonging'. This underlines how young people in different minority ethnic groups do not relate to citizenship in a single, undifferentiated, way.

Citizen identity

Over two-fifths of participants defined themselves unambiguously as citizens in all three waves of the research. This group included twice as many 'insiders' as 'outsiders' and more older and female participants. A further fifth who identified themselves as citizens at the third wave had earlier considered themselves either as partial citizens or not as citizens. Both 'outsiders' and females were over-represented in the last two groups and there was a clear age dynamic, with younger participants more likely to develop an identification with the status of citizenship over the lifetime of the project. Those who felt themselves to be partial citizens in the final wave were more likely to be 'insiders' and male. The four participants who did not consider themselves to be citizens at the third wave were all older white 'outsiders'. One of these, a 22 year-old white female, described herself as 'an insignificant little person' rather than a citizen and explained: 'I don't stand for anything. I haven't particularly achieved anything, so I don't feel like I'm a proper citizen'. Likewise, four out of the five who could not say whether they were citizens were white (younger) 'outsiders'. At each wave, 'outsiders' were less likely than 'insiders' to identify themselves as citizens. Ethnicity did not generally appear to be a distinguishing factor.

The extent to which the young people identified themselves as citizens reflected developments in their own lives, such as whether or not they had achieved waged employment and paid tax; been involved in their communities or undertaken voluntary work; or had voted. More subjective factors were also important. These included feelings about belonging, significance, respectful treatment, independence and whether they had had an effective say. Other studies in the programme, more specifically focused on 'disadvantaged young people', found that their sense of citizenship belonging and identity was rooted in families and communities (Youth, Citizenship and Social Change 2003b).

Different combinations of the models of citizenship described earlier underlay the young people's self-perceptions as citizens. Their assessment of changes in their sense of citizenship identity drew most frequently on the respectable economic independence model. This was followed by the constructive social participation model and then by the social-contractual and the right-to-a-voice models. Very few made reference to voting, but one 'insider' white female, eligible to vote for the first time, did so strongly:

> I do feel a greater sense of being a citizen than I did . . . I can't stop talking about the whole voting thing, which is quite bad, but it's given me a sense of being a citizen, being a member of the wider society, and being able to count as something.

In some instances, citizenship did not appear an attainable status. One 19 year-old 'outsider' white female said that the word made her think of 'old people and people who are like lawyers and people like that. Lawyers and social workers and things like that. They're citizens – people who are so high up'.

'First' and 'second class' citizenship

The potentially exclusionary implications of the respectable economic independence model implied by this quotation were reflected also in responses to the notion of 'first class' and 'second class' citizenship. First wave participants were asked what they thought of opinion polls which suggest that unemployed people are often made to feel like 'second class' citizens. There was considerable resistance to classifying people in this way. Nevertheless, the clear consensus was that unemployed people *are* regarded as second class citizens by society. A number of the 'outsiders' clearly saw the label as applying to them and placed themselves at the bottom of a hierarchical image of society. 'Lower than everybody else' was a phrase used more than once:

> It makes you feel like you *are* a second class citizen, cos you haven't got a job. I don't know what it means, but it makes you feel lower than everybody else.
>
> (22 year-old white male)

> You feel – like everyone else has got more of a say than you. You're just last – at the bottom.
>
> (19 year-old white female)

> Second class citizen, to me, means me really.
>
> (19 year-old white male)

The 'first class' citizen was overwhelmingly personified across groups by the educated homeowner with a secure job, family and car: in other words, the embodiment of the respectable economic independence model and of the socioeconomic status quo. Independence (from the state) and participation as workers and taxpayers were also the watchwords of 'first class' citizenship. Some typical examples of this exclusionary image, as articulated by 'outsiders', were:

> Well a job basically ain't it, and decent house. If you've got a council flat and signing on or on Social, then you're a dosser ain't you?
>
> (16 year-old white female)

> Someone who's got a respectable job and a nice house and good children at private school. BUPA [private health insurance] and all that bollocks.
>
> (22 year-old white male)

Other research in the programme also found that 'disadvantaged' young people perceive their own citizenship status as 'second class' and 'less weighty' because of their lesser life chances and widespread inequalities in society' (Youth, Citizenship and Social Change 2003a: 2, Harris *et al* 2001).

'Good' and 'bad' citizenship

Understandings of 'good' and 'bad' citizenship (explored in the first two waves) stood in vivid contrast to those of 'first class' and 'second class', drawing as they did on the constructive social participation model. This was epitomised in the observation of a 19 year-old 'insider' white female during the focus group held between the first and second waves:

> Money isn't always a good citizen. Sometimes the more money you've got, it seems as though you are a worse citizen . . . . Whereas the working class person on their estate can't do enough for their neighbour; they're a very good citizen.

The good citizen

All but 13 of the 110 first wave participants had ideas to offer as to what constitutes good citizenship. Most included a number of elements in their definition of good citizenship. The most common interpretation, offered by over two-thirds, involved a combination of the 'ordinarily' and 'extra' good (Conover *et al* 1991): a considerate and caring attitude towards others and a constructive approach towards and active participation in the community. The latter emerged particularly strongly. Female participants were more likely to refer explicitly to constructive participation in 'community' or neighbourhood. Generally, frequent references were made to doing 'one's fair share in the community', sometimes in an organized way, and sometimes more informally such as in 'looking out for' and 'helping' people in the neighbourhood. One 19 year-old 'outsider' white male explicitly emphasised the informal over the more formal:

> I wouldn't call a good citizen like the kind who goes out to do charity and trying to raise money. That's not my version of a good citizen. Mine's like they'll help you out. They'll lend you something if you need it, and that's the way I see a good citizen . . . . It's like your neighbours.

'Bad citizens' were defined as selfish, uncaring, lazy and lacking in respect. This was summed up by a 16 year-old 'insider' white male who saw a 'bad citizen' as:

> someone that's all take and no give, basically. Not participating in any way – just all for themselves . . . when somebody cares more about getting a car or whatever, than what's going on with the people who are say homeless on their doorsteps, you know?

Whether or not someone shows 'respect' was a criterion used by a number of 'outsiders'. One, a 22 year-old white male, talked of the good citizen as someone with 'a bit of respect for his surroundings and . . . respectful, polite. A bad citizen is someone who ain't got no respect for anybody . . . . Smashing this and that up; couldn't give a toss about where he lives'. Another, a 19 year-old white female, argued that:

people who have respect for each other and themselves are good citizens . . . . So I think good citizens are those that don't break the law, they respect, they have mutual respect for themselves and for people in their community and society. Whereas the bad ones are just, don't have any respect for anyone, not even themselves.

The importance that young people attach to respect when thinking about citizenship emerges from other research also (Harris *et al* 2001, Kerr *et al* 2003). One 'outsider' suggested, though, that respect was difficult when living in a poor environment. Here, respect was partly linked to not breaking the law. This reflected the second most common construction of the 'good' and 'bad' citizen overall: that of the law-abiding and non-disruptive versus the trouble-making citizen. A significant minority of first and second wave participants referred to abiding by the law or keeping out of trouble, although in most cases they referred also to other aspect of good citizenship. In a cross-national survey of 14 year-olds, obeying the law emerged as the most important facet of good citizenship (Kerr *et al* 2002).

Political conceptions of good citizenship were less frequently articulated. In our study, only four, all female 'insiders', mentioned voting. This is consistent with a 1999 Institute for Citizenship/Natwest MORI survey in which only nine per cent chose voting as important to being a good citizen. However, in the cross-national survey, seven out of ten 14 year-olds in England considered voting to be important (Kerr *et al* 2002). A very small number in the present study, mainly 'insiders', saw good citizenship in more active political or campaigning terms.

'Dissident citizenship'

Despite the link made with keeping within the law by a significant minority, a couple of 'insider' white males did question this from a political perspective, distinguishing between different kinds of law-breaking. Thus one of them suggested that someone who broke the law in the name of animal rights could be a good citizen while a car vandal would be a bad citizen. In the second wave, participants were asked whether it was ever justifiable or necessary for a citizen to break the law. Only 16 out of the 74 responded that it was never justifiable; 13 of these were 'outsiders' and the young Asians were disproportionately represented among this group. Most participants felt that citizenship status was not affected by certain illegal activities such as minor traffic offences; use of cannabis; stealing food out of necessity; and when part of a campaign.

A more specific question on whether it is ever justifiable or necessary for a citizen to break the law as part of a campaign or demonstration elicited a negative response from only nine participants. The most common justifications given were: the need to gain attention for an issue; the deservingness of the cause; the strength of feeling of the protesters; and the need to challenge an unfair law.

Sparks has suggested the notion of 'dissident citizenship' to describe 'oppositional democratic practices' through which 'dissident citizens constitute alternative public spaces' to pursue non-violent protest outside the formal democratic channels (Sparks 1997: 75). Such notions might help render citizenship a less oppressive notion for those who perceive it in terms of a status quo that excludes themselves. There was a sense, often not verbalised but expressed through tone, facial expression or atmosphere, that for some of the 'outsiders' questions about 'good citizenship' and their own involvement in citizenship-related activities carried such a potentially oppressive air (see also France 1998).

Voluntary work and good citizenship

In the first wave, the question of good citizenship was approached initially with reference to the UK government's promotion of volunteering as key to the development of 'responsible' or 'active' citizenship, particularly among young people. In the second wave they were asked more generally about any connection they saw between voluntary work and good citizenship.

Of the 74 participants in the second wave, 50 believed in such a connection; a number though qualified this by emphasising that it was neither an exclusive nor a necessary connection (an argument put also by those who opposed the idea). The two most frequently cited bases of such a connection were that both are about 'helping people' and about contributing to the community or society. In both instances, the young women and Asian participants were particularly likely to use such arguments. The small number of Asian participants in the second wave were also more willing to make the connection in the first place, but there were no obvious gender differences. 'Outsiders' were much less likely than 'insiders' to accept any connection.

There was less support in the first wave for the government's association of voluntary work with good citizenship. Some 'outsiders', such as this 16 year-old white female, also expressed a dislike of the idea of working without pay: 'No one's gonna get no medals to be a good citizen . . . . I think you'd be silly actually doing something for nothing'. 'Insiders' who opposed the idea tended to raise questions of motivation or to argue that not doing voluntary work does not mean that one is a bad citizen. One, a 16 year-old white female, demonstrated a shrewd understanding of the politically dominant citizenship philosophy when she observed that previously citizenship 'was an automatic thing but it seems now that you gonna have to work for your status in a way'.

Rights and responsibilities

New Labour's promotion of voluntary work as active citizenship is one example of its repeated emphasis on the need for a 'fresh understanding of the rights and responsibilities of the citizen' (Brown 2000), with the accent on responsibilities and obligations over rights. The general presumption appears to be that set out in the Cantle Report: 'the rights – *and in particular – the responsibilities* of citizenship need to be more clearly established' (Cantle 2001: 20, emphasis added).[3] Yet, the young people we interviewed found it markedly more difficult to identify their rights than they did their responsibilities.

Responsibilities

In line with their views about good citizenship, the most frequently mentioned citizenship responsibility referred to 'being constructive'. This included notions of 'giving back to the community', being responsible and courteous, respecting others, behaving in a socially acceptable manner. A 16 year-old 'outsider' white female summed it up as 'whether it's through taxes or helping in the community, just giving back something to society'. An 18 year-old 'outsider' white male responded: 'keep the country clean and that; help old people across the road, things like that. Being polite and courteous'.

Other responses referred to obeying the law; looking after oneself and one's family; being in work/paying tax; and voting. In the final wave, 'insiders' were about three times more likely than 'outsiders' to refer to employment/paying tax and were twice as likely to refer to being constructive; 'outsiders' were about three times more likely than 'insiders' to refer to looking after self or family. Female participants had a greater tendency to refer to obeying the law and to employment/paying tax and older participants to being constructive. The small number of Asian participants were more likely to refer to obeying the law.

The contrast between 'outsiders' and 'insiders' has a degree of resonance with the starker finding of Harris *et al* (2001) that African-Caribbean and Pakistani young people were only prepared to acknowledge obligations in relation to their own community, family and friends. However, the responses did not accord with those in Alan France's study in a deprived working class community, which found that some young people's acceptance of citizen responsibilities in both the community and the labour market 'had been undermined by experiences of exclusion and exploitation' (France, 1998: 108).

In contrast to the two studies just cited, when asked specifically about work obligations in earlier waves, the majority of 'outsiders' as well as 'insiders' signed up to the government's philosophy of paid work as a citizenship obligation, although sometimes with qualifications such as the state of the local labour market. Another qualification raised by some, most notably older 'outsider' white young women who had or were expecting children, was the presence of young children or pregnancy. When asked specifically in the second wave whether waged employment or parenting is more important to society, about half of both the young men and women answered the latter and most of the others felt they were of equal importance. Some articulated views that reflected the position of a number of feminist citizenship theorists that care should be acknowledged as an expression of citizenship responsibility alongside paid work (Knijn and Kremer 1997, Sevenhuijsen 1998, Lister 2003). For example, a 16 year-old 'insider' white female responded:

> I do see the value of working, I really do. But I think I'm going to have to side with a really positive important role – to stay at home, and raise the children. You're at home with them, and teaching them things: how to grow up to be good citizens.

Some participants, in particular both Asian and white 'insider' younger women, referred explicitly or implicitly to an underlying responsibility to be self-reliant and independent. In line with their general views about citizenship responsibilities, 'outsiders' were more likely to define paid work responsibility in relation to themselves and their families, whereas 'insiders' tended to talk more of a responsibility to the wider society, sometimes in addition to themselves and their families. A small group, mainly of 16 year-old 'outsiders', did not see employment as a responsibility and rejected the idea as coercive. One 16 year-old white male, for instance, rejected the idea as 'a load of rubbish . . . just pushing you to get a job, you know what I mean. Just trying to get you down so you say "sod this! I'm getting a job; don't want none of this stick"'.

The other area of particular concern to British politicians at present is voting, in the wake of the unprecedentedly low turn-out in the 2001 General Election, especially among young people. The 16th British Social Attitudes Survey found 'dramatic' age-group differences on the question of whether voting is a civic obligation: only a third of those aged under 25 saw voting as a duty compared with around two-thirds of those aged between 25 and 55 and nearly four-fifths of those aged over 55 (Park 1999).

Very few participants referred spontaneously to voting as a citizenship obligation. In the first wave, of 52 participants specifically asked, 12 were in favour and 34 opposed to the idea of voting as a social obligation, with the rest unsure. All but one of those in favour were 'insiders'; nine were female and none was Asian. The most forcefully put argument against voting as an obligation was, in fact, premised on a notion of responsibility that serves to problematise a simple equation of voting and sense of civic responsibility. A number of the young people believed strongly that it was more irresponsible to vote in ignorance – without knowledge of the candidates or issues at hand – than not to vote at all. A 16 year-old Asian female 'insider', still at school, who held the view that voting is important because 'one vote can make a full difference', believed strongly that the responsible citizen should 'not just vote for the hell of voting'. She suggested that 'if I was a bad citizen, I'd go to a voting poll and just tick any names. Not knowing what I was ticking – that would make me a bad citizen'. Such beliefs need to be read in the context of the acknowledgement by a number of participants, both 'insiders' and 'outsiders', of their lack of political knowledge both in terms of what the parties stand for and the mechanics of voting.

Rights

As noted, the young people were less fluent in the language of rights than of responsibilities.[4] When asked specifically about this in the third wave, around half struggled to identify their rights. Sixteen of these (of whom 15 were white 'outsiders') were unable to do so at all; in contrast, only one participant was unable to identify any responsibilities. Roughly a quarter of the remaining participants referred to political and social rights, respectively: the former in relation to the vote and the latter in relation to social benefits, housing, healthcare and education.

Two-thirds referred to civil rights such as freedom of speech, movement and worship and from discrimination. This included nine of the ten remaining Asian participants. One of them, an 18 year old 'outsider' male, spoke of 'freedom of speech; to be counted as equal; just to be treated equally really, like any other British citizen should be treated'. None of the 'outsiders' referred to social rights. Several participants (mainly 'insiders') also referred to employment as a right. The findings contrast with those of Conover et al, who remarked on the primacy given by British respondents to social rights of citizenship and their relative disregard of civil rights (Conover et al 1991; see also Dean with Melrose 1999, Dwyer 2000).

With regard more specifically to the right to social security, only a minority believed that they had an unconditional right to benefit, when questioned in the first wave. This small group referred to their right as a British citizen and/or the taxes paid by their parents or themselves. The majority, though, linked social rights with responsibilities, talking of benefit receipt as a conditional right, the most common condition specified being active job-seeking. A number questioned the fairness of taking money from people who are working and paying tax, without putting something back.

Others expressed some ambivalence about their own position. A 16 year-old 'outsider' white male, for example, spoke of a right to benefit in the face of the government's failure to supply jobs. Yet he also felt that in a way he did not have a right because:

> It's the taxpayer's money that we're having ain't it? When they pay tax it's coming towards us and we're just sitting on our arses all day and doing nothing, and in that way I don't think we deserve it, but like I say, I don't think we'd be able to survive without.

While on the whole opinions did not differ significantly between 'insiders' and 'outsiders', the most noticeable group to hold a distinct view was some older 'outsider' young white women who had or were expecting children. They believed that lone mothers with young children or expectant mothers should have an unconditional right to benefit.

Young people as citizens

Current political debate about young people's citizenship tends to focus on what young people do not do, creating an image of young people as deficient citizens (Eden and Roker 2002). When the focus shifts to what young people do do, a rather different picture emerges. In the present study, the great majority of young people had engaged at some time in some form of constructive social participation. There were a number of elements to this: formal, organized voluntary work; informal voluntary work (such as regularly helping elderly neighbours); informal political action (such as demonstrations) designed to bring about or prevent change; activities with political implications, although not explicitly political (for example involvement in a Hindu society which served to promote inter-cultural relations); awareness-raising (for instance challenging racism in conversation); altruistic acts (such as donating blood or giving to charity); and general social participation contributing to the strengthening of social capital (including reciprocal neighbourliness and membership of community or sports organizations).

Levels (although not patterns) of participation were similar among 'insiders' and 'outsiders'. Around half (more among 'insiders') had participated in formal voluntary work; nearly a quarter (more among 'outsiders') had experience of informal voluntary work. About a quarter (mainly 'insiders' and female 'outsiders') had some experience of informal political action (beyond signing petitions). Although the distinction was not sharp, 'insiders' were more likely to engage in less active, more global or national forms of action in comparison with 'outsiders', who were more likely to engage in more active, local forms (such as a demonstration to prevent the closure of a youth club).

Other research has also challenged the negative image of young people as apathetic and lazy. A study undertaken in three state schools in different parts of England found 'evidence of a much greater level of involvement in voluntary and campaigning activities than the common stereotype of young people would suggest', with 75 per cent of the sample classified as involved in some way (Roker *et al* 1999: 65). A follow-up study of youth social action groups revealed the diversity of young people involved, challenging the stereotypical image of 'mainly white middle class young people participating in social action' (Eden and Roker 2002: 38). In both cases, adult attitudes and behaviour were commonly cited as a major obstacle to effective participation.

With regard to formal political engagement, there was considerable fluidity in attitudes towards using the vote over the three years in our study. When it came to the 2001 General Election, about half voted. Although 'insiders' were twice as likely to have voted as 'outsiders', the differential had almost disappeared among the oldest participants. 'Insiders' and young women were more likely to give reasons for voting that reflected a sense of civic duty. Six (five of whom were female) said they were motivated to vote by the knowledge that the vote had been fought for. The main substantive reasons given for not voting among the other 33 referred to a perception of politics as boring or irrelevant; critical attitudes towards formal politics and politicians or the efficacy of voting; and lack of political literacy.

Conclusion

Young people take seriously the question of their relationship to the wider society. The overriding impression received from in-depth discussions on the meanings of citizenship is of a highly responsible group. The common assumptions of politicians that rights have been overemphasised at the expense of responsibilities and that young people, in particular, need to be made aware of their citizenship responsibilities are not borne out by the study. Indeed, the young people found it much more difficult to talk about rights than responsibilities and when they did identify rights they were more likely to be civil than political or social rights. Few saw social security rights as unconditional. The young people also tended to place a high premium on constructive social participation in the local community and many of them had engaged in such participation. It represented for many of them the essence of good citizenship and was one of two more responsibility-based models that emerged as prominent from general discussions of the meanings of citizenship. The most dominant model was, however, a less active one rooted in membership of the community or nation. Few thought about citizenship in social-contractual terms.

Together, these elements indicate that, of the three main citizenship paradigms developed in the literature, it is the communitarian to which the young people were most likely to subscribe (Bussemaker and Voet 1998, Delanty 2000).[5] They also displayed a belief in at least some 'civic virtues' (Dagger 1997) and the importance to citizenship of civility and respect

(McKinnon 2000) and giving to the community (Heater 1990). Liberal rights-based and civic republican political participation-based models did not figure prominently in their discussions. This suggests that they may have taken on board political messages about active citizenship and about responsibilities over rights (though not the related social-contractual model propounded by New Labour) that have become increasingly dominant over the past couple of decades in the UK.

Similarly, the young people's image of the first class citizen is redolent of the successful citizen promoted by Thatcherism and to a degree under New Labour: economically independent, with money, own home and a family. For some of those classified as 'outsiders', this meant that they themselves identified with the label of 'second class citizen', below everyone else. The respectable economic independence model of citizenship, which under-pinned such understandings, became more dominant during the course of the research. Its potentially divisive and exclusionary nature stands in ten-sion with the more inclusive universal, membership model, which was most dominant overall. It also stands in contradiction to T. H. Marshall's classic definition of citizenship as bestowing equal status on all full members of a national community (Marshall 1950). Instead of challenging class divisions, the respectable economic independence model of citizenship reinforces them.

This points to how everyday understandings of citizenship can have both inclusionary and exclusionary implications. Such implications need to be borne in mind by politicians and by educators responsible for citizenship education, introduced as a statutory subject in September 2002 in order to equip secondary school children with 'the knowledge, skills and disposi-tions for active citizenship' (Blunkett 2003: 12). The more that exclusion-ary models of citizenship dominate, the less likely it is that disadvantaged young people will identify themselves as citizens. The same is true if politi-cians, educators and others who work with young people promote a deficit image of young people's citizenship and impose a model that has no reso-nance with young people's own experiences (Kerr et al 2002, Youth, Citizenship and Social Change 2003a). Instead, they need to listen to young people's own views on citizenship and to acknowledge the existing contri-bution they make as citizens.

Endnotes

1 The study was funded by the Economic and Social Research Council (project L134 25 1039). References to the young people's ages all refer to their age at the time of the first wave. An earlier version of the chapter appeared in Citizenship Studies (2003) 7: 2, http://www.tandf.co.uk.
2 Apart from the above-average attrition of 'outsiders', anticipated in the construc-tion of the original sample, the final group broadly reflected the balance of the original. The analysis refers to the 64 who participated in all three waves except

where questions were confined to the first and/or second waves. In addition to the three qualitative interviews, a short factual questionnaire was administered at recruitment stage and a focus group of some of the participants was held after the first wave to help inform questioning in subsequent waves.
3 The Cantle Report was commissioned by the Government following disturbances in a number of Northern towns.
4 A MORI poll found that two-thirds of 15 to 24 year olds felt they knew little about their rights as citizens compared with half who felt the same about their responsibilities (Wolchover 2002).
5 The other two main paradigms are the liberal, which emphasises rights, and the civic republican, which promotes political participation.

References

Advisory Group on Citizenship (1998) *Education for Citizenship and the Teaching of Democracy in Schools*, London: Qualifications and Curriculum Authority.

Arnot, M. and Dillabough, J. (eds) (2000) *Challenging Democracy. International Perspectives on Gender, Education and Citizenship*, London: Routledge.

Blunkett, D. (2003) *Civil Renewal: A new agenda*, London: Home Office.

Brown, G. (2000) James Meade Lecture, 8 May, London.

Bussemaker, J. and Voet, R. (1998) 'Citizenship and gender, theoretical approaches and historical legacies', *Critical Social Policy*, 18(3): 277–307.

Cantle, T. (2001) *Community Cohesion: A report of the independent review team*, London: Home Office.

Conover, P. J., Crewe, I. M. and Searing, D. D. (1991) 'The nature of citizenship in the United States and Great Britain: empirical comments on theoretical themes', *Journal of Politics*, 53(3): 800–832.

Dagger, R. (1997) *Civic Virtues. Rights, Citizenship and Republican Liberalism*. Oxford: Oxford University Press.

Dean, H. with Melrose, M. (1999) *Poverty, Riches and Social Citizenship*, Basingstoke: Macmillan.

Delanty, G. (2000) *Citizenship in a Global Age*, Buckingham: Open University Press.

Dwyer, P. (2000) *Welfare Rights and Responsibilities. Contesting Social Citizenship*, Bristol: Policy Press.

Eden, K. and Roker, D. (2002) '. . . *Doing Something' Young People as Social Actors*, Leicester: Youth Work Press.

France, A. (1998) '"Why should we care?" Young people, citizenship and questions of social responsibility', *Journal of Youth Studies*, 1(1): 97–111.

Fulbrook, M. and Cesarini, D. (1996) 'Conclusion', in D. Cesarini and M. Fulbrook (eds), *Citizenship, Nationality and Migration in Europe*, London: Routledge.

Hall, T., Williamson, H. and Coffey, A. (1998) 'Conceptualizing citizenship, young people and the transition to adulthood', *Journal of Education Policy*, 13 (3): 301–315.

Harris, C., Roach, P., Thiara, R., et al. (2001) *Emergent Citizens? African Caribbean and Pakistani Young People in Bradford and Birmingham*, Birmingham: University of Birmingham.

Heater, D. (1990) *Citizenship*, London: Longman.

Hobson, B. and Lindholm, M. (1997) 'Collective identities, women's power resources, and the making of welfare states', *Theory and Society*, 26: 475–508.

Isin, E. F. and Wood, P. K. (1999) *Citizenship and Identity*, London: Sage.

Jones, E. and Gaventa, J. (2002) *Concepts of Citizenship, A Review*, Brighton: Institute for Development Studies.

Jones, K. B. (1994) 'Identity, action and locale: thinking about citizenship, civic action and feminism', *Social Politics*, 1(3): 256–270.

Kerr, D., Cleaver, E., Ireland, E. *et al.* (2003) *Citizenship Education Longitudinal Study First Cross-Sectional Survey 2001–2002*. London: Department for Education and Skills.

Kerr, D., Lines, A. Blenkinsop, S. *et al.* (2002) *England's Results from the IEA International Citizenship Education Study: What citizenship and education mean to 14 year olds*, London: Department for Education and Skills.

Knijn, T. and Kremer, M. (1997) 'Gender and the caring dimension of welfare states: towards inclusive citizenship', *Social Politics*, 4(3): 328–361.

Lister, R. (2003) *Citizenship: Feminist perspectives*, 2nd edn, Basingstoke: Palgrave.

McKinnon, C. (2000) 'Civil citizens', in C. McKinnon and I. Hampsher-Monk (eds), *The Demands of Citizenship*, London: Continuum.

Marshall, T. H. (1950) *Citizenship and Social Class*, Cambridge: Cambridge University Press.

Miller, D. (2000) 'Citizenship: what does it mean and why is it important?', in N. Pearce and J. Hallgarten (eds), op. cit.

Park, A. (1999) 'Young people and political apathy' in R. Jowell, J. Curtice, A. Park and K. Thompson (eds), *British Social Attitudes. The 16th Report*, Aldershot: Ashgate.

Pearce, N. and Hallgarten, J. (eds) (2000) *Tomorrow's Citizens. Critical Debates in Citizenship and Education*, London: Institute for Public Policy Research.

Roker, D. Player, K. and Coleman, J. (1999) *Challenging the Image*, Leicester: Youth Work Press.

Sevenhuijsen, S. (1998) *Citizenship and the Ethics of Care*, London: Routledge.

Shotter, J. (1993) 'Psychology and citizenship: identity and belonging', in B. S. Turner (ed.), *Citizenship and Social Theory*, London: Sage.

Sparks, H. (1997) 'Dissident citizenship: democratic theory, political courage, and activist women', *Hypatia*, 12 (4): 74–110.

Speaker's Commission (1990) *Encouraging Citizenship. Report of the Commission on Citizenship*, London: HMSO.

Stevenson, N. (ed.) (2001) *Culture and Citizenship*, London: Sage.

Turner, B. S. (1997) 'Citizenship studies: a general theory', *Citizenship Studies*, 1(1): 5–18.

Wolchover, J. (2002) 'Today's lesson: citizenship for beginners', *The Independent*, 18 April.

Youth, Citizenship and Social Change (2003a) 'Tomorrow's citizens: young people, citizenship and social participation', *Dissemination Report* 2, Brighton: Trust for the Study of Adolescence.

Youth, Citizenship and Social Change (2003b) 'Mind the gap! Education/training bridges into employability and citizenship, *Dissemination Report* 4, Brighton: Trust for the Study of Adolescence.

Postscript on citizenship

Tom Burke

I am a 19-year-old student currently studying for a BA (Hons) in International Relations with Development Studies at the University of Sussex. I have been active in youth participation projects for the past five years. It began with local projects and campaigning, but now includes involvement in national and international child rights advocacy projects. In these projects I have worked directly with young people and tried to help them express themselves. My own interests are based on which young people get the opportunity to participate and why, and what are the barriers to their participation, especially in decision-making processes My hobbies include clubbing and (when I get around to it!) reading.

This chapter by Ruth Lister *et al* offers a fascinating insight into some young people's views of their citizenship. It blows away the view of a homogenous British youth, showing how different young people have a different experience of citizenship depending on their education and their life prospects. Bravely, the authors claim that they will challenge representations of young people by the New Labour machine as 'deficient citizens'. Instead, they favour an understanding of young people as 'citizens in the making'.

I am compelled to agree that the concept of 'deficient citizens' is flawed. It raises questions as to 'what' young people are supposedly deficient of and who decides this. It is a label which neatly ignores a universal notion of citizenship. It ignores the barriers to young people's active participation in our society and helps to propagate the all too prevailing view of young people as somehow more generally 'deficient' or incomplete in comparison to their adult counterparts. Further, it is a deficiency that is the young person's own fault, often brought about through anti-social behaviour. This is a myth which this chapter helps to demolish.

However, in demolishing the myth of 'deficient citizens' they have created a new myth of young people as 'citizens in the making'. They turn from myth destroyers to myth makers in one short and degrading sentence.

The notion of 'citizens in the making' is just as fundamentally flawed as that of 'deficient citizens'. It perpetuates a passive view of young people who are idly waiting for citizenship, and if they are lucky, it will be bestowed upon them by others. It does not give young people their true credit as social actors in their own right nor does it recognise the contribution that young people are making to our society today.

I am not suggesting that the citizenship young people 'enjoy' is the same citizenship that adults have. The relationship between young people and adults is, like all social relationships, one based on power and in almost every circumstance young people have less power than adults and adult-run institutions, such as government. The difference between adult and youth citizenship is that the vast majority of young people are citizens whose citizenship is being violated by a government all too keen to criminalise young people and weaken their rights.

This government has consistently labelled the vast majority of young people as troublesome because of their apparent anti-social behaviour. Child prostitutes are legally seen as criminals and not as victims. Children as young as ten are tried in adult Crown Courts. The UK continues to lock up more children and young people than any other country in Europe. The recent Sexual Offences Bill criminalises two consenting under 16s to kiss! The Anti-social Behaviour Act has given police powers to disperse groups of two or more young people and take any unaccompanied under 16 home to their parents after 9 p.m., creating a de facto national curfew. It also allows the public disclosure of those given an Anti-social Behaviour Order, making the 'naming and shaming' campaigns of children a real possibility.

The criminalisation of young people in the media, in the majority of schools and education institutions, the criminal justice system and through the government's spin machine has been so strong that young people themselves have started to believe it: believing the hype and propaganda that they are second class and, as noted above, somehow not citizens. This is creating a self-creating prophecy where young people become so hopeless that even the few opportunities that are open to them become out of reach due to a lack of aspiration. There is a famine of hope for too many young people which must be reversed.

I would argue that the inequality in power between young people and adults prevents the vast majority of young people from fulfilling the dominant notion of being a citizen. When the participants in Ruth Lister *et al*'s study were asked if they identified themselves as citizens, the 'outsiders' were less likely than 'insiders' to do so. I would suggest that all the young people in the study, and our society, should be viewed as citizens. The difference between the two groups' view of their citizenship identity is one of perception. The 'outsiders' have recognised that their rights and entitlements are being denied but the 'insiders' perceive that these rights and entitlements are being fulfilled. If they are 'typical' of most British young people, then the 'insiders' perception is inaccurate.

We need to ensure that young people do know their rights and how to claim them, based on a pedagogical process, formal and informal, which sees all young people as citizens now and aims to give them the knowledge and skills to enable them to take up their rights. In the research by Ruth Lister *et al*, twice as many 'insiders' than 'outsiders' identified themselves unambiguously as 'citizens'. Such a pedagogical process would highlight to the 'insiders' just how badly society treats them as well as 'outsiders':

- Their right to an adequate living standard is violated, with one in three children living below the poverty line; three million living in poor housing.
- Their right to education is violated: during 2001/02 there were 9535 permanent exclusions from school, and of these 82 per cent were young men.
- Black African-Caribbean children are three times more likely to be excluded than white children.
- Inequalities in achievement remain with those in receipt of free school meals, who are likely to have the lowest achievement levels in schools.
- Only 15 per cent of primary schools and 7 per cent of secondary schools are fully accessible to disabled pupils.
- Teenage women in Britain are more likely to get pregnant than teenage women in any other European country.
- A postcode lottery for funding for youth services has emerged with huge inequalities in funding across the country.

I am not a citizen in the making. I am a citizen today. We must view *all* young people as citizens today. We must create a society where *all* young people identify themselves as citizens. Citizenship is something which every young person is automatically entitled to and not something which needs to be earned or taken away. Citizenship is a right not a charitable act. As Ruth Lister *et al* note, citizenship must be inclusive not exclusive.

Margaret Thatcher is (in)famous for pleading that 'Young people should not be idle. It is very bad for them'. I completely agree. We must not be idle when we are being criminalised and our rights eroded.

Chapter 4

Beyond rhetoric: Extending rights to young people

Michael Freeman

It is all too obvious to us today that we cannot debate issues of exclusion and inclusion without introducing and emphasising rights. After all, we now live in a rights-conscious culture, the most striking evidence of which is the incorporation of the European Convention on Human Rights into United Kingdom law in 1998. But it was not always thus. I can think of no rights that adults enjoy today that were 'given' to them: all were fought for and often bitterly contested. We have also become increasingly conscious of the wrongs of discrimination, with protection and rights now accorded (or at least mooted) to disabled people, to gay people and even to such an unlikely group as transsexuals.

The 'young' have not found it as easy. There is little talk even today of the rights of the 'young'. True, there is rather more discussion of children's rights – the arbitrary dividing line between 'children' and 'adults' being 18 – but there is also complacency. Fifteen years ago, in 1989, the world wallowed in the glory of the Children's Convention: the United Nations (UN) Convention on the Rights of the Child. And who can forget the World Summit for Children a year later, and Margaret Thatcher's statement '. . . children come first because children are our most sacred trust'? The question is rhetorical, for if no one else forgot this, she certainly did. She presided over a steep rise in child poverty and deprivation which New Labour has done little to reverse. And, whatever the state of deprivation, of exclusion, of children and youth in Britain, it is nothing as compared with much of the world, with the young dying of starvation and AIDS in much of Africa, of radiation in the Ukraine and other parts of, what I like to call, the Soviet Disunion, being used as slave labour in much of Africa and Asia (and increasingly in the West) and living in shanties, refugee camps, and as prostitutes for Western tourists in many countries of the Third World (the latter a problem being increasingly exported to the West).

Why rights?

This chapter is about rights. Why, it may be asked. There are some who believe we have been taken in by 'the myth of rights' (Scheingold 1974, Kerruish

1991). Rights are characterised by some as vacuous, competitive and abstract. To one leading critical thinker, rights discourse is a 'trap', because 'it is logically incoherent and manipulable, traditionally individualist and wilfully blind to the realities of substantive inequality' (Kennedy 1992: 57). Now, it must be admitted that rights can be all these things. It is very easy for the powerful to agree to the enactment of rights, as, of course, has happened to a very large extent with the UN Convention on the Rights of the Child, and then do very little to make them a reality. Agreeing to rights is relatively easy: putting them into practice, so that they have an impact on lives may be inconvenient, troublesome or costly (or all three). As Monrad Paulsen commented (in relation to laws mandating the reporting of child abuse), 'no law can be better than its implementation, and implementation can be no better than resources permit' (Paulsen 1974: 48). But it requires more than this: it requires the will to commit the resources, the political decision – often, it may be said, a gamble since there are no votes in prioritising children or youth – to advance interests of those who would otherwise remain on the margins. Rights require not just resources but also need to be tied into effective remedies. To this end, the importance of representation hardly needs to be stressed. And it is representation not just in the obvious forum, the courts, where the legality of state and local state actions can be challenged, but also before policy-making bodies. It is a pity that the row over Margaret Hodge's appointment as Minister for Children (in June 2003) should have diverted attention away from the so much more important issue of what a Minister of Children was there to do, and whether a Minister, rather than the more obvious Children's Commissioner (or Ombudsperson) was the best way of ensuring children's rights were promoted. But given that at virtually the same time the Prime Minister ruled out once again an anti-smacking law, it may be doubted whether promoting children's interests is really on his agenda.

Rights are a 'militant concept', part of an 'ideology in a campaign for social change' (Cohen 1980: 52). Critics, referred to already, believe that rights can atomise. They can, and they can deflate social struggles. But this need not necessarily happen. Rather than seeing rights in individualistic terms, rights can be emphasised as 'relational' (Nedelsky 1989; see also Gilligan 1982). Rights can, rather obviously, only exist in relation to others, and thus within the framework of responsibilities. The existence of a right does not mean it should necessarily or always be exercised. Responsibility to others dictates that we do not invariably insist upon our rights. Furthermore, our responsibilities can trump our rights. The close inter-relationship of rights and responsibilities has only come to be recognised recently, but it is important. And it does not make rights any less significant.

Rights remain important for they are 'valuable commodities' (Wasserstrom 1964: 629). In Bandman's words, they 'enable us to stand with dignity if necessary to demand what is our due without having to grovel, plead or beg' (Bandman 1973: 236). It is instructive to reflect upon what a society without rights would look like. Such a society would be morally impoverished. It might well be a benevolent society in which people were treated well, but they would have no cause for complaint if standards were to fall. A world with a claim on rights by contrast is 'one in which all persons are dignified objects of respect. . . . No amount of love and compassion, or obedience to higher authority, or *noblesse oblige,* can substitute for those values' (Feinberg 1966: 8).

Marginalised groups have only come to be regarded as rights-holders in the relatively recent past. This is not just the case with children: in the perspective of history it will surely seem odd how women, in particular married women, were excluded from the *polis* and all that this involved in many spheres until well into the last century. It is a badge of the marginalised that they are deprived of rights, such that others (the privileged) have rights over them. In the case of slaves, they were *res* (literally property): in the case of children it was as if they were property. Who can forget Mia Kellmer-Pringle's graphic censure of those for whom the birth of a child was like the acquisition of a consumer durable: like a TV or fridge – these were the examples of 30 years ago – they completed a family? (Kellmer-Pringle 1976: 156).

Why rights for the young?

But in the case of the young, is it necessary to emphasise rights? In relation to children at least four arguments have been made to suggest that an emphasis on rights is unnecessary or exaggerated. These arguments apply with less force to older adolescents and young people but their force cannot be discounted here either.

There is first an argument, best articulated by Onora O'Neill (1988). This does not question the view that children's lives are a public concern, rather than a private matter. Nor does it question the aim of securing positive rights for children. But it does question whether children's positive rights are best grounded by appeals to fundamental rights. She claims that 'children's fundamental rights are best grounded by embedding them in a wider account of fundamental obligations' (O'Neill 1988: 445–6). It is her contention that 'we can perhaps go *further* to secure the ethical basis of children's positive rights if we do *not* try to base them on claims about fundamental rights' (ibid: 446, emphasis in original). In the specific case of children, she believes that taking rights as fundamental has 'political costs rather than advantages' (ibid: 306).

I have several differences with O'Neill. She cannot envisage a children's movement. But, of course, there have been prototypes: school unionisation, NAYPIC (the National Association of Young People in Care) and movements on behalf of children and young people (as there were and are movements to propagate the interests and advance the causes of other marginalised groups). Secondly, she thinks the dependency of children is 'very different' from the dependency of other oppressed groups. She gives four reasons for believing this:

1. it is not artificially produced, though she concedes it can be artificially extended;
2. it cannot be ended merely by social or political changes;
3. others are not reciprocally dependent on children, whereas slave-owners, for example, need their slaves; and
4. in the case of children and the young, the 'oppressors' usually want the dependency to end.

Of course, there are some differences, but I do not think children's dependency is quite as different as O'Neill would have us believe. To some extent it is (cf. point 1) artificially produced: both the lessons of history (Ariès 1962) and our own experiences and intuitions tell us that many children have the capacity to be less dependent than many adults. As far as point 2 is concerned, some – clearly not all – can be ended by political, if not by social, change. The reciprocal dependency argument point 3 can also be overplayed: think of the parent who needs to be loved and shown affection by his child or the enormous input made by young carers which generally goes unrecognised and certainly unrewarded (see, for example, Chapter 13 this volume). And it is patently untrue that all parents want the dependency of the young to end (cf. point 4).

A third difference I have with O'Neill stems from the second. She sees children as a special case. Although she concedes that the fact that children cannot claim rights is no reason for denying them rights, the claiming/waiving dilemma seems to be at the root of her thinking. She is wedded to the 'will theory' of rights. But I think the interest theory is both more coherent and has greater explanatory power. Children have interests to protect before they develop wills to assert, and others can complain on behalf of younger children when those interests are trampled upon. This argument anyway weakens the older a child gets, and in the context of this book has little force. It cannot be right, as O'Neill states, that the child's 'main remedy is to grow up': first, because the meaning of 'growing up' is a social construction – those who define can so easily infanticise; secondly, she underestimates the capacity and maturity of many children. To some extent English law recognises this with the so-called *Gillick* principle (see *Gillick* v. *West Norfolk and Wisbech Area Health Authority*, 1986), and, more spectacularly, by imposing criminal responsibility on children as young as ten years old. This was graphically illustrated in the *Bulger* case in 1993, which has had such terrifying consequences. Thirdly, what O'Neill ignores is the impact on adult life that parenting and socialisation leave. Thus, a child deprived of the sort of rights accorded by the UN Convention will grow up very differently from one to whom such rights are granted.

O'Neill's essay must be contended with by those who espouse children's rights. But she is not alone in deflecting our attention away from rights for children. There is also the argument that the importance of rights and rights language itself can be exaggerated. There are other morally significant values such as love, friendship, compassion and altruism, and these raise relationships to a higher plain than where the goal is duty – compliance to uphold rights. But children and the young cannot rely on these virtues. They are particularly vulnerable, and need rights to protect their dignity and integrity. Of course, when you give any group rights, there is likely to be conflict, and this is no less so with children and the young generally. They will complain, make claims (not all of which will be legitimate) and challenge authority. Were they not able to do so, life would be easier for parents, teachers, social workers, the police, etc. But there would still be conflict which would simmer below the surface, only occasionally boiling over. Think of our treatment of prisoners who have few rights (though these have increased recently) and of the riots which periodically erupt.

Another argument commonly adduced is related to the last one. It assumes that adults already relate to children in terms of love, care and altruism, so that the case for children's rights becomes otiose – or so the argument runs. But this idealises adult–child relations. It emphasises that adults (and parents in particular) consider only the best interests of children. There is thus a tendency for those who postulate this argument also to adopt a laissez faire attitude towards the family. Goldstein *et al*, in a series of books starting with *Beyond the Best Interests of the Child* (Goldstein *et al* 1973) and culminating in *The Best Interests of the Child* (Goldstein *et al* 1996), claim almost the only right which children have is the right to autonomous parents. That children prosper within such a private space is clearly not always the case.

The final argument against rights for children equally rests on a myth. It sees childhood as a golden age, the best years of our life if we but only knew it. Childhood becomes on this view synonymous with innocence. It is the time when, spared the rigours of adult life, we enjoy freedom and experience play and joy. The argument runs: just as we avoid the responsibilities and adversities of adult life in childhood, so there should be no necessity to think in terms of rights, a concept which we must assume is reserved for adults whose lives are so much more difficult. Unfortunately, far too many children do not live in this mythic 'walled garden of Happy, Safe, Protected, Innocence, Childhood' (Holt 1975: 152). They are rather more likely to experience it as deprived and abused, with few systems in place to put their interests first.

Which rights?

One cannot discuss rights in this context without examining the provisions in the UN Convention on the Rights of the Child. True, its scope is limited to those under 18 years old, but many of its provisions resonate with the problems of young people who are older than what is now seen as the conventional age of majority. Ironically, if pressure for a Convention had succeeded earlier – the declaration was as early as 1959 – it would undoubtedly have embraced all under 21 years of age. The Convention may be seen as an 'advocacy tool' (Veerman 1992: 184), and one that promotes the welfare of children as an issue of justice, rather than as one of benevolence or charity. We may look at it in this way and in doing so examine its relevance to the young above 18 years old as well as to those below this age. We will see the Convention has its limits (and see Freeman 2000), even when applied to 'children', and some of those limits may become clearer when we focus on the wider group.

Participation rights

Perhaps most significant is that the Convention recognises the right for children to 'have a say' in processes affecting their lives. In this way the child is, and probably for the first time, regarded as a 'principal' (Pais 1992: 76). This comes out most clearly in Article 12 which requires State Parties to 'assure to the child who is capable of forming his or her own views the right to express those views freely in all matters affecting the child'. In particular, it is stressed, the child is to be given the opportunity to be heard in any judicial or administrative proceeding either directly or through a representative. It is acknowledged that this is a right that becomes more meaningful as the child gets older and maturer. This is also acknowledged in English law, at least in theory, with the *Gillick* principle, first formulated in 1985 and now also embedded in legislation (the Children Act 1989 and the Children (Scotland) Act 1995) (Fortin 2003).

Participation is a key to inclusion. It is emblematic of what being a person is. But children and young persons (even when technically 'legal persons', a status acquired at 18 years of age) all-too-often remain social problems rather than participants in social processes. Participating rights are about being proactive, about making decisions and about being genuinely consulted. Less maturity and less experience may mean more mistakes – it does not follow that it will, and we know that the most experienced amongst us and the most 'mature' make mistakes – but central to any true understanding of rights is that they include the right to do what we (in this case 'adult society') think is wrong. We must respect the capacity of the young to take risks. Of course, they will make what we and what they subsequently think are mistakes, but we would not be taking rights seriously if we only respected autonomy when we considered the agent was doing the right thing.

And paternalism?

But does paternalism have a place? Amongst those who espoused children's liberation, particularly in the 1970s, the answer was 'no' (Farson 1978, Holt 1975). A fortiori, their arguments would apply to young adults. I am not comfortable with paternalism, but I think there must be limits to autonomy, and I think these must go beyond the Millian 'harm principle'. (Mill, of course, excluded those under 21 from his famous principle anyway, but a critical examination of his principle is not apposite here.) In seeking to find these limits, it is worth examining part at least of the context of social exclusion. It cannot be ignored, though some I know would want it to be, that there are some clear correlates of social exclusion. Unemployment and low-status employment are two very obvious ones. We cannot ignore the close inter-relationship between employment prospects and educational success. Thus, it is important to recognise, as the UN Convention does in Article 28, the right to education. Can compulsory education thus be defended even where it interferes with what the child wants? I think so, but in saying this I would draw attention to the way education is conceived of in the Convention. Article 29 states the objectives of education. Thus, it is to be directed to the development of both cultural identity and values, and national values as well as those of civilisations different from the particular child's. It is also to be directed towards the development of the child's personality, the development of respect for human rights and the preparation of the child for responsible life. These purposes need not be written in stone and we would do well to be flexible, but they are important, and the right to education thus conceived is one into which I would wish to opt every child.

A right to education

By contrast, it is worth noting that our legislation has shamefacedly refused to acknowledge children's rights in the area of education. There is no right to education as such, and the messages conveyed by legislation are very clear: education is to be centrally directed and market-driven, and the consumers of education are the parents, and not the children (Freeman 1996, Jeffs 1995). Schools have been said to operate in ways that 'express contempt for the values of a free society' (Strike 1982: 147). Pupils excluded from school are denied the right even to 'make representations' to the body deciding whether they may be re-admitted to school. Until the mid–1980s, there was a trend towards increased student involvement in decision-making processes at school, but this policy was reversed by the Education Act 1986.

Government education policy, with its emphasis on centralisation, constrains the scope for any extension of children's rights within education (Ranson 1992). And, as Best put it ten years ago (Best 1993: 125), the goal is now 'a mass, standardised product'. Jeffs is surely right to observe that the 'right of children to a broad-based, intellectually stimulating education has been sacrificed on the high altar of competition' (Jeffs 1995: 35). At least the cane has now gone, though this was still allowed and used until the late 1990s.

This education example was introduced to suggest that there are limits to autonomy, but other insights have emerged from it: the content and scope of education, the importance of self-government and the value of giving the recipients of education an input into it. Like other examples I could give – the use of drugs or the refusal to eat – it is controversial and papers could be written examining as case studies each of these examples, and many others. But there is a general point, and I will content myself by addressing it (as I have done previously: see in particular Freeman 1983).

And freedom?

Too often writers of children's rights have dichotomised: there is either salvation or liberation, either nurturance or self-determination. But to take children's rights seriously requires us to take seriously both protection of children and acceptance of their autonomy. The view I espouse is premised on the need to respect individual autonomy and to treat persons as equals. It is not dependent on actual autonomy but on the capacity for it. It draws on Rawls (1971): it is the normative value of equality and autonomy which form the substructure of the Rawlsian conception of the social contract. Rawls's principles of justice cannot be stated in detail here, but for our purposes they confine paternalism without totally eliminating it. Parties to a hypothetical social contract would know that some human beings are less capable than others, and they would know how the actions of those with limited capacities might thwart their autonomy in a future time when their capacities were no longer limited.

These considerations would lead to an acceptance of interventions in people's lives to protect them against irrational actions. But what is to be regarded as 'irrational' must be strictly confined. Subjective values of the would-be protector must not intrude. Irrationality must be defined in terms of a neutral theory capable of accommodating pluralistic visions of the 'good'. And we should only be prepared to dismiss an action as irrational when it is manifestly so and is severe and systematic, when taking the action will lead to major irreversible impairment of interests. I would maintain the use of hard drugs or the refusal to attend school come into this category. Significantly, as I have indicated, they are also correlates of exclusion.

The question we should ask ourselves is: what sort of action or conduct would we wish, as children, to be shielded against on the assumption that we would want to mature to a rationally autonomous adult and be capable of deciding our own system of ends as free and rational beings? We would, I am convinced, choose principles that would enable us to mature to independent adulthood. One definition of irrationality would be that which precluded action and conduct which would frustrate such a goal. And within the constraints of such a definition we would defend a limited version of paternalism. This is not paternalism in its classical sense – this would give little scope for children's rights at all. Furthermore, it must be emphasised that this version of paternalism, which I call 'liberal paternalism', is a two-edged sword in that, since the goal is rational independence, those who exercise constraints must do so in such a way as to enable children to develop their capacities.

All paternalistic interventions require moral justification. In many cases it is not difficult to adduce sufficient convincing, reasoned argument. Thus, it is not difficult to present the case for protecting children against actions that may lead to their death, serious injury or psychological harm. Teenage girls have the rights to expect us to protect them from those who would push them into the sex industry. Children have the right to expect us to protect them from paedophiles. There are clear dangers that the suggestion of Farson (1978), Holt (1975) and others that a child's right to self-determination includes a right to a sexual relationship with whomsoever he or she pleases could so easily become a charter for exploitation and degradation.

What should legitimise all interferences with autonomy is, what Gerald Dworkin (1972: 122) has called, 'future-oriented consent'. The question is: can the restrictions be justified in terms that the child would eventually come to appreciate. Looking back, would the child appreciate and accept the reason for the restriction imposed on him, given what he now knows as a rationally autonomous adult? The dichotomy drawn above is thus to some extent a false divide. Dichotomies and other classifications should not divert us away from the fact that true protection of children does protect their rights. Thus, those who emphasise what tends to be called child-saving and those who argue for children's liberation are both right: both are correct in pointing out part of what needs recognising, but both are wrong in failing to see the value in the claims of the other side. To take children's rights seriously requires us to take seriously not only nurturance but also self-determination and demands of us that we adopt policies, practices and laws which both protect children and protect their rights. Hence, the *via media* I have long advocated (Freeman 1983).

Let us now look at some of the rights which are of greatest significance to older children and to young people generally. What emphasis one adopts here is dependent on the economic and social context: in developing countries, for example, there can be few more important rights than what the UN Convention recognises in Article 24 as 'the enjoyment of the highest attainable standard of health'. But our focus is on the United Kingdom and on older children and young adults. The right to education is fundamental:

this has already been considered. I would, however, add, using the language of the UN Convention (see Article 28), the emphasis on taking measures to 'encourage regular attendance at schools and the reduction of drop-out rates'. Expressed thus, there is no imputation (or any necessary imputation) that truancy and dropping-out are the pupil's fault, but rather a recognition that it is a problem that must be tackled.

Child labour

Article 32 of the UN Convention addresses the problem of child labour and what it says can be generalised to embrace the work environment of young people as a whole. It recognises 'the right of the child to be protected from economic exploitation and from performing any work that is likely to be hazardous or to interfere with the child's education, or to be harmful to the child's health or physical, mental, spiritual, moral or social development'. Although usually perceived as a problem in the developing world, it is clear that our attention needs to be directed to 'economic exploitation' too. It is easier to tackle this within the formal sector, but its elimination at the informal, irregular level is much more difficult. Those on the margins are more likely to work on the margins, where conditions are poorest and remuneration at its lowest. And if they work within the family environment, not only may the exploitation be at its most severe and sustained but also the level of protection is likely to be at its weakest. Even the 'minimum wage' – anyway at its reduced level – is unlikely to bite. Far too few young workers are unionised, and the trade union movement has done far too little to recruit them as members. Only in recent years have we come to recognise the work done by 'young carers' (Becker 2000), a veritable army of unpaid workers, and the sacrifices they make, but their rights, even after legislation, are few.

Sexual exploitation and abuse

The Convention (in Article 34) addresses also the problem of sexual exploitation and abuse. We have awoken all too slowly to the sexual abuse of the young in institutional settings (Myers *et al* 1999). Given the close relationship between an upbringing in care and social and economic exclusion, this is particularly troublesome. But, surprisingly, less concern has been expressed about sexual exploitation, although much more attention is now being focused on this. The Convention expects States Parties to take all appropriate measures to prevent the 'exploitative use of children in prostitution and other unlawful sexual practices' and the 'exploitative use of children in pornographic performances and materials'. We have done far too little to implement these provisions. It took until the end of 1998 for guidelines to be published recommending that child prostitutes be treated as victims of crimes rather than as offenders, and we still await the decriminalisation of child prostitution (see Ayre and Barrett 2000). Far too little has been done to target paedophiles and other sex offenders. At times this has created a moral panic – for example, major protests in Portsmouth in 2000. The young deserve better: there can be few clearer indicia of social exclusion than being treated as a sex object. Not only does sexual exploitation endanger welfare but it also clearly undermines human dignity. Where children have been sexually exploited, there is a duty under the Convention (Article 39: see also Article 16 of the Convention for the Suppression of Traffic in Persons and of the Exploitation of the Prostitution of Others 1949) to provide for recovery and reintegration. Do we meet these obligations? Or do the victims just drift further into deeper black holes? There is more than a suspicion that it is the latter.

The drugs issue

Other forms of exploitation are also targeted by the UN Convention. Thus, Article 33 requires measures to be taken to protect children from the 'illicit use of narcotic drugs and psychotropic substances' and 'to prevent the use of children in the illicit production and trafficking of such substances'. Guidance on the type of effective measures to take is found in a recommendation of the Parliamentary Assembly of the Council of Europe. It observed that children in difficulties frequently reject traditional institutions, such as psychiatric hospitals. And so it recommends the development of therapeutic communities able to meet social, psychological and health needs, and which are also able to listen 'actively' to children (Recommendation 989, 1984). It also recommends a prohibition on the sale of glue and solvents to children. There is an obligation here too to promote the recovery and reintegration of those who have abused narcotics or substances. This is a duty to which we pay far too little attention.

Social exploitation

The Convention also included the catch-all Article 36, which imposes an obligation on States Parties to protect the child against 'all other forms of exploitation prejudicial to any aspects of the child's welfare'. This is usually (see Van Bueren 1995) understood to focus on 'social exploitation', and is therefore important in our context. Amongst those most at risk of social exploitation are those abandoned by their families (in which category we may also include those deprived of satisfactory aftercare upon leaving the care of institutions and substitute families) and street children (see Ennew 2000). These two categories are obviously closely intertwined. It will also include children who are refugees and asylum seekers (Candappa 2002; see also Chapter 10 this volume) and disabled children (Middleton 1999).

A rights agenda

This chapter has emphasised the centrality of rights. It has been stressed that this fits well into contemporary culture, particularly in a world which so readily took to heart the UN Convention (only Somalia and the United States have not ratified this). The Convention only applies to those under 18 years old but the principles and arguments underlying so very many articles can be applied by analogy to young people in general: indeed, many of them apply with equal, or almost equal, force to the whole population.

Rights are important because they are inclusive. But, as indicated already, we must get beyond rhetoric. Rights without remedies are of symbolic importance only. Remedies themselves require the injection of resources and a commitment on behalf of all of us that we regard rights with respect and that we want them to have an impact on people's lives (on all people's lives, and not just the privileged).

Rights are an important advocacy tool, a weapon to use in battles to secure recognition. Giving people rights without access to those who can present those rights without the right of representation is thus of little value.

Rights offer legitimacy to campaigns, to pressure groups, to the disadvantaged and to the excluded. They offer a way in; they open doors.

Rights are a resource. They offer a reasoned argument. They put a moral case. Too often those who oppose rights can offer little in response (I'm reminded of those who 'argue' the case against anti-smacking laws by saying 'it never did me any harm'!).

Rights offer fora for action. Without rights the excluded can request, beg and rely on others being nice or cooperative or generous, but they cannot demand. The most important right, though this is rarely articulated, is the right to possess rights (Arendt 1986).

And rights are 'trumps', as Ronald Dworkin (1977: 189) so eloquently reminded us. They cannot be knocked off their pedestal because it would be better for others were these rights not to exist. It would be easier for the powerful if those below them lacked rights. It would be easier to rule: decision-making would be swifter, cheaper and more convenient.

We must therefore see our future agenda as structured by rights. This will lead us to adopt laws, practices and institutions which will enable those on the margins of society to participate more meaningfully. It is also a path to a more just society. And this has consequences for all of us, not just the young.

References

Arendt, H. (1986) *The Origins of Totalitarianism*, London: Andre Deutsch.
Ariès, P. (1962) *Centuries of Childhood*, London: Jonathan Cape.
Ayre, P. and Barnett, D. (2000) 'Young people and prostitution: An end to the beginning', *Children and Society*, 14: 121.

Bandman, B. (1973) 'Do children have any natural rights?' *Proceedings of the 29th Annual Meeting of the Philosophy of Education Society*, 234.

Becker, S. (2000) 'Young carers', in M. Davies (ed.), *The Blackwell Encyclopaedia of Social Work*, Oxford: Blackwell.

Best, J.H. (1993) 'Perspectives on the deregulation of schooling in America', *British Journal of Educational Studies*, 41 (2): 122.

Candappa, M. (2002) 'Human rights and refugee children in the UK', in B. Franklin (ed.), *The New Handbook of Children's Rights*, London: Routledge.

Cohen, H. (1980) *Equal Rights For Children*, Totowa, New Jersey: Littlefield, Adams.

Dworkin, G. (1972) 'Paternalism', in R. Wasserstrom (ed.), *Morality and The Law*, California: Wadsworth.

Dworkin, R. (1977) *Taking Rights Seriously*, London: Dackworth.

Ennew, J. (2000) 'Why the Convention is not about street children', in D. Fottrell (ed.), *Revisiting Children's Rights*, The Hague: Kluwer.

Farson, R. (1978) *Birthrights*, Harmondsworth: Penguin.

Feinberg, J. (1966) 'Duties, rights and claims', *American Philosophy Quarterly*, 3: 137.

Fortin, J. (2003) *Children's Rights and the Developing Law*, London: Butterworths.

Freeman, M. (1983) *The Rights and Wrongs of Children*, London: Frances Pinter.

Freeman, M. (1996) 'Children's education: A test case for best interests and autonomy', in R. Davie and D. Galloway (eds), *Listening To Children In Education*, London: David Fulton.

Freeman, M. (2000) 'The future of children's rights', *Children and Society*, 14: 277.

Gilligan, C (1982) *In A Different Voice*, Cambridge, Mass: Harvard University Press.

Goldstein, J., Freud, A. and Solnit, A. (1979) *Beyond The Best Interests of the Child*, New York: Free Press.

Goldstein, J., Freud, A. and Solnit, A. (1996) *The Best Interests of the Child*, New York: Free Press.

Holt, J. (1975) *Escape From Childhood*, Harmondworth: Penguin.

Jeffs, T. (1995) 'Children's educational right to a new ERA' in B. Franklin (ed.), *The Handbook of Children's Rights*, London: Routledge.

Kellmer-Pringle, M. (1980) *The Needs of Children*, London: Hutchinson.

Kennedy, D. (1992) 'Legal education as training for hierarchy', in I. Griggs-Spall and P. Ireland (eds), *Critical Lawyers' Handbook*, London: Pluto Press.

Kerruish, V. (1991) *Jurisprudence As Ideology*, London: Routledge.

Middleton, L. (1999) *Disabled Children: Challenging social exclusion*, Oxford: Blackwells.

Myers, J., O'Neill, T. and Jones, J. (1999) 'Preventing institutional abuse: An exploration of children's rights, needs and participation in residential care', in Violence Against Children Study Group, *Children, Child Abuse and Child Protection*, Chichester: Wiley.

Nedelsky, J. (1989) 'Reconceiving autonomy: Sources, thoughts and possibilities', *Yale Journal of Law and Feminism 7*.

O'Neill, O. (1988) 'Children's rights and children's lives', *Ethics*, 98: 445.

Pais, M.S. (1992) 'The United Nations Convention on the Rights of the Child', *Bulletin on Human Rights*, 91(2): 75.

Paulsen, M. (1974) 'The Law and abused children', in R. Helfer and C. Kempe (eds), *The Battered Child*, Chicago: University of Chicago Press.

Ranson, S. (1992) *Local Democracy for the Learning Society*, London: National Commission for Education.

Rawls, J. (1972) *A Theory of Justice*, Cambridge, Mass: Harvard University Press.

Scheingold, S. (1974) *The Politics of Rights: Lawyers, public policy and political change*, New Haven: Yale University Press.

Strike, K. (1982) *Learning and Liberty*, London: Martin Robertson.

Van Bueren, G. (1995) *The International Law on the Rights of The Child*, Dordrecht: Martinus Nijhoff.

Veerman, P. (1991) *The Rights of the Child and the Changing Image of Childhood*, Dordrecht: Martinus Nijhoff.

Wasserstrom, R. (1964) 'Rights, human rights and racial discrimination', *Journal of Philosophy*, 61: 628.

Postscript on rights

Ellen Leaver and Regan Tammi

My name's Ellen Leaver. I am 20 years old and come from Scotland but I am now studying in London. I have had an interest in children's rights for a long time and joined Article 12 in Scotland at the age of 13. I was involved in many projects through Article 12 both in Scotland and with an international outlook. In 2002 I was one of the two young people on the government's delegation to the UN Special Session on Children, one of the most amazing experiences of my life. My interests extended to human rights and I am now studying law at Queen Mary University in London with a view to specialising in rights and environmental concerns. I believe that children are a special group of people who have needs which are both common to all humans and are specific to them. The UNCRC was a step forward but after the Special Session and the pre-ceding Children's Forum it is clear that there is a very long way to go, but if the young people I have met are anything to go by, and they don't loose their passion and determination, I believe the world and its children have a brighter future.

I am Regan Tammi, I'm 18 years old and live in Montrose, Scotland. I have had an interest in animal and environmental rights since an early age and have been a member of Greenpeace for the last four years. My interest and involvement with human rights came as a direct result of my negative experiences of secondary education, which ended at 16 when the school rector suggested that, with my views and appearance, I would be better off studying elsewhere. Although I was devastated at the time and shocked that an educational establishment should seek to exclude a young person because they held strong views and chose not to wear a school uniform, looking back this was the best thing that could have happened to me as it made me all the more determined to achieve my aims. Since leaving school I have spent time studying biol-ogy, english and genetics at college, held down a number of part-time jobs ranging from forestry worker to supermarket check-out assistant and since March 2004 I have been working for LBV-Unterfranken in Germany, a national society for the protection of wildlife and the environment.

The ratification of the United Nations Convention on the Rights of the Child (UNCRC) was a monumental occasion for all the world's children. The UK is one of 191 states that have ratified the Convention but we have not as yet made it legally binding. In 2001 statistics were paraded in front of the UN Special Session on Children, that demonstrated the successes achieved. It must be recognised that these were only the first steps and that much remains to be done. Many of the statistics relate to standards in health care and the numbers of children receiving a basic education. Most presume that these are not problems that we need consider here in the UK and as a result it becomes more difficult to defend the notion of rights for young people. Although to some extent this is true, it must be noted that many children in the UK live in poverty, and there are groups who find themselves excluded from education and many other areas of life.

Young people and children play a much more vital role in society than is often realised. Michael Freeman mentions the role of young carers which is unrecognised and grossly undervalued. It is perhaps a cliché to say that children are the adults of tomorrow; on the other hand, like so many clichés it is the simple truth. It is, therefore, the duty of adults to help us grow and learn, in order to become adults capable of looking after the world and our own children.

In the UK and other Western countries, those articles in the UNCRC relating to education must not be disregarded as already fulfilled. Freeman believes that compulsory basic education can be defended on the basis of defending the child's interests: that is to say that in order to promote social inclusion and a better future it may be necessary to enforce school attendance. This is all very well, but among the groups of children so often excluded from society and education are those who suffer learning or behavioural difficulties. These young people are treated as problems and many find themselves entirely excluded from school; little is done to reintegrate them and often they find themselves in specialised environments designed to 'deal' with them. Other groups isolated from education in the UK include young travellers. These young people find themselves excluded from society behind the veil of labels. The system has done too little to recognise the importance of finding a way to integrate them into education.

Our communities are ever-expanding today with the influx of refugees and asylum seekers. Many are young people also face discrimination and exclusion from the system. Michael Freeman also noted that Article 29 extends the purposes of education beyond reading and writing. It has struck us that the most important of these goals of education today is the development of respect for human rights and 'for civilisations different from his or her own'. It is the idea of promoting tolerance and understanding through education which is most in need of a fresh boost, with France having reinforced their ban on religious signs being worn in school, thus isolating the Islamic community and all others who wear signs as a matter of great importance (Article 14 on freedom of thought, conscience and religion may be considered on this point). Does such a ban help tolerance? There are arguments on both sides we need not delve into, but it must be noted that in the West we are not necessarily the guardians of rights and freedoms.

Michael Freeman points out that where rights exist, complaints and challenges will be made. Yes, he is right, it would be easier for all if children were not to possess this right to complain. Perhaps it would make it more difficult to exercise power over the young; they would question the legitimacy of new police powers to impose curfews. Although we do not deny that some young people do cause problems and that youth crime is an issue, can this power be defended because we don't like to see groups of young people 'hanging around.' We question the fact that such a power to impose curfews does not come hand in hand with resources and programmes directed at creating a stimulating and enjoyable community for all, especially young people. In September 2002 the UN Committee on the Rights of the Child recommended that the government commits more resources to involving children and young people and to youth organisations in promoting awareness of rights.

As Michael Freeman points out '[R]ights without remedies are of symbolic importance only'. Getting beyond the 'rhetoric' means setting up, and monitoring, systems that empower children, young people and adults to voice their opinions and to have those opinions and their best interests taken into account when decisions are being taken, whether at local and community level (including schools) or at national level. These systems should be flexible and allow people of all ages and abilities to participate on equal grounds. Those who are most in need often lack the confidence or energy to challenge rights abuses. For these people the support of advocates is crucial. The recently appointed Children's Commissioners should play a pivotal role in these processes.

It is clear to us that the most important right for enforcement in the UNCRC is Article 12 – the right of the child to express an opinion on all matters affecting him or her. It is active and valuable participation together with active listening that is vital to move forward. Also as Freeman states, the most important right 'is the right to possess rights' and the young should not be excluded from this.

It is easy to see why Michael Freeman begins with the idea of 'rhetoric'. A Convention was signed, promises made and the word 'rights' is used so frequently one wonders whether we have forgotten the true meaning. Despite all of this pageantry, there exist no real enforcement and no effective dissemination of information. As we have seen too many times in recent years it is the young who truly suffer silently in this system.

Chapter 5

Education and learning for social inclusion

Greg Mannion

Introduction

The current policy framework surrounding young people's educational transitions is shown to be driven by a focus on 'tackling social exclusion'. A number of critiques and effects of this approach are outlined. In light of these arguments, this chapter suggests that there is potential for thinking afresh about educational youth policy in terms of social inclusion.

Conceptual and analytical approaches to researching transitions have been deployed in order to try to cross the structure–agency boundary in the analysis of data. In other fields, actor network theory (ANT) provides an additional non-dualistic framework for analysis (Clarke 2003). Here, ANT provides an alternative way of thinking about structure and agency during transitions. The ANT perspective suggests that the interaction of a wide range of human and non-human entities are seen to mutually constitute each other and produce the social world. Empirical data from a completed research project on youth transitions is analysed anew in light of ANT's contribution.

Common to many studies on youth transition is a sense that uncertainty, discontinuity, reversals and seesaws characterise young people's lives. But little work has been done to capture the nature of how and what young people *learn* during the transition experience. Again, ANT provides an alternative way of theorising how learning takes place during transitional phases. This chapter considers how we might conceptualise 'learning for social inclusion' and how schooling might engage with the networks of connections that appear to be important in making young people's social inclusion possible not just in their future lives but *while young people are still young*.

Social exclusion and educational solutions

Social exclusion has been used by the UK government as a shorthand term for a 'condition' brought about when people or areas suffer from a combination of linked problems such as unemployment, poor skills, low incomes, poor housing, high crime, bad health and family breakdown (Social Exclusion Unit 2001). Because the UK is seen to have high levels of social exclusion, tackling social exclusion, promoting social inclusion and reintegrating the 'excluded' back into services and working to address problems in a 'joined-up' manner have become critical aims for the current Labour government. In particular, some issues that are seen to be the indicators of social exclusion – school exclusion and truancy, sleeping rough, teenage pregnancy, and the practices of young people 'at risk' – come in for specific attention. As far as education is concerned, policy usually centres on school attendance and achievement. The extant presumption is that social inclusion equates with or is strongly connected to future employment needs rather than current educational need. Because of this, young people's social *in*clusion is framed as an outcome to be realised when or if they find work later in life. Policy makers, commentators and academics seem to buy into the 'tackling social exclusion' paradigm and by default fail to focus on young people's current needs or their need for engagement in diverse aspects of society. Numerous examples of this rationale can be found. The following comes from the Scottish context:

> By improving educational attainment, by making the education system more inclusive, and by integrating support for children and families around the school system, the prospects of all children can be improved. But some children face special difficulties which, if not addressed, could all too easily consign them to exclusion in later life.
>
> (Scottish Office 1999, Section 6)

More recently, in a discourse laden with references to poverty and joblessness, the UK government's *National Action Plan on Social Inclusion* (UK Government 2003) spans a range of interventions and integrated service delivery approaches. Here too, youth-specific educational strategies which are designed primarily to target those 'at risk' of becoming socially excluded may miss the mark because they overemphasise outcomes, deficits and 'deviancy' (Edwards *et al* 2001).

Aspects of the rationale at play here need scrutiny and have been noted by other commentators (Jeffs and Smith 2001, Mannion 2002). First, the indicators of social exclusion may not necessarily be what need addressing at all. For argument's sake, we might consider what the policy landscape might look like should we be focusing on alternative practices such as voting levels among the young or participation in the arts or relevant work-based learning. Indeed, even if 'tackling issues' was the right way forward, the selected features of social exclusion (school exclusion and truancy, sleeping rough, teenage pregnancy, etc.) may not be the only social practices that need attending to. Secondly, we cannot be sure that full employment would in itself lead to an inclusive society. Thirdly, the complexity of knowing what it means to be included or excluded and the normative dimensions of its definition mean that there is likely to be no one simple solution or obvious 'root' causes. But the strongest criticism is far-reaching in that it calls into question the framing of the 'problem' in terms of exclusion: tackling social *exclusion* may be entirely different to supporting and enhancing young people's social *inclusion*. Inclusive practices are not simply the opposite of exclusionary ones; they are likely to transcend entirely the inclusion/exclusion dichotomy (Edwards *et al* 2001).

In summary, a paradigm of 'tackling social exclusion' permeates numerous policy statements and youth-specific interventions. The main effect is a narrowly focused view of what counts as social inclusion for young people. As far as education is concerned, this takes the debate away from what education might offer in terms of supporting and enhancing young people's social inclusion and civic engagement. The narrowing of the focus is brought about by:

- conflating inclusion with employment;
- limiting the scope for current social inclusion (where education is concerned this is by focusing the debate on attendance and school-based achievement); and
- being concerned with 'at-risk' children and young people.

Some of the effects which result include:

- deferring young people's social inclusion until adulthood;
- emphasising deficits by positioning people as recipients of services;
- individualising the debate on problem youths; and
- not recognising the importance of the process of becoming socially included.

The evidence cited here describes how young people learned to participate in networks in a way that enhanced their chances of becoming more socially included. This learning, however, needs to be understood using alternative frameworks to those usually used to shape policy and professional practice. As we shall see, social inclusion or integration is an ongoing process that affects young people both now and in their future lives.

Researching transitions, revisiting data

It has been proposed that youth transition research has been using outmoded models and concepts (Jeffs and Smith 2001). This is because people generally move in and out of education more freely at any age because they are obliged to retrain (Field 2001). As youth-like transitions and lifestyles begin to permeate the life course, and as youth transitions become extended and more complex, we could argue that young people's lives will be affected by the same or similar risks, paradoxes and insecurities as any adult's life. Yet, with the ongoing interest in the role of education in preventing the risk of exclusion, particularly around school-leaving age, it can be argued that the youth phase is still a key target area for policy makers and researchers alike. Transition studies have moved on from looking for linear school-to-work trajectories and are now open to include other features (e.g. domestic, financial or interpersonal). Now, a critical and more holistic approach to researching transitions is advocated (EGISR 2001). In parallel, while the conceptual and analytical approaches have in the past often focused on either structural or cultural aspects, more recent work has sought to cross this boundary using a variety of sociological approaches and heuristic tools.

Researchers tend to put the analysis of the *reproduction of inequality* alongside processes of *individualisation* (see, for example, Furlong and Cartmel 1997, Rudd and Evans 1998). Bourdieu's concept of the 'habitus' (Bourdieu and Wacquant 1992) is seen by many as a pertinent way of looking at taken-for-granted values and assumptions in everyday practice through bringing together the interactions of personal beliefs and dispositions alongside the structural and material factors. Hodkinson (1998) draws on Bourdieu (1984, 1993) to get beyond simply seeing career decision-making as either structurally determined or rationally individualistic. Similarly, Raffo and Reeves (2000) draw on more than one theorist in order to effect this bridge between what resistance young people can put up to the forces that determine their lives and their own ability to have choice and agency. Raffo and Reeves (2000) also build on Bourdieu to offer a typology of individualised systems of social capital. Others position young people's strategies of 'staging' and 'presenting' themselves in between processes of structuration and agency: life is expressed at the same time as its structural limits are explored and extended (EGISR 2001). There is now a growing recognition that structure and agency are mutually specifying or co-implicated. In this respect, ANT provides an additional take on these ongoing debates.

ANT has described change and interaction in terms of networks. Centrally, ANT asserts that the human and the non-human are mutually specifying and that humans are themselves effects of networks. It is through networks that we derive our human attributes that are always best seen in relation to other humans and non-human entities (Law 1992, Clarke 2003). Thus, ANT advocates a form of generalised symmetry by seeing 'the social [as] nothing other than patterned networks of heterogeneous materials' (Law 1992: 2). ANT, therefore, offers a way of overcoming the structure–agency boundary issues by always seeing entities (including humans) as features of ever-emerging networking. In this respect it offers a way of understanding data about interacting features or factors in social and material processes.

ANT is sometimes described as a sociology of translation (Callon 1986) that involves paying attention to a variety of 'actors' (which can be social or material) and focuses on the ways in which identities of implicated actors emerge. ANT is likely to be of particular use in transition research, because it encourages us to focus on ever-emerging 'translation' or displacement processes and asserts that identities are never fixed (Callon 1986). 'Translation', not unlike transition, involves a set of overlapping 'moments' during which 'the identities of actors, the possibility of interaction and the margins of manoeuvre are negotiated and delimited' (Callon 1986: 203). A network reading of youth transitions enables the phase to be seen as a form of 'translation' or shift in the interactions within and between networks that are spread across space and time and, distinctively, include a role for inanimate entities (Miettinen 1999). The study of young people's transitions informed by ANT highlights some aspects (or effects) of an ongoing translation or 'displacement' of youth identities. ANT provides an alternative and quite holistic approach, shifting the debate away from both the individualised psychological and narrow sociological perspectives that are commonly deployed.

The study

The data cited in this chapter come from a completed case study research project entitled 'Patterns of Progression and Participation in Post-16 Education and Training'. The early analysis of the data (Canning and Mannion 2000) foregrounded the structural determinants of post-16 transitions while still continuing to acknowledge the importance of 'agency'. In doing so, the project follows the efforts of numerous researchers in this field who similarly try to take account of structure and agency in the analysis.

A case study methodology was used to gather data within one local authority area in Scotland. The research project took the view from the outset that transitions were likely to be more than simple linear and rationally planned journeys from school to work (Coles 1995). Data was collected in a way that respected that transitions were likely to include interaction between many diverse events and people and materials within the time frame chosen. The data pertain to a time frame from mid-year in S4 (approximately aged 15 years old in Scottish secondary schools when they usually take Standard Grades) until the time of interview, when respondents were aged between 16 and 19 years old. This period of time in the life of a young person contains a series of potentially critical 'turning points' (Hodkinson and Sparkes 1997: 38–39) that provide insight into the processes that include or exclude. The case study set out to answer three specific research questions:

- What information sources did young people draw upon in their decision-making processes leading up to and following the end of compulsory schooling?
- Who and what were the important influences in the decision-making
  process?
- What are the key factors that affected the transitions?

The data are drawn from interviews with a theoretically sampled cohort of
young people aged 16–19 years old during autumn 2000. Two discrete
groups within the study were 42 new college entrants who had begun full-
time National Certificate (NC) courses in eight subject areas in one college
and 71 trainees in a variety of local employment sectors who attended any
of four local colleges and training centres part-time. Many of the new
entrant college students began NC courses soon after leaving school, mostly
after their fourth year. The trainees tended to be older, having made a more
circuitous route into training, with many not coming directly from school.
Focus group interviews were conducted with small numbers of young people (three to seven) from the cohort. Four participatory appraisal techniques using written and verbal feedback techniques supported and
encouraged the respondents to elaborate upon their experience of transition
within four areas of inquiry:

- sources of information;
- influences;
- choices made; and
- factors affecting transition.

Transcriptions were made of the tape-recorded interviews and records
were kept of the respondents' written responses using categories generated
by the authors (see Mannion 2002 for further detail on methodology).
Two related sets of data result: a set of transcribed evidence and sets of
ratings for each of the above four areas of enquiry. A coding system was
used to reflect the popularity of similar types of mentions (both written
and oral). Presented here are some of the transcribed data (drawn mostly
from the exercises on information sources, influences and factors affecting
transition) as they pertained to the roles of guidance teachers and careers
advisers in enabling the process of becoming tied to different organisations
and communities. Elsewhere (Mannion 2002), other evidence is explored
which suggests that schooling, as a system, was being experienced as
exclusive at the level of culture and values. School practices that were
critical included the way rewards were allocated and mechanisms of control and socialisation enacted. The exclusive cultures along with the lack
of curricular relevance were shown to combine to make schooling
problematic.

Findings

The kinship network

The written and transcribed data on information sources provided ample evidence that both trainees and new college entrants used the kinship network as their single most popular source of information. Young people destined for college attached a high importance to the richness and reliability of written/text-based information but often the young people and their families were proactive in acquiring it. Extended family and 'neighbourly' networks were the most popularly mentioned sources of 'influence' on both subgroups:

M(CE)[1]: Well, ma Dad's been in the Army eh, and he was asking me to go to it so I was finding out things about it. [. . .] ma Dad helped me the most because when I was at school and that he went and got the information, all the books and that. [He] just like come down to college and picked up like just all the different [information].

Some quite fluid and weak ties were created through the 'outreach work' of the kinship network, making it a potent information source:

F(CE): Well, ma Dad told me to speak to some of the Policemen cause one of my neighbours was retired so things have changed so he told me just to phone up and ask. [. . .] I phoned up the Police Headquarters and asked if there would be anybody there to help coach me and tell me things. [. . .] there was a Policewoman as well, she came to my house and spoke about this course and things that we were gonna be doing.

The kinship network drew on relatively strong ties with varying degrees of trust and reciprocation to provide crucial information for aspiring trainees:

M(T)[2]: My cousin worked for the company that I'm working with and she just says that they were needin' apprentice painters.

M(T): My Dad's friend works in the dockyard and he's quite high up and he tell't me about it and got me the forms for it. I got a reference from him as well.

Because of the strong role played by parents as central players, young people's trajectories often seemed complicit with the expectations and aspirations of their parents; those who chose not to comply, had to resist their influential force. The data reveal how the repertoire of schemata contributing to young people's dispositions (their emergent habitus) towards formal education and work served to replicate social patterns:

M(CE):   They just constantly kept on telling me what I should do and what was good for me and that. [. . .] what courses I should take and they wanted me to be the total best that I could be and I just thought it was too hard.

F(CE):   Well, they wanted me to stay on at school. They didn't want me to leave but I just left anyway.

For the trainees, parents and close family/partners were often influential in encouraging these young people to get a job that would enable them to gain a qualification or a trade. Influence could be 'felt' in subtle yet powerful ways as the 'rules' of the game became apparent through interactions with significant others at and connected to home:

M(T):   My Dad's a metal worker hi'self so, eh, I mean obviously he was, eh, quite interested in pushin' me in the same direction as him.

M(T):   Well my next door neighbour. . . eh, I got on well wi' them. [. . .] Aye well the boy next door to me, he's the, he's in the building trade. [. . .] I just blethered to him about that.

Guidance teachers

In Scotland guidance teachers have a role in guiding pupils in their personal, curricular and vocational areas of concern. They are involved in helping pupils with problems such as bullying or behavioural difficulties (personal guidance), helping pupils make informed subject choices and monitoring their progress across all subjects (curricular guidance). In addition, they should assist pupils in making choices about careers and further or higher education (vocational guidance). In the study, mentions of 'Guidance Teachers' were second only to 'Relations' as a category for the new college entrants. A minority of respondents had positive comments to make about their role in information provision but their role was not always as supportive as many young people would have liked:

F(CE):   Just some of the Guidance Teacher's, like, they care but they don't really care, if you know what I mean. It's just like, 'well, if you want to go to college just go to college', but like ma Guidance Teacher he sat with me for about an hour. [. . .] he would look up, he would send me booklets and things like that about it.

M(CE):   Ma Guidance Teacher didn't give me a lot of information, she just tell't me to do what I want. [. . .] she thought I'd be better going tae college cause I wasnae getting, well . . . I didnae like school.

Some guidance teachers did not provide relevant information at all times. Evidence suggested that guidance teachers had competing demands on their services:

M(CE): They weren't very helpful; my Guidance Teacher didn't really speak to me much about it. She was mostly concentrating on people who wanted to dae Highers.

F(CE): I think they want, like the best for their school rather than the best for us. I think they're going on the popularity [of the school].

Two-thirds of college students mentioned their guidance teacher as a source of information, while less than one-third of the trainees did so. Guidance teachers' role in transition into training must be seen as definitively weak. The role of guidance teachers seemed constrained by having to concentrate on attendance, pastoral care, discipline and subject choice:

M(T): They just guided you through the school.

F(T): My Guidance Teacher [. . .] he used to like put my attendance slips in and make sure I got them signed in all my classes and that, eh, and my behaviour and that.

It seemed that many guidance staff were often not actively supportive of those considering positions of employment and training:

M(T): They were very negative towards me wantin' to be a mechanic.

M(T): I was told I wasn't allowed to do Higher Still. [. . .] he said I was too disruptive.

F(T): Em, they just guided you the wrong way, [. . .] whatever you wanted to do, they said you wouldn't be able to do it.

F(T): [. . .] I just didn't feel they helped me very much, they just agreed wi' what I had to say and just never really encouraged me.

Some felt their guidance teachers encouraged departures once exam 'failure' was the assessment:

F(T): My Guidance Teacher was waiting for me outside my last exam with my leavers form all signed and told me that I didn't have to hand it in I just had to sign it and that was it. [. . .] I do think that young people who don't want to go university or whatever should leave after fourth year but I do think that schools also have to change.

Careers services

The role of a careers adviser is to provide counselling, advice, guidance, information and support to young people both inside and outside education. They work with young people to assess their abilities, interests and potential, and to identify barriers with respect to entering employment, education and training. There is an emphasis on working with clients at risk of 'social exclusion'. One student distinguished the differing role of the careers adviser from the guidance teacher:

F(CE): A Guidance Teacher is supposed to help you with all your problems. If you're getting bullied then you just go to see your Guidance Teacher whereas your Careers Adviser, she's helping you with your future plans and trying to get you instead of being, like, home without a job and without any other education, she'd rather you went into education or got a job.

Careers services played a small but important role in school–college transitions. In contrast to guidance teachers, the careers adviser was a very significant source of information and influence for the trainees:

M(CE): Well, she was a good influence, she showed me what it could be like at college and it was a brighter better atmosphere.

F(T): Eh, she [Careers Adviser] was quite good. I just told her that I wanted to go into Childcare and she looked up, like, em, loads of different things I could do like HNC and that but I wouldnae be able to do that the now. She said, em and I would have to do that later on and she just gave me information about the Skillseekers and that.

The following trainee felt there was space for a greater input by careers services in facilitating awareness raising about choices post-16:

M(T): If Careers were more about going in [to school] and tell you what was going on you would have more of a wider [set] of options open to you.

Factors affecting transitions

Factors that had most strongly affected new college entrants' transitions were categorised as 'experiences of schooling'. 'School experiences' were multifaceted and overwhelmingly negative in their tenor for those who had gone to college. Repeatedly, college students mentioned the same types of experiences in their accounts. Some felt they were bored or disliked school. Others reported degrees of curricular irrelevance when set alongside their goals ('I wanted to study tourism'). Others reported having poor relations with staff or that 'school was far too strict'. A perception that they had grown out of school and that there was a desire for a 'more relaxed, mature environment' pervaded other accounts. Still others reported being asked to leave. In addition, schooling appeared to provide these young people with experiences of an examination system that served as a negative consolidation of weaknesses rather than any celebration of personal strengths at this critical time in their lives. But departure from school was simply one part of a set of factors, as this account describes:

MI: Eh, I wasnae enjoying school and had tae get out o' school. [. . .] So I like had to come to college because being a Christmas leaver [. . .] I just thought I'd give like fifth year a shot . . . [. . .] the teachers and everything, I wasnae getting on with them so I just. . .[. . .] my Mum and Dad were really wanting me to do something wi' ma career so [. . .] and some of my friends were coming to college.

In contrast, trainees did not feel as strongly influenced by their school experience as much as new college entrants. The three most commonly mentioned written factors for trainees were:

- career/job/work;
- independence/money; and
- qualifications/gaining a trade.

These factors show how future career goals were strongly connected with short-term needs for disposable income, an interest in 'learning by doing' and the felt need to activate a career with prospects. In some cases, they commented that work experience placements were not in the domain of work they wanted; other trainees felt that school work placements were not long enough and only happened once a year:

M(T): The schools didn't really prepare you for work cause it's a totally different world eh. [. . .] [You're] protected a lot at school fae things but work, your just on your aen, well, so to speak. [. . .] [School] builds your character up. [. . .] It gae's you determination, drive and a real will to go out and dae something [. . .] but the thing is when you're at school [. . .] you can't think beyond school, you cannae. / Ken, you're at school and you're like 'oh, this is it, I'm gonnae be here for the rest o' my life', it seems like forever.

Schools were not providing obvious transition experiences for work or learning beyond the school gates. One college student commented that the school library 'never had up-to-date stuff about [the] college' while 'getting on with life' meant leaving the school environment for most trainees:

F(T)1: All, by the time you get into fourth year, all the that you've ever done is go to school, go to school and you just want to. . .
F(T)2: See the world, get on with yourself.
M1: You just want to get out there, get some money, your house, get a car.
F(T)1: Get qualified, get some experience in what you want to do.
F(T)2: In fourth year, you're 16, you've spent 11 years of 16 years in school.
GM: Mmm hmm.
F(T)1: You really do just want to leave it.
GM: Right.
F(T): . . .and get on wi' your life really.

Discussion

Having considered the data in this thematic and categorical way, any number of avenues of further interpretation present themselves. Space does not permit the full exploration of all the consequences for separate professional groups such as careers services or guidance teachers, nor does the chapter seek to be comprehensive in narrating the 'whole story'. Readers are reminded that the sample does not include the voices of those who opted out of education, training or employment ('status zer0' youth) or data on those who stayed on. Suffice to say there appeared to be no systemic structured approach to delivering information to *all* young people about *all* post–16 choices and destinations. Information was being provided late in the compulsory schooling years and on demand rather than as a right.

For the purposes of this chapter, the data are considered 'in the round' for what we can garner to be relevant to young people's social inclusion. The next level of analysis seeks to use a heuristic tool – namely the 'habitus' – to highlight some of the relational and material aspects of young people's transitions and to offer a tentative exploration of what learning for social inclusion might involve. Elsewhere (Mannion 2002), the analysis focused on the reasons why so many respondents explained the transitional phase in terms of having to leave school. How can we understand and theorise this finding when placed alongside the data on kinship networks and professional guidance and advice? The heuristic tool of the habitus is proposed to be of use here because it allows us to read structure and agency into the data in a way that connects them intimately. Alongside this, the ANT perspective suggests that an explanation in terms of networks is also possible.

We could say that the habitus of these young people did not predispose them to availing of professional forms of support, but this does not explain the positive role played by careers services. Another reading suggests that because of young people's dispositions, they did not feel the need to generate ties with school-based professionals. Put another way, we could argue that for the mainly working class youths in this research, because supportive ties were mainly found inside the family and not among school-based professionals, this may have disposed them to exit from formal schooling. Because 'getting on with school staff' was also important, we could frame the stories as accounts of failed relations between pupils and teachers. But interpersonal relations do not account for all factors. ANT reminds us that things and people, as well as identities, spaces and stories, are all implicated in power relations. So while the habitus explains much here, interpersonal relations and the networked roles of both human and non-human entities were also significant. Non-human 'actants' such as information, examinations, school rituals, timetables, money, qualifications, uniforms and so on coalesced within professional–pupil interactions in attempts to bring people, events and activities together into the stable network of identities associated with 'staying on' or 'leaving'.

For the new college entrants, one might say that their habitus was about 'staying on' to the extent that they remained in formal education. But school was no longer 'a place for them' because of a range of factors that included inanimate entities. An overarching aspect of the accounts was the way in which the choice of leaving or staying on was strongly framed by judgements made about examination results. School failure was finally ritually instituted through these largely academically oriented hurdles, which were used to separate out stayers from leavers. Not only did the school network of devices and strategies fail to be attractive to them, it appeared to actively encourage departure. Features of college life that made it attractive (by default for many) included the opportunity to study particular and fewer subjects, work part-time and study in a more relaxed and 'mature' environment.

For the trainees, their habitus may have meant that an early engagement in a career was likely but the workings of a range of other social relations, activities and materials were important too. Money and independence were key factors as well as the prospect of 'respected' qualifications and a future career. Space and geography were also important. Where they lived, who the local employers were, what their parents worked as and who their neighbours were all affected transitions, especially once the network of schooling failed to continue to enrol them as pupils. For trainees, their work-based experience contrasted sharply with the relative irrelevance of formal school-based devices (curricula, culture, examinations, information provisions and support).

After 'tackling social exclusion'

For both trainees and new college entrants, the out-of-school network was the arena in which they learned how to become socially included in ways that were different to those framing the policy discourse of 'tackling social exclusion'. What does this finding say to us about the framing of youth policy around the idea of 'tackling social exclusion' through joined-up services?

First, we should note that non-professionals were more commonly mentioned in terms of information and influence. We have shown how kinship groups are the contexts within which the management of negotiation (decision-making) takes place (see also Ahier and Moore 1999). This finding serves to highlight the possible irrelevance of the drive for 'joined-up' inter-professional approaches. It would appear that there is a need for greater openness about the competing demands being placed on some professionals dedicated to the support of young people before effective inter-agency working can be realised. The Connexions Service (DfEE 2000) epitomises the 'tackling exclusion' paradigm with a sustained emphasis on the 'condition of the socially excluded' and the perceived need to redeem those 'at risk' (see Hughes and Morgan 2000). Some doubt there can be really effective inter-agency working in the Connexions Service because of the strong leadership of Careers (Watts 2001; see also Chapter 2 this volume), whereas others worry about the potential partiality of the personal advisers if they are to be appointed by headteachers.

Secondly, we can see from the data that the process of starting careers was merely part of a complex multifaceted set of problems, experiences, tasks and strategies for these young people. Yet, within the educational policy discourse, school-based attainment and achievement are central concerns needed to ensure young people's future inclusion via employment. But being employed, per se, was never the sole goal. 'Qualifications', 'prospects' and the learning context were important aspects of a range of factors.

Thirdly, we can say that young people's social integration did not appear to be a deferred concern. The sense of urgency about 'getting on with life' in their terms reflects a concern with gaining new rights and responsibilities (via work or going to college) *while they were still young*. As such, social engagement was an emergent property of multiple strategies and activities taken on during transitions. These were ongoing processes often unconnected to the world of schooling and not solely driven by the 'need for work'. This finding is dissonant with the policy discourse that frames social exclusion as a risky future outcome for those who truant from school. A moot point here is that becoming socially included was not the inverse of being socially excluded.

Given the dissonance between the young people's terms of reference and what some professionals and schooling appeared to offer, what can we say about formal education, learning and professional approaches? Is there anything distinctive about learning that advances social inclusion? Are there particular and identifiable strategies and practices associated with this form of learning? To address these questions, this chapter concludes with explorations of social inclusion, social capital and transitions as concepts to help us understand the process of 'learning for social inclusion'.

Learning for social inclusion

The European Commission's definition of social exclusion provides a helpful starting point. For the Commission, social exclusion is defined as the multiple and changing factors which result in people being excluded from the normal exchanges, practices and rights of modern society (Commission of European Communities 1993). It suggests that social inclusion is about the process of actively gaining rights and obligations of mainstream society and having these rights and responsibilities recognised. In the same vein, social capital, in Bourdieu's terms, refers to 'contacts and group memberships which, through the accumulation of exchanges, obligations and shared identities, provide actual or potential support and access to valued resources' (Bourdieu 1993: 143). These definitions find resonance with young people's accounts, because inclusion is not limited to schooling or deferred until some future time. Taking these ideas on board, Learning for Social Inclusion (LfSI) can be initially conceived of as the process of coming to know how to capitalise on various forms of social ties with a view to gaining the rights and obligations of society and having them recognised.

But social capital is seen as a precursor to the acquisition of other forms of capital, such as human capital (skills and qualifications), economic capital (wealth), cultural capital (ways of perceiving and valuing) and symbolic capital (personal qualities related to prestige). Likewise, ANT demands 'that machines, animals, micro-chips and people, as well as identities, categories, spaces and stories, all have politics and all are implicated in power relations' (Clarke 2003: 112). Our conceptualisation needs some amendment. We need to attend to the related ways in which all of Bourdieu's sociological forms of capital (social, economic, cultural and symbolic) and material resources are generated since these can be so mutually specifying. Therefore, learning for social inclusion will involve the generation of diverse forms of capital (social, human, economic and symbolic) as well as the acquisition of material resources (for example, a home or a mobile phone).

To put it another way, LfSI for young people in transition can be conceived of as knowing how to capitalise socially, but also materially, culturally and spatially, on various forms of social ties and heterogeneous networks with the broad purpose of gaining rights and obligations and having them recognised. But young people's accounts must leave us concerned about where and which rights and obligations were being gained and who was recognising them. The normative dimension of LfSI is exposed in the dissonance between the learning these leavers enacted informally outside of their school lives and formally within it.

Schooling and learning

Evidence here on youth transitions suggests we should consider how schools and school-linked professionals might engage with the networks of connections that young people regard as important in making social inclusion possible not just in their future lives but *while they are still young*. First, schools do not appear to be functioning as effective sites of LfSI as many of these young respondents saw it. This is because schools appeared to have an inward focus on progression and viewed achievements mostly in school-related terms. Schools generally had weak links with colleges and very poor links with the world of work. Work experiences organised by school provided only a limited experience of workplaces. The concentration on teaching nationally set curricula meant that local cultures, knowledge about employment opportunities and a holistic view of the young person's career path were often neglected. Schools appeared to be functioning as sites of translation of youth in school terms through the labelling of success, deviancy and 'otherness'. A restricted construction of 'pupil' meant that many young people reached school-leaving age before having had the chance to explore alternatives or having their efforts in the exploration of alternative identities recognised. Youth transition research requires us to think also about an outward focus on relations beyond the school. Beattie's report (Beattie Committee 1999) is important here because 'inclusive schooling' must also allow for 'inclusive' exits and onward movements from compulsory schooling into other provisions. Thus, LfSI builds on 'inclusive education' discourse but calls for us to look at learning as a feature of social practices that occur within and beyond the boundaries of schooling. If schools wished to support these young people's LfSI, they would need to have been places where pupils learned to capitalise socially, but also materially, culturally and spatially, on various forms of social ties and heterogeneous networks. Social inclusion will mean different things to different stakeholders. It is not simply enough, as policy discourse suggests (EGISR 2001), to differentiate between 'the integrated' and 'the excluded'.

Making a place for learning that promotes the social inclusion of younger children has been demonstrated to be characteristically challenging in relational, political and spatial terms (Mannion 2003). LfSI of young people in secondary schools is similarly challenging, requiring new flows between networks of a range of somewhat unconnected professionals, families, institutions and other entities. Supporting transitions and changing the nature of the translation of youth identities may mean allowing for new forms of knowing to be realised within a rejuvenated, more equitable organisational culture, via the delivery of more appropriate curricula and enhanced inter-agency working between a range of players (both human and material). If schools are to be more than 'enclosures separated from the world, quasi-monastic spaces where they live a life apart' (Bourdieu 1993: 96), they must embrace such changes.

There are far-reaching implications for school-based and school-linked professionals and the development of new forms of inter-sectoral communication between schools, colleges, training providers and employers. More than joining-up services and 'tackling social exclusion' is required. It will mean schools taking on board a more outward and onward focus, especially for those young people choosing to leave upon reaching compulsory school-leaving age, many of whom find schools currently render them 'socially out of play' (Bourdieu 1993: 96). Evidence provided by young people suggests that this is a time of acute adjustment that will continue to need special support. The impact of acknowledging schools' roles and responsibilities in supporting LfSI will be felt as much by adults as by young people. But any change to models of supporting transitions will need careful planning. Shifting policy away from 'tackling social exclusion' towards a focus on 'supporting social inclusion', especially on young people's own terms, may require a more fundamental change than some may be ready to embrace. It will likely involve stakeholders who are not commonly found in and around schools and the reconstruction of curricula around the process of not only gaining rights and obligations but also having them recognised.

Endnotes

1 M(CE) refers to a male college entrant. F(CE) refers to a female college entrant.
2 M(T) refers to a male trainee. F(T) refers to a female trainee.

References

Ahier, J. and Moore, R. (1999) 'Post-16 education, semi-dependent youth and the privatisation of inter-age transfers: Re-theorising youth transition', *British Journal of Sociology of Education*, 20(4): 515–530.

Beattie Committee (1999) *Implementing Inclusiveness: Realising potential*, Edinburgh: Scottish Executive Stationery Office.

Bourdieu, P. (1984) *Distinction: A social critique of the judgement of taste*, London: Routledge and Kegan Paul.

Bourdieu, P. (1993) *Sociology in Question*, London: Sage.

Bourdieu, P. and Wacquant, L. J. D. (1992) *An Invitation to Reflexive Sociology*. Chicago: The University of Chicago Press.

Callon, M. (1986) 'Some elements of a sociology of translation: domestication of the scallops and the fishermen', in J. Law (ed.), *Power, Action and Belief: A new sociology of knowledge*, London: Routledge and Kegan Paul.

Canning R. and Mannion, G. (2000) *Patterns of Progression and Participation in Post-16 Education and Training – Final report*. Stirling: Institute of Education, University of Stirling, pp 1–132.

Clarke, J. (2003) 'A New kind of symmetry: Actor-network theories and the new literacy studies', *Studies in the Education of Adults*, 334(2): 107–122.

Coles, B. (1995) *Youth and Social Policy*. London: UCL Press.

Commission of the European Communities (1993) *Background Report: Social exclusion – poverty and other social problems in the European Community*, ISEC/B11/93. Office for Official Publications of the European Communities.

DfEE (2000) *Connexions: The best start in life for every young person*. London: Department for Education and Employment.

Edwards, R. Armstrong, P. and Miller, N. (2001) 'Include me out: critical readings of social exclusion, social inclusion and lifelong learning', *International Journal of Lifelong Education*, 20(5): 417–428.

European Group for Integrated Social Research (EGISR) (2001) 'Misleading trajectories: Transition dilemmas of young adults in Europe', *Journal of Youth Studies*, 4(1): 101–118.

Field, J. (2001) 'Lifelong education', *International Journal of Lifelong Education*, 20(1/2): 3–15.

Furlong, A. and Cartmel, F. (1997) *Young People and Social Change. Individualization and Risk in Late Modernity*, Buckingham: Open University Press.

Jeffs, T. and Smith, M. K. (2001) 'Social exclusion, joined-up thinking and individualization – New Labour's Connexions strategy'. Available at: *http://www. infed.org/personaladvisers/connexions_strategy.htm* (accessed March 2003).

Hodkinson, P. (1998) 'Career decision making and the transition from school to work', in M. Grenfell and D. James (eds), *Bourdieu and Education: Acts of practical theory*, London: Falmer Press.

Hodkinson, P. and Sparkes, C. (1997) 'Careership: a sociological theory of career decision making', *British Journal of Sociology of Education*, 18(1): 29–44.

Hughes, D. and Morgan, S. in association with Watts, A. G., Hartas, D., Merton, B. and Ford, G. (2000) *Research to Inform the Development of the New Connexions Service*. Derby: Occasional Paper from Centre for Guidance Studies. Available at: http://www.derby.ac.uk/cegs (accessed March 2003).

Law, J. (1992) 'Notes on the theory of the actor-network: ordering strategy and heterogeneity', *Systems Practice*, 5(4): 379–393.

Mannion, G. (2002) 'Open the gates an' that's it 'See ya later!': School culture and young people's transitions into post-compulsory education and training', *Scottish Educational Review*, 34(1): 86–100.

Mannion G. (2003) 'Children's participation in school grounds developments: creating a place for education that promotes children's social inclusion', *International Journal of Inclusive Education*, 7(2): 175–192.

Miettinen, R. (1999) 'The riddle of things: activity theory and actor-network theory as approaches to studying innovations', *Mind, Culture and Activity*, 6(3): 170–195.

Raffo, C. and Reeves, M. (2000) 'Youth transitions and social exclusion: Developments in social capital theory', *Journal of Youth Studies*, 3(2): 147–166.

Rudd, P and Evans, K. (1998) 'Structure and agency in youth transitions. Student experiences of vocational further education', *Journal of Youth Studies*, 1(1): 39–62.

Scottish Office (1999) *Social Inclusion – Opening the Door to a Better Scotland*, Edinburgh: Scottish Executive Stationery Office. Available at: *http://www. scotland.gov.uk/library/documents-w7/sima–03.htm* (accessed July 2002).

Social Exclusion Unit (2001) *Preventing Social Exclusion.* Report by the Social Exclusion Unit, London: Her Majesty's Stationery Office. Available at: *www. cabinet-office.gov.uk/seu/index.htm* (accessed March 2003).

UK Government (2003) *United Kingdom National Action Plan on Social Inclusion 2003–15*, London: Her Majesty's Stationery Office.

Watts, A. G. (2001) 'Career guidance and social exclusion: A cautionary tale', *British Journal of Guidance and Counselling*, 29(2): 157–176.

Postscript on education

Heather Barnshaw and Mary Ho

I'm Heather Barnshaw, aged 19. I come from London and am currently a third year geography student at the University of Edinburgh. From quite early on in secondary school I had decided that I wanted to go to university and chose to stay in school to take my A Levels rather than going to college.

I'm Mary Ho, aged 20 and a third year Honours Business Studies student at the University of Edinburgh. I was educated in Fife, Scotland and have a varied experience of education, incorporating state secondary school, college and now university. Throughout my pathway, I have greatly benefited from advice from those around me and from school and such widening access schemes as LEAPS (Lothians Equal Access Programme for Schools) in my transition from school to higher education. Although LEAPS can be viewed as an organisation working towards diminishing the social exclusion of certain groups, they are more than that. They work to promote equal opportunities but also operate towards the social inclusion of young people, albeit in an indirect sense. I have benefited greatly from this scheme and, subsequently, I have become a volunteer with them, not only helping the next generation of young people to realise their potential but also contributing something back to my local community and moreover society.

First and foremost, we broadly agree with Greg Mannion's chapter and recommendations for the social inclusion of young people through education. From our personal experiences and observations of the current education systems within the UK, we have several comments and recommendations of our own to contribute to this discussion.

In addition to the documented input of friends and family, we have both benefited from advice from teachers. We feel that the teacher who knows the young person best should have the most involved role in explaining the *full* range of options open to them post-16, catering for their individual needs and capabilities. In Scotland, this would be the guidance teacher and in England their form teacher – the role of whom should be much greater than at present. This may involve a shift in focus of guidance teachers away from tackling truancy (which would be made the responsibility of, say, a registration teacher) towards trying to harness and develop young people's options for future development. Furthermore, an earlier intervention by careers advisers can first of all facilitate a greater awareness of future options or careers paths and secondly provide relevant and appropriate information on how to reach their chosen goal. In England, Connexions offers useful advice to young people but is mainly targeted at those aged 16–19 years old, and could be made far more effective if it were publicised more strongly to those aged 14–15 years old.

A more specific recommendation for the schools curriculum would be greater availability of vocational and work-related training within school, so that young people can pursue both vocational and academic options together if they wish. There have been recent changes to include more work experience, which is helping pupils to make more informed choices. However, caution must be taken to avoid an overemphasis on either vocational options or academic studies; that is, the avoidance of 'pushing' all young people within a particular school towards one or the other. Young people should be able to exercise free choice in what they want.

As discussed in Greg Mannion's chapter, those who advance to further education colleges perceive this environment as being more mature and as an initial step towards social inclusion. Contrary to the belief that college is a better environment for relevant learning and social inclusion than school, this is not necessarily the case. The general perception within society is that social inclusion equates with employment and social exclusion is anything outwith this circumstance, but we feel that social inclusion should encompass making any contribution to society. This need not be financial but could include, for example, voluntary work within communities. Although radical, the prerequisite to the social inclusion of young people may be facilitated by a shift in societal views and perceptions of young people and the contributions they make – whether it is through taxation or continuing their education.

This could be achieved through the edification of communities and society and challenging the current counterculture to staying on at school as a 'soft option', especially in Scotland. It must be noted that there are obviously regional differences in viewpoints on this issue. Furthermore, we praise the recent introduction of 'paying' young people to stay on in schools in Scotland – as this in a way equates the options of staying on for young people relative to starting work or going to college. In other words, staying on will be viewed by them as a way of earning as well, albeit in their educational futures.

Moreover, as an initial step, the current education system, and in particular the role of social education to young people, should incorporate learning about citizenship and in effect promoting social inclusion. We feel that informing young people about the political system, their worth or value to society and the importance of contributions to the community is an important prelude to changing views on this issue. Additionally, a greater recognition by communities of the contribution made by young people to society is necessary. By establishing links between schools and the local community, perhaps in areas such as charity work or conservation, young people in schools would feel less excluded from society.

On a related point, in recent years positive discrimination has been used increasingly in an attempt to reduce social exclusion, particularly with respect to widening access to university for young people who are considered to be socially excluded or 'at risk'. Such a policy, however, carries with it a number of real dangers in that it actually fails to treat everyone equally – even if its origins are merited in promoting equal opportunities for all.

Often future potential is equated with previous academic attainment, although this is often not the case. There are discrepancies between what an individual is capable of in reality and in what is shown by past school achievements for a variety of reasons, including shortcomings within the school curriculum offered to them. I (Heather) think that less emphasis should be placed on previous examination achievement in favour of potential for future success; a student with an enthusiastic justification of their reasons for wanting to study a subject at university with fewer or lower qualifications should be viewed as a stronger or equally strong candidate as a student who has better qualifications but less enthusiasm for the subject. This would be particularly true for subjects not commonly taught in schools.

In an ideal world, problems such as shortcomings within the school curriculum on offer due to resource limitations would not exist and all young people would be offered an exceptional education by state schools, regardless of the area they live in. Although I (Heather) appreciate the reluctance of the general public to accept increased taxation in order to pay for improving schools, it should be acknowledged that investing in the education of future generations offers benefits to the whole country, not just those receiving that education. This can also be extended to university education; a central argument for recent increases in tuition fees is that students should regard this as investing in their own futures, especially in increasing their future earnings. It is, however, noted less often that by investing in their own futures, they are also investing their own time and money for the benefit of the nation in the future.

We believe that all young people should be socially included, regardless of what they choose to do in terms of continuing with their education or training or entering paid employment. But in suggesting that policy makers should concentrate more on social inclusion, we must not detract from the positive benefits accruing from schemes that aim to help the socially excluded. I (Mary) am a beneficiary and strong supporter of widening participation within society and in promoting the empowerment of young people. I feel that by empowering young people at the earliest time possible through intervention in the education system, they will be more aware of their options and perhaps be more proactive in seeking to be included themselves.

This leads us to our final point that, despite the current debates on how to make young people socially included, some young people do not have the inclination themselves to want to be socially included. More should be done to encourage young people to 'care' about their communities and society as a whole. I (Mary) believe that if young people are taught more about citizenship, then this will lead to more consideration for their local communities and, naturally, lead to them making contributions and thus being socially included. This, however, is not a panacea. There are two sides to this problem and society in general needs to socially include and accept young people as well. Thus, this begs for a wider cultural shift in attitudes and changes to the way society views young people.

Chapter 6

The inclusive illusion of youth transitions

Monica Barry

Introduction

Many discourses on youth transitions imply a transition that culminates in social inclusion – inclusion as a 'full' citizen, having attained all the trappings of so-called 'adulthood'. However, as this chapter will highlight, this is not always the case. Many young people move through the various phases of transition but do not attain all the expected goals, and certainly not in the time scale or order suggested by most models of youth transition. Although individual young people are increasingly being seen as 'choosing' their own transitional pathways, they are still held back by structural constraints: partly, it is argued here, because of discrimination by age and status. This chapter outlines the standard model of transition in relation to disadvantaged young people and draws on the findings from two recent qualitative studies undertaken by the author – one of young people's experiences of offending (the Offender study) (Barry 2004) and the other of young people's experiences of growing up (the Transitions study) (Barry 2001a, 2001b, 2002). Both sets of young people (in the age range 15–30 years old) were in the process of reassessing their lives, reshaping their identities and modifying their attitudes in the transition from childhood to adulthood. Both groups experienced disadvantage and poverty in both childhood and youth. And both groups struggled with the potentially discriminatory attitudes and practices of those with whom they came into contact during this critical phase in their lives.

The chronology of transition

Models of youth transitions have tended to focus on the three chronological phases of the life course – childhood, youth and adulthood, the youth phase being roughly the ten year period from age 15 to 25 years old. Because of the nebulous nature of youth transitions, such research still tends to adhere to a differentiation by chronological age: namely, 'childhood' (0–14 years old), 'youth' (15–24 years old) and 'adulthood' (25+ years old) (see, for example,

Jones 1996). With no obvious alternative frameworks currently available to sociologists of youth, these phases of transition are often used as markers of change or distinction but it is acknowledged that these three transitional phases, described below, are zigzagging, overlapping and contentious (Coles 1995, MacDonald *et al* 2001, Wyn and White 1997).

Childhood

Early definitions of childhood suggest that children need to be protected for moral as well as educational reasons. Aries (1962: 412) describes children as being 'subjected to a special treatment, a sort of quarantine', and even though recent Children's Acts and the UN Convention on the Rights of the Child have attempted to diffuse the 'quarantine' effect that the term 'childhood' implies, the term still differentiates children from adults in terms of risk, protection and rights and emphasises the 'otherness' of children (Brown 1998, Franklin 2002). Children are increasingly constrained by legal processes which separate them out from their older counterparts and which both enable and restrict their access to rights and responsibilities as citizens (Barry 2001a, 2001b).

For many children from disadvantaged communities, 'childhood' does not offer the same type of protection that it offers young people from more affluent communities. It is likely that middle class children may gain a greater amount of protection against, for example, marginalisation or poverty through the income and associated benefits accruing from their families (Allatt 1993). Children deprived of such opportunities, however, may suffer more from denial than from a lack of protection per se (denial of rights to an adequate standard of living and to developmental and other opportunities). Many such children may also experience greater degrees of responsibility – for example, in having to care for themselves or others within the family (Barry 2001a, 2001b; see also Chapter 13) or in helping out in family businesses (Morrow 1999) – thus questioning the traditional image of childhood as being a time of innocence and positive dependence.

Children are almost totally confined, in a legal sense, to the care of adults, in particular their families or carers, but once they reach school age, this dependence on families dissipates (albeit often temporarily) as the school milieu takes over, not only in terms of education and daytime supervision but also for leisure and social interaction. It is within the school environment that children increasingly relate to other children rather than family members for leisure activities, identity and friendship. Nevertheless, since all children, by dint of their age and status (as well as their size), occupy a relatively powerless and protected position in society, much of their collective activity involves pushing the boundaries of that environment in ways that may be considered antisocial or illegal (Morrow 2001). For more disadvantaged children, many of the opportunities and values of mainstream society often elude them through conventional means; thus, they may resort to unorthodox means (through offending, for example) of gaining success, money, power or social identity. This recourse to 'anti-social behaviour' may also exacerbate their existing problem of 'otherness'.

Youth

The term 'youth' is a concept which has attracted increasing sociological interest since the 1980s in understanding the extended and fragmented period that young people may go through before attaining full 'adult' status (Chisholm 1993, Coles 1995). 'Youth' has become an additional bridging stage between childhood and adulthood to exemplify the protracted transition brought about by tighter labour market restrictions on school leavers, extended education and often compulsory training (Bynner *et al* 1997). It thus offers a convenient sociological bridge between the widening poles of childhood and adulthood in the Western world. However, it is acknowledged that not all cultures or ethnic groups easily fit this mainly white, Western European image of youth.

The youth phase, taken to be in the age range 15–24 years old (Jones 1996), is the phase during which most but not all of the age-related rights and responsibilities that young people gain as emerging adults come to fruition[1]. However, youth could be described as a time of distancing from, initially, the family environment and, subsequently, the school environment and, a time of experimentation with identities, autonomy and attitudes. The main milieu within which young people congregate is the friendship group, both within and outwith the school environment.

According to Coles (1995: 4), youth is 'an interstitial phase' between childhood and adulthood, during which young people are treated 'neither as children nor as adults' (Cole 1995: 6). Musgrove (1964) is more specific in suggesting that youth are an oppressed group, rejected by adults, and that their exclusion from 'adulthood' has been engineered for adverse rather than benign reasons. As Cohen and Ainley (2000) imply, this has more recently had as much to do with political expedience as with economic downturn:

> The enlargement of adolescence, its encroachment on childhood, and prolongation into what used to be adulthood is . . . both culturally driven and required by the economic collapse of earlier strategies (Cohen and Ainley 2000: 90).

Adulthood

All individuals aged 25 and over are deemed to come under the rubric of 'full adulthood', irrespective of their competence, since from the age of 25, all legal rights to full 'adulthood' are in place, culminating in eligibility for full state benefits (Jones 1996). At the age of 25, individuals have full responsibilities as citizens: they are expected to support themselves through paid employment or other income – although they are also eligible for state benefits, and they are liable to pay taxes towards services for themselves and others. In this respect, adulthood is seen as an 'end point' when specific rights and privileges are bestowed.

Thomson and Holland (2002) drew on young people's views in identifying two models of adulthood which challenge the conventional definition:

- an individualised model (feeling mature and autonomous) and
- a relational model (stressing responsibility and caring for others).

The key factors which young people equate with adulthood also mirror those identified by Coles (1995). These are parenthood, a home of one's own and stable employment, but these vary in importance for young people, depending on social class, race and gender (Jones 2002, Thomson and Holland 2002).

Understanding the process of youth transition

All models of youth transition imply a linear, psychosocial development starting in late childhood, which progresses in a piecemeal fashion towards the conventional goals of adulthood. The main transitional pathways or 'careers' identified by sociologists in the 1980s and early 1990s have been summarised by Coles (1995) as follows:

- the transition from full-time education and training to a full-time job in the labour market (the school-to-work transition);
- the transition from family of origin to family of destination (the domestic transition); and
- the transition from residence with parents (or surrogate parents) to living away from them (the housing transition) (Coles 1995: 8).

Such a model of transition assumes a predictable linear progression to a mainstream end-point – adulthood. However, Wyn and White (1997), amongst others, note that there are multiple routes along the continuum to adulthood, and no obvious point of arrival. Indeed, one's route to adulthood can be a continual maze of cyclical, reversible and uncertain pathways (Stephen and Squires 2003). Jones (2002) also notes that transitions no longer follow a normative or sequential pattern, and nor is adulthood so clearly defined nor as secure as it might have been some 50 years ago.

Wyn and White argue that although the term 'transitions' offers a 'metaphor for the process of growing up' (Wyn and White 1997: 98), it is a misleading concept, not least in contemporary societies where the bound-aries between youth and adulthood are blurred, employment is insecure and often temporary and the conventional markers of adulthood (for example, marriage or child rearing) are often purposefully delayed. The focus is also very much on the end point of that transition continuum, rather than the processes involved in the intermediate stages.

Yet, at the start of the transitions continuum, namely childhood, many young people highlight the fact that their responsibilities as children often made them *feel* 'adult', but without the associated benefits of 'adulthood'. This end of the continuum tends to be given scant attention in the transi-tions literature and the fact that young people speak of feeling adult in childhood causes some consternation within the transitions debate where *adulthood*, rather than *being or feeling adult*, is taken to be the end point. As the findings from the recent studies cited in this chapter suggest, taking on responsibilities as children can make young people feel adult at an early age, whereas to these young people, adulthood per se is about rights and status, irrespective of responsibilities.

Young people are increasingly seen as proactively defining, negotiating and making sense of their own transitions. Many recent accounts of young people's experience of youth transitions (Holland *et al* 1999, Barry 2001b, amongst others) suggest that their transition to adulthood is determined as much by personal agency and responsibility as it is by structural con-straints. It is young people's own narratives that have recently made aca-demics question the linear approach to transitions which had hitherto been the norm. As James and Prout (1997) argue, growing up nowadays involves several transitional processes rather than a one-off initiation process: youth transitions extend 'over considerable periods of time rather than being concentrated into ritual moments' (James and Prout 1997: 248).

Nevertheless, 'ritual moments' were the key to understanding transitions in earlier anthropological literature on the 'rites of passage' that children and young people progress through in preparation for adulthood. Whilst the terminology in such anthropological studies was different from that deployed in the sociological literature on contemporary youth transitions, nevertheless three elements in the concept of 'rites of passage', identified by Van Gennep (1960; cited in Turner 1967), equated with the sociological concepts of childhood, youth and adulthood. These were:

- Separation – 'symbolic behaviour signifying the detachment of the indi-vidual or group either from an earlier fixed point in the social structure or a set of cultural conditions.
- Margin – 'during the intervening "liminal" period, the characteristics of the ritual subject (the "passenger") are ambiguous; he passes

through a cultural realm that has few or none of the attributes of the
past or coming state.

- Aggregation – 'the passage is consummated. The ritual subject . . . is in a stable state once more and, by virtue of this, has rights and obligations vis-à-vis others of a clearly defined and "structural" type' (Turner 1967: 94–95).

Turner (1969) describes individuals within the second 'liminal' phase as 'persons or principles that (1) fall in the interstices of social structure, (2) are on its margins, or (3) occupy its lowest rungs' (Turner 1969: 125). In describing the 'liminal phase', Turner identifies equality as being a strong factor in relationships between individuals in transition: 'The liminal group is a community or comity of comrades' (Turner 1967: 100). He argues that this bonding amongst young people in transition reflects their lack of status in society:

> Transitional beings . . . *have* nothing. They have no status, property, insignia, secular clothing, rank, kinship, position, nothing to demarcate them structurally from their fellows.
>
> (Turner 1967: 98–99, emphasis in original).

Whilst the anthropological literature on 'rites of passage' has tended to be ignored in recent sociological debates about youth transitions, the framework identified by van Gennep and Turner, and notably the category of 'liminality', are seen here as particularly helpful in understanding the lack of parity between young people and their older counterparts in contemporary society. However, whilst for Turner's small-scale traditional societies liminality was a planned-for and brief stage pending a 'new beginning', for many disadvantaged young people in Britain this phase in the life cycle is extended, holds no status and offers few supportive structures to guide their transition to adulthood. This lack of support in the liminal phase leaves young people between the two stools of protected children and autonomous adults (Barry 2002).

Constraints on full 'adult' identity

It is in this 'liminal' phase of youth that young people can experience the worst effects of both autonomy and regulation at once. On the one hand, they have left the relative protection of childhood and gained greater independence from their families, but on the other hand, they have entered a new sphere of legal and social constraints which delay or deny their full attainment of adulthood. For many young people, these constraints on a full adult identity are associated not only with structural barriers but more importantly perhaps, with the discriminatory or prejudiced attitudes of their older counterparts, and the resultant denial of responsibility and opportunity for personal development. These latter constraints are explored further below from the perspective of young people themselves.

Adults' attitudes

People of all ages gain status and identity through interaction with and feedback from other people, and for young people in particular, the views and reactions of significant adults in their lives are an important spring-board to adulthood. Family, friends, professional workers and employers all have a key role to play in building that sense of identity and 'belonging' that young people value so highly, but these sources of social capital (Bourdieu 1977, 1986) are often misplaced and can have adverse rather than benign effects on young people's experiences of transition.

For young people from unsettled or disadvantaged family backgrounds, relationships with parents can often be traumatic and conflictual as well as supportive and trusting. For many of the young people in both the Transitions and the Offender studies, parents had been discouraging, dis-trusting or emotionally cold, often having problems of their own which pre-cluded their giving appropriate care or attention to their offspring. Abuse or neglect for these young people as children were frequently cited barriers to a close-knit family unit in later years:

> There is still a lot of insecurity there. I mean, I still think sometimes when I go over to my mum's, 'shit, what am I going into? Are they going to be OK? Are they going to be fighting or what's going on?' . . . . It's hard to overcome and it's something I'll never ever forget.
>
> (21 year-old woman, Transitions study)

> . . . my mum being an alcoholic and then she battered me. She couldn't be bothered. Going with all different men. She just didn't care . . . she's still hurting me. She doesn't really give a damn about anybody or any-thing . . . . I just cannae trust her.
>
> (25 year-old woman, Offender study)

Professional workers were also more likely to be cited as obstructive than as supportive. For example, young mothers in the Transitions study often spoke of the attitudes of teachers or the biological father of their child as being either prejudiced or dismissive, whilst those who had been in care often found social workers unsupportive. As one young man succinctly put it:

> I don't believe in social workers. . . . They don't help people. I'm not the sort of person that will sit and talk and express themselves. If I did, it wouldn't be to a fucking social worker, I can tell you that.
>
> (15 year-old man, Transitions study)

Equally, for many respondents in the Offender study, the police and other criminal justice agency workers were often deemed to be a barrier rather than an incentive to rehabilitation. Continued harassment was often mentioned as an example of an inherent mistrust or discrimination of certain young people by the police, even once those young people had stopped offending for a prolonged period:

> . . . when you're walking through the town, you can put your finger up and say 'come and search us if you want' . . . . I'm not doing it any more, [but the police] choose not to believe that and they choose just to keep tarring me with that same brush.
>
> (20 year-old woman, Offender study)

> I had enough of going around and getting lifted by the police and that. Everything what was happening, I was getting blamed for, even when I was in the jail they were coming [to my house] saying that I had been seen, they said 'we saw your son walking down the street with a telly'. I was in the jail!
>
> (22 year-old man, Offender study)

One's reputation more generally within the adult community was often a source of anxiety for young people as they grew older, as exemplified by the criminal reputations of the Offender study sample. They spoke of not being trusted to take on responsibility or of not being able to overcome discriminatory attitudes and practices of potential employers, the police or the local community. One 27-year-old woman who had stopped offending three years prior to interview still felt she had a bad reputation locally: '. . . everyone would look down on me, they still actually do. . . and names stick . . . even so now'. Another young man described the effects he still had on neighbours in his home town:

> See when I go [home], everyone locks their doors and locks their cars, they'll board up their windows and that. Have you ever seen that Western where you see them walking into town – the whole town shuts up? That's what [town] is like when I walk in!
>
> (19 year-old man, Offender study)

A denial of responsibility

People from disadvantaged backgrounds often have had the experience of working, either formally or informally, as children, either in part-time work or as young carers of a family member (Barry 2001b). For example, in the Transitions study, many of the respondents talked of caring for others or themselves as children. If one or other parent was suffering from a mental or physical illness, young children often became self-supporting as well as carers of that parent. However, whilst these young people described taking

on responsibilities as children, these skills were rarely acknowledged or cap-
italised on in youth and early adulthood. Those young people who entered
the care system in their teenage years following a high degree of responsibility within their families as children were often then divested of their competencies and skills, as social workers, residential workers and foster carers
took over the role of ensuring their care and protection. Several young people in care talked of being treated as 'incompetent' children rather than as
people with existing skills and responsibilities:

> I just want them to listen to me. I'm at the stage where, you know, I
> think I'm an adult and . . . they should be listening to me. But they still
> treat me like a child.
> (16 year-old woman, Transitions study)

> I mean, [if] you think you're mature and you think you can handle your-
> self, then you should be given a chance, not to be told every five minutes.
> (15 year-old man, Transitions study)

For young people with disabilities, whilst independent living may be their
ideal preference, they are often treated as dependent children for longer
because of a concern by parents or carers about their ability to live on their
own (Hendey and Pascall 2001).

The vagaries of the youth labour market meant that few of these young
people had experienced employment in early adulthood, irrespective of
their work experience as children. Yet many spoke of their preference for
'honest money', as one young man in the Offender study described it,
through legitimate means – and certainly many offenders suggested that if
they could receive an income from gainful employment, they would have no
reason to offend. For several drug-dependent women, who because of their
drug addiction or the lack of child care facilities could not find employment, being prescribed methadone (and therefore not having to fund their
habit through theft) was often the impetus to them stopping offending.

Many young people from disadvantaged backgrounds are limited in their
opportunities for employment. Often the skills and competencies they learn
in childhood (for example, through being a young carer or working part-
time) are ignored by potential employers, their reputation or criminal record
is held against them or they feel unprepared, educationally or practically, for
the world of work:

> I think in a way education in schools can be quite sheltered . . . . I mean
> I've obviously got like my facts, my knowledge from school, but if I just
> had that and went out into the world with that, I'd be a lost cause
> really.
> (16 year-old woman, Transitions study)

> I was working last year for a week. That was really about it. . . it's really because of my reputation as well, you know, with being in jail all the time and all that.
>
> (23 year-old man, Offender study)

Nevertheless, young people's overwhelming aspiration in the transition to adulthood is to acquire a full-time, permanent and meaningful job (Barnardo's 1996, MacDonald 1997, Williamson 1997). Whilst for people with disabilities, employment is often a secondary consideration given their primary wish for independent living (Hendey and Pascall 2001), it is nevertheless the overriding concern of many able-bodied young people. Not only does employment provide a stable and independent income but it also offers one the opportunity to keep occupied, to take on responsibility and to feel trusted:

> I've got a job . . . . I've got something to look forward to when I get up in the morning.
>
> (22 year-old man, Offender study)

> I've got keys to the shop, I open up the shop and shut up shop, and it's brilliant, they trust me.
>
> (29 year-old woman, Offender study)

> The good things [about working] were just feeling like you've got money, they give you money, you've earned that, you've earned that respect and you've earned that money, do you know what I mean? I gained respect.
>
> (17 year-old woman, Transitions study)

Whilst young mothers do not readily have the opportunity to work because of restrictive child care arrangements, their role as young mothers offers them a strong sense of responsibility and competence. Not only did the raising of children furnish many of the young mothers in the Transitions study with skills of parenting and housekeeping, but often their caring roles as children (for younger siblings or ill parents) had put them in good stead for motherhood. Being a young mother not only gave them responsibility but also heightened their sense of maturity:

> You have to grow up very, very fast because you have another life to look after and you need to make decisions quicker and stick with them.
>
> (21 year-old woman, pregnant at 18, Transitions study)

> . . . knowing you were pregnant, you had to grow up too fast . . . . Like 17 or 18, I jumped maybe by five years.
>
> (22 year-old woman, pregnant at 17, Transitions study)

I had all these skills at a very young age anyway, and I did things when I was pregnant. Like I worked part-time, and bought prams and put stuff away . . . . I was very organised with money. I . . . spent the nine months preparing for the responsibility of having her.

(21 year-old woman, pregnant at 16, Transitions study)

Several respondents, both male and female, in the Offender study also talked of the responsibility of having children as an impetus to stopping offending and 'growing up'. Having the desire, capacity and opportunity to take on responsibility for the care of one's children may explain, in particular, young women's reduced offending:

I've got a responsibility to myself, to keep myself out of trouble and off drugs and I've got my baby on its way . . . . I'm 27 and I'm getting older. You're not young forever.

(27 year-old woman, Offender study)

Reasons for stopping? Well the kids, know what I mean. To try and make a family . . . . I just didn't want to hurt them anymore. I knew I had hurt them enough.

(27 year-old woman, Offender study)

. . . having a son. Once he was born, then I really put the foot down . . . . Because I had someone else I had to look out for other than myself . . . my son, he was too young to look after himself. That's my job.

(24 year-old man, Offender study)

A criminal reputation

The Offender study explored young people's views of the criminal justice system as part of their experience of offending and desistance, and their involvement in this system was identified as a potential barrier to a smooth transition to conventional 'adult' status mainly because of the stigma attached. The criminal justice system has long been doubted as being a proactive and rehabilitative support system for young people involved in offending (Coles 2000). Whilst for many young offenders, the fear of court appearances and imprisonment are seen as an impetus to stopping offending, the lengthy delays involved in the system often result in an inability to sustain a non-offending lifestyle through legitimate means. Coles (2000) has argued that the youth justice system in particular has a poor track record in preventing further offending amongst young people, with over three-quarters of young male offenders being reconvicted within two years of a custodial sentence. One of the main problems for the young people in the Offender study was their lack of opportunities for a 'clean slate' because of pending court cases. This was exacerbated by having a criminal record and being subjected to further, seemingly unwarranted police 'harassment', coupled with a general lack of encouragement by control agents in the process of desistance. Having a criminal record, awaiting further court cases and being incarcerated also highlighted the futility for some of applying for jobs, wanting to adopt a more conventional lifestyle and wanting to improve their reputation.

According to Bromley (1993), a bad reputation can cause anxiety and guilt, whereas a good one can bring self-worth and security. Bromley suggests that disempowered or alienated individuals tend to focus on their immediate group for the development of a good reputation, not least because they are excluded from a wider, more conventional social network: 'Membership of a minority group of like-minded individuals can be an effective buffer against a hostile majority' (Bromley 1993: 33). To break this vicious circle of being dependent for social identity on those with an equally unfavourable reputation, Bromley suggests that:

> If people wish to break free from a particular social identity, they need to break free from the constraints of social circumstances, and the influence of particular people.
>
> (Bromley 1993: 57)

However, for young offenders and young people more generally in the liminal phase of transition, with few opportunities for inclusion and integration, breaking free from the constraints of social circumstances is not easily achieved without the proactive support of significant adults in their lives. Without such support, young people may resort in the meantime to the inclusive company and attention of peers and peer group activities which merely exacerbate their already deteriorating reputations. Offending is one means of gaining status and other forms of capital with peers in the liminal phase and can provide one with money, drugs, a sense of excitement or purpose and a means of consolidating much needed friendships. However, the benefits of offending are often short-lived as the constraining effects of the criminal justice system and an increasingly negative reputation take over.

Discussion and conclusions

The transition from childhood to adulthood is often portrayed as a transition from dependence to independence. However, such a model of youth transition rarely incorporates the lived reality for disadvantaged young people – what it means to grow up in a society which often denies them the opportunities, skills and responsibilities afforded to 'adults'. Yet, the vast majority of such young people have conventional aspirations which mirror those of the wider society. Wyn and White (1997) thus argue that disadvantaged young people should not be seen as any different from other age groups: '. . . in many cases the 'resistance' exerted by 'disadvantaged' young people is not necessarily *against* mainstream institutions but constitutes struggles for a place *within* them' (Wyn and White: 92, emphases in original).

However, the essentialist nature of the term 'youth' emphasises young people's 'otherness'. The concept of 'youth' segregates and problematises young people to the exclusion of the wider social and political environment of which they are a part. Jeffs and Smith (1998: 45) argue that youth 'has limited use as a social category, is gender-blind and views those so named as being in deficit and in need of training and control'. They go further in suggesting that concepts of youth transition share 'a desperation to hold fast to notions of an imagined mainstream in which the majority of young people neatly go forward in a unidirectional way towards some magical moment when adulthood is conferred' (Jeffs and Smith 1998: 53), when in reality all ages are prone to: '[B]acktracking, re-visiting, revising and . . . reversing' earlier life decisions (Jeffs and Smith 1998: 54). Indeed, youth culture is changing so rapidly that it no longer necessarily relates to 'youth' per se nor to different factions (by age, class, gender and race) within it.

However, the social construction of age, and the impact of postmodern thinking regarding individualisation (Beck 1992, Young 2002), have lessened the impact of class inequalities and resulted in young people generally viewing failure in the transition to adulthood as a personal problem rather than a public issue (Bates and Riseborough 1993). Such an internalisation by young people of their limited capacities and marginal status in society is encouraged by those in positions of power as a means of 'deflecting attention away from the structural reasons for poverty and unemployment' (Wyn and White 1997: 135).

My contention is that whilst the concept of 'youth' is a useful heuristic device for understanding, from a chronological viewpoint at least, the middle phase of transition between childhood and adulthood, the notion of 'liminality' suggested by the anthropological literature holds greater relevance. Liminality takes the burden and focus away from the individual and towards the state. It re-emphasises the need to acknowledge social, political and legal constraints on young people by dint of their age and status. Jeffs and Smith (1998: 47) suggest that: '[T]here can be no acceptable reason for controlling people on the grounds of their age any more than on the basis of their race or gender'. Whereas ageism as a form of discrimination usually relates to 'the elderly' by 'adults' (Thompson 1993), at the other end of the life-course, the political and social power imbalances inherent in the liminal phase of youth are denying young people the rights and opportunities more readily available to their older counterparts.

Overall, the young people in both studies cited here had a positive image of themselves as being mature and able to cope in difficult circumstances, and were generally, although often misleadingly, optimistic about their futures despite a lack of opportunities, rights and encouragement. From these two studies, it would seem that disadvantaged young people have few 'pull' factors to encourage them in the transition to adulthood. For those in the Offender study, offending was often seen as the only means available to them of gaining social recognition at a time when few socially recognised means of legitimating their stake in the social world were available to them. Equally, for those who had stopped offending, many did not have employment or a stable relationship – factors which are often seen as a major incentive to desistance – and yet they had still managed to desist (Barry 2004).

This chapter has highlighted the views and experiences of young people about their aspirations, their perceptions of responsibility and competence, and the importance for them of reciprocal and reinforcing relationships with adults throughout the transition to adulthood. The concept of liminality in transition has demonstrated the importance of emphasising young people's connectedness to, rather than separateness from, society and the importance of having access to sources of social, economic, cultural and symbolic capital (in Bourdieu's terminology) in that critical period of their lives. There should be a greater emphasis in policy terms on reducing the constraints of structural inequalities for young people which relate to their age and status. These young people were experiencing structural constraints due to discontinuity, instability and liminality in youth. Many spoke of changing family structures, moving home area on a regular basis and living within families marred by illness, violence or poverty. But their self-determination enabled them to accumulate forms of capital, however 'entrepreneurial' in nature and often against all the odds, in an attempt to feel a part of, and have a stake in, the wider society. Nevertheless, self-determination on its own is not enough to ensure a smooth transition to full societal integration. Until there is a reciprocal and constructive approach taken by society to the problems faced by its young people, then the inclusive nature of that transition will continue to remain illusionary.

Endnote

1 There are two obvious exemptions: the age of criminal responsibility (eight in Scotland) and the age at which part-time work is allowed (13 in Scotland).

References

Allatt, P. (1993) 'Becoming privileged: The role of family processes', in I. Bates and G. Riseborough (eds), *Youth and Inequality*, Buckingham: Open University Press.

Aries, P. (1962) *Centuries of Childhood*, London: Jonathan Cape.

Barnardo's (1996) *Young People's Social Attitudes: Having their say – the views of 12–19 year olds*, Ilford: Barnardo's.

Barry, M. (2001a) *A Sense of Purpose: Care leavers' views and experiences of growing up*, London: Save the Children/Joseph Rowntree Foundation.

Barry, M. (2001b) *Challenging Transitions: Young people's views and experiences of growing up*, London: Save the Children/Joseph Rowntree Foundation.

Barry, M. (2002) 'Minor rights and major concerns: the views of young people in care', in B. Franklin (ed.), *The New Handbook of Children's Rights: Comparative policy and practice*, London: Routledge.

Barry, M. (2004) *Understanding Youth Offending: In search of 'social recognition'*, unpublished PhD thesis, Stirling: University of Stirling.

Bates, I. and Riseborough, G. (1993) *Youth and Inequality*, Buckingham: Open University Press.

Beck, U. (1992) *Risk Society: Towards a new modernity*, London: Sage.

Bourdieu, P. (1977) *Outline of a Theory of Practice*, Cambridge: Cambridge University Press.

Bourdieu, P. (1986) 'The forms of capital', in J. G. Richardson (ed.), *Handbook of Theory and Research for the Sociology of Education*, Westport, CT: Greenwood Press.

Braithwaite, J. (1989) *Crime, Shame and Reintegration*, Cambridge: Cambridge University Press.

Bromley, D. (1993) *Reputation, Image and Impression Management*, Chichester: Wiley.

Brown, S. (1998) *Understanding Youth and Crime: Listening to youth?*, Buckingham: Open University Press.

Bynner, J., Chisholm, L. and Furlong, A. (eds) (1997) *Youth, Citizenship and Social Change in a European Context*, Aldershot: Ashgate.

Chisholm, L. (1993) 'Youth transitions in Britain on the threshold of a 'New Europe', *Journal of Education Policy*, 8(1): 29–41.

Cohen, P. and Ainley, P. (2000) 'In the country of the blind?: Youth studies and cultural studies in Britain', *Journal of Youth Studies*, 3(1):

Coles, B. (1995) *Youth and Social Policy: Youth citizenship and young careers*, London, UCL Press.

Coles, B. (2000) *Joined-up Youth Research, Policy and Practice: A new agenda for change?*, Leicester: Youth Work Press.

Franklin, B. (2002) (ed.) *The New Handbook of Children's Rights: Comparative policy and practice*, London: Routledge.

Hendey, N. and Pascall, G. (2001) *Disability and Transition to Adulthood: Achieving independent living*, Brighton: Pavilion.

Holland, J., Gillies, V. and McCarthy, J.R. (1999) Living on the edge: Accounts of young people leaving childhood behind, paper presented to the ESA Conference, Amsterdam, August.

Hollands, R. (2002) 'Divisions in the dark: Youth cultures, transitions and segmented consumption spaces in the night-time Economy', *Journal of Youth Studies*, 5(2): 153–172.

James, A. and Prout, A. (1997) 'Re-presenting childhood', in A. James and A. Prout (eds), *Constructing and Reconstructing Childhood*, London: Falmer Press.

Jeffs, T. and Smith, M. (1998) 'The problem of "youth" for youth work', *Youth and Policy*, No. 62: 45–66.

Jones, G. (1996) Deferred citizenship: A coherent policy of exclusion?, *Young People Now*, 26 March.

Jones, G. (2002) *The Youth Divide: Diverging paths to adulthood*, York: Joseph Rowntree Foundation.

MacDonald, R. (1997) 'Youth, social exclusion and the millennium', in R. MacDonald (ed.), *Youth, the 'Underclass' and Social Exclusion*, London: Routledge.

MacDonald, R., Mason, P., Shildrick, T. *et al* (2001) 'Snakes and ladders: In defence of studies of youth transition', *Sociological Research Online*, 5(4): http://www.socresonline.org.uk/5/4/macdonald.html (accessed July 2003).

Morrow, V. (1999) 'Conceptualising social capital in relation to the well-being of children and young people: a critical review', *The Sociological Review*, 47: 744–765.

Morrow, V. (2001) 'Young people's explanations and experiences of social exclusion: retrieving Bourdieu's concept of social capital', *International Journal of Sociology and Social Policy*, 21(4–6): 37–63.

Musgrove, F. (1964) *Youth and the Social Order*, London: Routledge and Kegan Paul.

Roberts, K. (2003) 'Problems and priorities for the sociology of youth', in A. Bennett, M. Cieslik and S. Miles (eds), *Researching Youth*, Basingstoke: Palgrave Macmillan.

Stephen, D. and Squires, P. (2003) 'Adults don't realise how sheltered they are': A contribution to the debate on youth transitions from some voices on the margins', *Journal of Youth Studies*, 6(2): 145–164.

Thompson, N. (1993) *Anti-Discriminatory Practice*, Basingstoke: Macmillan.

Thomson, R. and Holland, J. (2002) *Inventing Adulthood: Young People's Strategies for Transition*, Swindon: ESRC.

Turner, V. (1967) *The Forest of Symbols: Aspects of Ndombu ritual*, Ithaca, NY: Cornell University Press.

Turner, V. (1969) *The Ritual Process: Structure and anti-structure*, Chicago: Aldine.

Williamson, H. (1997) 'Status Zer0 youth and the 'underclass': Some consideration', in R. MacDonald (ed.), *Youth, the 'Underclass' and Social Exclusion*, London: Routledge.

Wyn, J. and White, R. (1997) *Rethinking Youth*, London: Sage.

Young, J. (2002) 'Critical criminology in the twenty-first century: critique, irony and the always unfinished', in K. Carrington and R. Hogg (eds) *Critical Criminology: Issues, debates, challenges*, Cullompton, Devon: Willan.

Postscript on youth transitions

Lindsay Kelly and Jackie Mooney

Lindsay Kelly

My name is Lindsay Kelly and I am 23 years old. I have lived in Edinburgh for five and a half years, having moved here from Argyll to attend University. Since graduating with a BA in Law, I have worked in education in an administrative capacity – first for the University of Edinburgh, and currently at Lothian Equal Access Programme for Schools (LEAPS). My own transition, from 'childhood' to where I find myself now, as the research would term me, 'youth', was aided by a supportive network of family and friends and for that, I know, I am extremely lucky. My interest in this project ties in with LEAPS and the students we work with. I am interested in their progression and the economic, social and educational barriers they face during these periods of transition.

Personally, I progressed from school to university with relative ease, but the process was gradual and I was fortunate to have a childhood which protected me and preserved my innocence. My work as a Young Leader with Brownies was extremely significant as it was a chance for me to be treated, and trusted, as an adult, and I gained the respect of my elders within the Pack. I have perhaps not had as much relevant experience as youngsters who have had to care for a relative in the home, whose work comes with no qualification or thanks, and does not bring the benefits of 'adulthood'. This seems very unfair and I am not sure how work like this could be measured in a way that would be able to benefit the youth in an official capacity, but it is something that should certainly be considered. Young people in this situation obviously have to grow up very fast and I found this chapter very interesting in that respect, as it was something I had not given proper consideration to in the past.

I find myself now in an 'in-between' stage where I feel too old to be a youngster but am too young (and don't want!!) to be an adult. I hate being told what to do, but have the maturity to accept that this is part and parcel of the workplace and of life and would not moan about it.

I personally sometimes feel more mature than I actually am but, to be honest, that worries me more than it pleases me these days! The work I do now, with LEAPS, attempts to give chances to young people who have perhaps not had all the support they deserve and attempts to 'level the playing field' of education. I would not agree with Turner's idea that 'Transitional beings . . . have nothing' as I think young people move through the stages of their life taking each responsibility and right as it comes along: 16 years old, smoking and sex; 17 years old, driving; 18 years old, voting; and so on. These ages are obviously irrespective of personality and experience and there are people who feel ready to do these things at an earlier age, whether through peer pressure, circumstance or personal choice. I believe the law (in general) is there to protect young people, not hinder them, but it cannot advocate for the personalities of individuals. The laws that protect children have perhaps failed to take into account the fact that young people are growing up faster than they used to, as divorce and other events become more and more the norm, forcing children to realise responsibility at a younger age.

I do occasionally feel discriminated against in the workplace because of age, and think this is very unfair. I think that all too often people look at age and judge people on it, when they should look at the person, and judge them on who they are. I am a confident, positive young woman with almost four years of good administrative experience behind me, yet am often passed over for jobs as a result of my 'lack of experience'. This is frustrating as I cannot get experience if no one will give me a chance, but you can't get the chance without the experience – vicious circle!

I think there are huge differences between 'feeling adult' and 'being adult'. My family is very loving and supportive but when we get together, we can be the silliest, most immature bunch! One of my friends and I agreed recently that we couldn't imagine the other person in work because we only see each other socially and are completely mad, but accepted that we are both probably pretty normal in work, having a separate 'work persona'. I think this is key in maturing into an adult. I have never felt, as a 'youth', that I have no responsibility or status. I can be impatient in some ways in that I want everything NOW but I have realised that it is better to wait for some things. I love that I can go to work every day, do my job, get on with colleagues, be treated well then go out with my friends and have a laugh. I do remember the routine of 'stop treating me like a child' and the retort of 'only when you stop acting like one' but the truth is I never will! My parents and sister are also like this and my Mum says of Dad 'he'll never grow up – he'll just get older' which sums it up for me very well! This isn't meant in a nasty way but in the way that he is a little boy at heart and it's something I love and hope I can hold onto – the young spirit.

Jackie Mooney

I am 17 years of age and live in Fife, Scotland. I am currently at a local college studying for my Highers (English, Maths, Psychology and Sociology). I decided that the school might not be right for me because of the way I interacted with staff and other pupils in school and I believed that I would perform better if I had a look to see what the college had to offer. I would eventually like to go to university to study social sciences. I wanted to write this postscript because I think it's a really good idea to ask young people themselves what they think about issues, because you really do get left out, and politicians and policy makers tend to assume certain characteristics about you. Hopefully this book will make people realise that young people can and should have some control over issues that affect them.

Education or the move into work is one of the most important aspects of the transition from childhood to adulthood. Messages, such as 'staying on at school will get you a decent job' and 'you need qualifications to go far these days', seem to be getting more common in households with adolescents. This, to me, has the possible reverse effect to the one intended as this exerts extra pressure on you to pass exams. This extra pressure can lead to stress and even the burning out of many young people.

There are many minor incidents that can leave many young people feeling discriminated against. I am sure that most youths have experienced a watchful eye from shop assistants. I do realise that there are many teenagers that do occasionally slip the odd item into their bags but I do not think that there is any reason for all the glaring. It makes you feel uneasy and to lose the will to pick up items to look at more closely in case you get accused. Obviously, this is not going to happen all the time but the feeling can force you out of the shop.

As far as being listened to as a child or adolescent, does anybody else have memories of being told 'not to be stupid'? In all my memories of it, the case was that nonsense poured out of my mouth. Possible scenarios could include that children may learn to isolate themselves, as they may feel that they would just get told to be quiet. I have also experienced adults who consider their view to be the 'be all and end all'. Anything that exceeds this is absurd. This channels this one way of thinking into the listening youth's mind.

As Monica Barry suggests, I think that 'being adult' is different from 'feeling adult'. But these also differ from 'being seen as adult'. 'Feeling adult', to me, is when the young person thinks they are adult. 'Being adult' is when the laws allow youths to participate in certain activities (age of consent). 'Being adult' can also mean responsibility of an adult nature. This can be like having a child, the responsibility of a job, etc. However, 'feeling adult' can only come from inside the young person. This internal overwhelming emotion can come from almost anything that can give the adolescent status: from meeting up with friends to have a 'proper meal out'; deciding what to do next year (school/college/university/work); paying for things out of your own pocket; or even simply reflecting on all this after a year.

Youth has often been described as a 'no-man's land' between childhood and adulthood. To an extent, this is true. It ties in with the 'being/feeling adult' distinction. If a youth 'feels adult', then youth is going to be a limbo. In my experience, I have met this dilemma many a time. You want to do things because you're 'that age' but you cannot do them because you're 'that age'.

All the events that an individual goes through during the transition can be supported (encouraged and even praised) or hindered (barricaded and restricted). This can depend on the personality of the adult (parents/staff), and it could go either way. The direction also depends on what is being encouraged. For example, a youth may be encouraged to study hard and do well in school, but be restricted when it comes to wanting to consume alcohol at the weekend. The hindering does slacken, though. As the young person displays responsibility and the ability to make better decisions, adults, in my experience, tend to open the boundaries. When I took on the responsibility of college and working hard, I found that my parents gave me more guidance than rules.

When job hunting, skills that are learned by young people in the home are more or less ignored. I have never attended an interview that has asked me about my home life. However, I do think that the responsibilities taken on in the home can be a good indication if the person is right for, or can manage, the job.

There is only one thing that I can think of that really holds back young people from being full adult citizens: that is the vote. I think that it is a shame that young people under the age of 18, who are perfectly capable of comprehending factors that affect their society, cannot be part of this system by which they are very much affected.

Chapter 7

Youth, leisure and social inclusion

Ken Roberts

A theme of this book is the contrast between what young people themselves want and what governments believe they need; between young people's own assessments of their circumstances and the official view. There are usually big differences. Accordingly, this chapter contrasts young people's own leisure problems to which they want solutions with the government's priorities. We shall see that these are completely different. No surprise here! However, the chapter opens with a review of how young people's uses of leisure have changed since the mid-twentieth century, which leads into an examination of the main differences and divisions among young people at leisure today. The chapter then proceeds to compare current government priorities with young people's own issues, and asks whose agenda is most likely to work. We shall see that leisure is an instance where young people tend to be wiser than their rulers.

Youth cultures across the generations

Pre-World War II

Before 1945 there was little commercial leisure aimed primarily at young people. The reason was simple: young people had little money. The dance halls were young people's places but the cinema, radio, the fashion industries, popular music and spectator sports catered primarily for adult tastes and audiences.

Middle class youth attended secondary schools at least up to age 16. These schools offered extra-curricular activities and required homework. Much of the free time that remained was spent in the young people's relatively spacious homes. Some joined sports, hobby and church-based clubs. Some pioneered flying and driving as exciting new leisure activities. The rags of university students and the exhibitionism of flappers and suchlike were treated as harmless fun.

The main problem group at the time was believed to be the young people who left elementary schools at age 14, whose lives were less firmly controlled by their families, and who were vulnerable to the temptations of the street. These were the young people who were targeted by the youth services – the uniformed organisations and the social clubs that churches and local authorities supported. Some of the voluntary organisations had their own local bases. Otherwise, they were most likely to meet in school or church halls. The inter-war years were the heyday of Britain's traditional youth services which, at that time, aimed to recruit mainly young people aged 14–21 years old: those who were between the end of schooling and the traditional 'age of majority'. These youth services never reached the majority of young people but they were the highest profile leisure provisions targeted at the age group. The young people who joined tended to be from the same respectable middle and working class families which sent their children to Sunday School. Those considered most at risk were harder to reach. They were described as 'unclubbable'.

Post-1945

Economic growth and full employment soon created the affluent young worker and commercialised youth cultures followed. Young people with money to spend were targeted by producers of fashion clothing, music and much else. The young people who were the first to become part of these scenes were the old unclubbables – early school-leavers who entered non-skilled employment in which they could advance rapidly to full adult earnings. Respectable working class and middle class youth were kept, or chose to keep themselves, apart from teddy boy and kindred youth scenes. The values of on-scene youth were found to be diametrically opposed to middle class values which approved of academic achievement and deferred gratifications (Coleman 1961, Sugarman 1967). In popular discourse the new commercialised youth cultures were linked to the rising rates of juvenile delinquency and the rising rates of teenage sexual activity. Civilisation was believed to be at risk! The traditional youth services were manifestly unable to compete with glamorous commercial facilities (Albermarle Report 1960). Before long, youth workers were quitting their clubs and seeking clients in the young people's own places.

By the 1960s middle class youth were developing their own youth cultures. Beatniks, hippies and the flower people were born. Commentators were agreed that these youth cultures were very different from their working class counterparts. The middle class youth cultures were more individualistic, less aggressive and more political. By the 1970s sociologists were arguing that the teddy boy, rocker, skinhead and similar youth cultures were working class not only in terms of the social origins and destinations of the young people who became involved but also in the values that the youth cultures embodied – toughness, loyalty to mates and a willingness to defy 'them'. Sociologists based at Birmingham University's Centre for

Contemporary Cultural Studies argued that the post-war working class youth cultures could be construed as primitive forms of working class 'resistance' (Hall and Jefferson 1976).

Mainstreaming commercial youth cultures

Since the 1970s there have been major changes. Young people have been remaining longer in full-time education, and present-day cohorts pass their eighteenth birthdays before over 50 per cent have left. They are now aged over 20 before over 50 per cent have left education and entered full-time employment (Organisation for Economic Co-operation and Development 2000). Another change is that different classes of young people are no longer as clearly separated as formerly. Most 11–16 year olds now attend comprehensive schools. Up to age 16 they all follow the same national curriculum. Sixth form and further education colleges now cater for young people from all social class backgrounds, who are heading towards all levels of employment. A further change is that young adults are typically marrying and becoming parents later than formerly: in their late-20s rather than their early-20s. Most female university graduates (roughly a third of the age group today) pass age 30 without having become mothers. There is now a post-adolescent, young adult, young singles life stage. The life space thus created has been partly filled by new social practices pioneered by young people – living singly, in shared housing, and cohabitating, for example. Few young people now leave the parental home, marry and commence life in a new family home, simultaneously.

In the 1920s and 1930s the youth club was the leisure place most clearly associated with the age group. The traditional youth clubs and uniformed organisations still exist. Indeed, some are thriving, but they have stayed in business only by catering for children rather than young people. Most present-day young people have been members of a youth club or organisation at some time or another, but by age 15 they are most likely to have decided that they are too old for such places (Department for Education 1995). In the 1950s and 1960s the street and the town centre became youth cultures' main sites, though the terraces of football grounds were also adopted as suitable meeting places by participants in certain youth cultures: thus, the problem of football hooliganism was born. Since the 1980s the introduction of all-seater stadiums has changed the composition of football crowds, and the street and town centre are no longer the places where on-scene youth are most likely to be found. Their favoured haunts are now the pub and the club. Segments of the licensed trade (the venues and the beverages) target young consumers. There are particular pubs and wine bars which are meant for the young singles. Any older voyeurs are clearly outsiders. Virtually all present-day young people participate in these scenes. Friday nights and Saturday nights are their leisure highlights (Hollands 1995). As many as 90 per cent of young adults drink alcohol, 80 per cent go to pubs and over 50 per cent go to clubs at least once a month (Hollands and Chatterton 2002). These scenes appeal to males and females, from all social class backgrounds. The cultures (the places, the music and the related fashions) have been mainstreamed, meaning that they are now served by major business corporations and considered respectable, and they serve young people from all social backgrounds. Even skinhead and punk styles are now presented and accepted by the public as respectable fashions. The family television audience is invited to select the nation's next pop idols, and millions vote. Drug use has now been 'normalised' among young people (Parker *et al* 2002). Most young people from all social backgrounds now have some experience as users, and the vast majority go regularly to places where they know that drugs are available, have friends who are regular users and accept all this as simply normal.

Young people's (and children's) leisure is now far more commercial than in the mid-twentieth century. The early pop festivals were cultural rather than commercial events. At the first Glastonbury in 1970 the 1500 who paid £1 for admission were entitled to free milk from the farm as well as the entertainment. Nowadays, Glastonbury attracts crowds of 100,000 who pay £100 each for admission (milk not included).

Divisions and differences

Blurred distinctions

Alongside the above developments, class and gender divisions among youth at leisure have become blurred. There are still age differences in young people's leisure, but these are clear-cut only among the under-18s who experience rapid shifts from adult-led, to casual peer group-based, then to commercial leisure (Hendry *et al* 1993). Although it is possible to identify lifestyle clusters (activities that tend to be done by the same individuals such as playing sport and watching sport), it is not the case that young people divide neatly into those who play sport, those who are into clubbing, and so on. Often it is the same individuals who do both. The main class differences now are not about 'what' so much as 'how much' young people do or 'how often' they participate. Young people on middle class trajectories tend to do most (Roberts and Parsell 1994). Like middle class adults, they have become leisure omnivores – they enjoy and do most things (Erikson 1996, Peterson and Kern 1996). Young people no longer divide into those who like pop and those who enjoy classical music. Most of the young people who go to classical concerts also enjoy rock. Middle class young people no longer defer gratifications (in any sense). They raise sufficient money from parents, part-time jobs and loans (while they remain students) to lead full and active leisure lives. Recent analysts have agreed that youth cultures are no longer class-based: particular scenes attract young people drawn from, and who are heading towards, all social levels (Bennett 1999, Karvonen *et al* 2000, Muggleton 2000).

Culture-based distinctions

Nowadays, young people from all social classes, males and females, are involved in the same kinds of scenes and activities, but this does not make everyone's leisure the same as everyone else's. Indeed, youth cultures are all about making distinctions. There is less 'resistance', symbolic or otherwise, or any other statement-making to adult society, than in the 1950s and 1960s. Youth cultures today are more about signifying differences vis-à-vis other crowds of young people, and today these distinctions do not map squarely onto the traditional social indicators – age, sex and social class (Bugge 2001).

The industries that produce and market beverages, venues and music know that none will appeal to all young people. This is impossible. It is realistic only to target specific market segments. The crowd attracted to a pub may depend initially on the décor, the location and the type of music that is played, and thereafter by whichever crowd of young people the place is adopted. It is difficult, probably impossible, for quantitative surveys to capture these distinctions, but they are portrayed vividly in qualitative enquiries.

Present-day popular music and club scenes are highly differentiated. Specific clubs, nights of the week and DJs attract their own crowds on the basis of the mixes of music that are played and the kinds of atmosphere that are created. The entertainment may be rap, hip-hop, soul, bass and drums, rhythm and blues, a techno, a retro or metallic sound, goth, acid, reggae or a particular kind of house or dance music. Clubbing is a very special experience, difficult to describe to the totally uninitiated. Whether a club is in a cellar or above ground, the outside world is always blacked out. The club offers a total sensory experience. The experience is unavoidable. The lights flash and the music is loud and continuous. Alcohol and whatever other substances are being used contribute to the atmosphere. Everyone in attendance should be enjoying the experience, and evidently so. The experience is one of diffuse friendliness, even incredible sociability. Crowds form on the basis of their attraction to a particular scene. These crowds are not based on any other social divisions – by neighbourhoods, education, occupation or gender – but every crowd is likely to feel that it is somehow different from others (see Malbon 1999, Thornton 1995).

Clubbing is a profit-making industry. Those who attend realise this. Even so, they still regard it as somehow underground and subversive. They distinguish between the 'serious' or 'authentic' rock that is played for them and the commercial mainstream of Radio 1 and the Top 40. Once past age

15, young people typically express disdain for the manufactured boy and girl bands that play kiddie pop. Who says that the older young people's music is more authentic? Just the performers and their audiences. In practice, of course, the entire popular music business (including so-called 'serious' rock) is commercial. The 'major' and 'indie' segments have a symbiotic relationship. Sounds and performers move readily from the so-called underground into the big time, if and when they can. Popular music is now a major industry, and an important export industry for Britain, yet the culture of the business heaps ridicule on any politicians or other 'straights' who attempt to align themselves with 'cool Britannia'.

Reputation-based crowds, ordinary and spectacular youth

There are different kinds of pubs and clubs, and there are different types of young people (so they say) who are identified on the basis of the places they frequent, the things they do, the clothes that they wear, their hairstyles, their musical preferences, and so on. School and college students readily identify the crowds that they know, if asked, though they may not necessarily place themselves in any. Some crowds are identified by internationally known labels – goths and skins, for example. Then, in any school, there are likely to be crowds known as computer geeks, designer label groups, a sports crowd, and so on (Kenvyn 2000, Thurlow 2001). These are not necessarily real interacting groups of people. Individuals can be identified and can align themselves with reputation-based crowds on the basis of their choices of clothing, music or whatever the crucial signifier might be. Whereas in the 1950s and 1960s groups of young people from particular neighbourhoods and schools adopted particular styles, nowadays it is the styles that create the crowds. These formations have been described as 'new tribes' and 'neo-communities' (to distinguish them from communities with deeper roots). Present-day crowds are often short-lived. A crowd can form then disintegrate within the space of a single summer (Thornton 1995).

   Now it is interesting that although most young people will readily apply labels to others, the majority refuse to attach any labels to themselves. All the relevant studies, from the 1950s to the present day, have found that most young people decline to identify with any particular style or crowd and prefer to describe themselves as just 'normal' or 'ordinary' (Brown 1987, Jenkins 1983, Hendry et al 2002b, Shildrick 2002). The crowds that individuals name may be real or imaginary. Either way, they enable young people to insist on their own ordinariness. Most do not dress to conform to any particular style. Most say that they like more than one kind of music. Most visit pubs and clubs which attract different crowds. By virtue of the mixtures of fashion that they wear and the performers and kinds of music in their personal collections, ordinary youth express their individuality.

They aim to 'stick out' as well as to 'fit in' within the range of tastes considered normal by their own ordinary friends (Miles 2000).

Ordinary youth are self-defined by who they are not. They are not extreme, and do not stand out spectacularly in their dress, coiffeur or musical tastes. They are not conformists. They are not slaves to any one style. Rather, they are 'cool' individuals who are able to appreciate and enjoy a variety of scenes. Studies in educational settings (for example, Brown 1987) find that ordinary youth also distinguish themselves from swots, ear 'oles, squares or straights (the labels vary from school to school and college to college). The swots (or whatever) may be a purely imaginary other. No study has found young people identifying themselves as members of such a group, but their use as a negative reference group enables ordinary young people to stress that they are no longer 'under the thumbs' of parents and teachers, that they know how to enjoy themselves, that they are streetwise, and that while they want to get on they have no urge to be ahead of everyone else. Ordinary youth's other negative reference group is the rems (remedials), dropouts or junkies (again, there appears to be a wide collection of labels). The stereotypes may again be imaginary, but the labels are applied to actual young people. In some girls' private schools anyone not aiming for higher education may be regarded as weird (Roker 1991). In comprehensives the 'dropouts' are usually the pupils in school classes where no-one is expected to achieve anything better than lower-grade GCSEs, who have poor attendance records and/or exclusion orders against them, who have been in trouble with the police, who often come from poor households and/or live on those council estates where most residents have not become owner-occupiers. Ordinary out-of-school youth make a similar distinction between themselves and the slapheads, doleites or dossers. Once gain, the labels vary tremendously and the stereotypes are never accurate portrayals, but the labels are applied to real young people – those who are not progressing further in education or training, and who are not holding down regular jobs.

All the relevant studies have found that unemployed young people have low rates (the lowest in their age group) of participation in the leisure activities that feature on survey checklists. There are two main ways in which young people can access organised leisure. One is by paying market prices. The other is via education where free to use or subsidised facilities, and lots of age peers, are always readily available. The unemployed are heavily disadvantaged (Hendry et al 1984, Roberts et al 1987, 1990). They also experience less social contact than any other members of their age group. Social contact is good for people's sense of well-being and self-esteem. Most social contact occurs routinely and predictably but is unarranged. Full-time students experience the most encounters, followed by young people in jobs, and the unemployed are the most isolated (Emler and McNamara 1996). Ordinary youth appear content to leave things this way. They do not wish to be involved with young people who are notorious for their trouble with the police, thieving and, sometimes, violence.

So 'excluded' youth develop their own social practices, often based in the neighbourhoods where they live. They hang about on the streets beyond the age when ordinary youth have abandoned this juvenile way of passing time (Shildrick 2002). Know-how on how to get by and how to get on without a regular job is passed on through local social networks: how to maximise benefit entitlements and how to access fiddly jobs; how to shoplift, how to pickpocket and how to dispose of stolen goods; and what to do and what to say when picked-up by the police (Craine and Coles 1995). Ordinary youth may regard drug use as normal, but not the so-called underclass's daily contact with dealers, heroin and solvent use (Shildrick 2002).

What government wants

So much for the trends and divisions among present-day youth at leisure. We now turn to the problems identified by recent governments. What do they want to change? Unambiguous nowadays: governments have sought to use leisure to include the excluded (the so-called rems, dolites, slapheads, etc.). The UK government (like all others) has additional aims in supporting leisure provisions for young people, but combating social exclusion tops the current agenda. There have been some amazing continuities in governments' and voluntary organisations' stated aims. The inclusion terminology is new but not the intention. Rescuing 'at-risk' youth was the prime aim when the uniformed youth movements were created a century and more ago. Inclusion does not head the agenda in all areas of current state leisure policy. For instance, the main objective in media policy is to maximise UK-based business and employment. Youth leisure provision, in contrast, has been incorporated into the government's inclusion agenda.

Today's main problem groups are said to be young people from disadvantaged families (where unemployment is high and incomes low), especially those from families where there is evidently a lack of parenting skills, and most of all those from neighbourhoods with concentrations of such families where so-called 'underclass' subcultures are likely to be bred (Murray 1990, 1994). We know that children from such backgrounds tend to be low achievers and early leavers from education. They often leave prematurely having been excluded, or persistent or spasmodic truants, before age 16 (Bynner et al 2002). They leave school without useful qualifications and are then at risk of becoming 'status zer0' or NEET (not in education, employment or training). These young people are then at risk of long-term floundering and failing to progress in the labour market; of long-term welfare dependency; of trouble with the police and courts, leading to custodial sentences which always exacerbate difficulties in obtaining employment; and of early parenthood, with the girls becoming single mums and the males absent fathers, thus rearing another generation of disadvantaged children (Bynner *et al* 2002, Jones 2002).

How might leisure provisions help? The government's aim is to involve at-risk youth in acceptable and satisfying uses of free time, to involve them in social relationships with included young people and adults, thus generating beneficial forms of social capital. In such milieux, members of the at-risk group are supposed to assimilate mainstream values and aspirations, leading to improved performances in education and better outcomes in the labour market.

As already acknowledged, this has never been the sole aim of non-commercial provisions for young people's leisure. Governments have always at least acknowledged a responsibility to facilitate the social development of all young people. From time to time additional concerns have risen up policy agendas. A battery of subsidiary concerns is currently included beneath the banner of 'health promotion'. The government is concerned that too many young people are indulging in unsafe sex, abusing drugs, tobacco and alcohol, failing to eat healthily and failing to take sufficient exercise. Britain's youth have certainly become flabbier. Too many are said to be couch potatoes. The free time (outside school and work) of Britain's 8–18 year olds is actually less active than that of the over-65s (Fisher 2002). The answer is believed to lie in encouraging young people to play more sport, though young people's sport participation has not declined: in fact it is much higher today than in the 1950s and 1960s (Roberts 1995). The main reasons for the decline in children's and young people's fitness are their diets and the motor car, which has ended the use of streets as playgrounds, reduced the amount of walking when all age groups go out and transformed the bicycle from a means of transport into a children's toy. However, promoting sport is easier than restricting the availability or appeal of confectionery, snacks and convenience foods, or reducing car use, and the promotion of youth sport is supposed to lead to other benefits. The government wants more young people with sporting talent to become top-level performers and win glory for the country. Sport is also one of the activities whereby it is hoped to include the excluded. The arts (making music, painting, crafts, drama, and so on) can also play a part, but sport is known to have a wider appeal.

We know that, by creating the right systems, governments can increase their countries' chances of sporting success (Green and Oakley 2002), and that, by providing more and better facilities, levels of youth participation in sport can be boosted (Roberts and Brodie 1992). We also know that trying to use leisure provisions to include the excluded simply does not work. A strong clue as to why this should be so can be found in the divisions (identified above) that young people at leisure form among themselves. The inclusion via leisure agenda has been tested to destruction. We have over a century's experience of these efforts. If the medicine worked there would no longer be a problem to address. The kindest recent reviews of the evidence conclude that we still lack convincing proof that the 'leisure solution' can work on a wide scale (Centre for Leisure and Sport Research 2002, Coalter *et al* 2000, Collins 1999, Shaw 1999, Witt and Crompton 1996). However, Williamson and Middlemiss (1999) are probably more perceptive (as well as more critical) in noting how frequently projects massage statistics and some-times invent evidence of success in order to sustain their funding. Promising to solve otherwise intractable social problems remains the leisure services' best way of winning government money. The Department for Culture, Media and Sport (1999) knows that it needs to address wider political priorities if its exchequer grant is to be raised (or even maintained). Voluntary associa-tions and local councils know from experience what they need to promise in order to attract central government funds. For their part, governments appear to feel that they need to be seen to be 'doing something' to tackle high-profile problems, and leisure projects are typically non-controversial, cheap and produce visible outcomes (new facilities) even if these do not lead to the intended impacts. Everyone seems happy to let this roundabout continue. Disadvantaged people have never been the principal users of leisure facilities provided by either the state or the voluntary sector. The better-off appear well pleased to lobby for funds to tackle the lack of facilities for disadvantaged people, then use those facilities for their own enjoyment.

What young people want

So much for the government's intentions. We can now turn to the leisure problems that young people themselves would like their societies to address. Young people have never spoken in unison, but some of their leisure requests have been repeated by generation after generation.

Things to do, places to go

This is among young people's long-standing wishes. Nowadays, it is voiced mainly by younger young people, typically the under-16s who feel too old for youth clubs and family leisure, but who are still too young and/or lack the money to access pubs and other adult facilities. Young people who live in outlying suburbs and rural areas often feel disadvan-taged vis-à-vis city youth, while the latter complain about the absence of affordable leisure. The under-16s spend a great deal of time just hanging about, doing nothing in particular. Nothing seems to change in this respect (Hendry *et al* 2002a, Jephcott 1967, Leigh 1971). What provisions do these young people want? They say that they want sports centres and meeting places where any supervision is unobtrusive (presumably as in university student unions). It is hard to decide whether young people are reflecting on their own first-hand experience or merely repeating what they have heard and read when they blame delinquency and drug abuse on the absence of alternative things to do.

More leisure time?

Nowadays, some young people have an entirely different complaint: a shortage of time. This predicament is most common among the over-16s, especially among academic young people (those studying for A levels and degrees), but also among some on training schemes, who combine part-time evening and weekend work with their main 'occupations'. When travelling time is included, the work weeks of these busy young people can exceed 70 hours (see Allatt and Dixon 2002). They find that there are insufficient hours in the week to study/train, earn, keep in touch with their families, meet all their friends, engage in all their preferred pastimes and still have literally spare time when they can relax on their own.

Access to adult opportunities

This is another age-old yearning, still typical among younger young people. It appears that they have always looked forward to the time when they will cease to be too young. Too young to do what? The details of the yearnings have changed alongside changes in young adults' lifestyles. Nowadays, younger teenagers want to be able to go to pop concerts, weekend pop festivals, pubs and clubs, on holiday just with friends and to live independently. Motor transport is high on present-day teenagers' wish lists (Carabine and Longhurst 2002). Car ownership is eagerly anticipated. When achieved, there is a sense of liberation: a massive widening of leisure opportunities.

Staying young

Once again, however, nowadays, there is a contrary wish, common among older young people who want to stay young (at least in a lifestyle sense). As we have seen, over the last 30 years youth cultures have merged with young singles scenes, and many 20-somethings, even 30-somethings, do not wish to relinquish the lifestyle (Hollands 1995). Youth was once called a brief flowering period. It is no longer brief. Youth has been extended. The attractions of the young adult lifestyle are not the only reasons why the typical ages when people marry and become parents have risen. Today's young adults are circumspect: they want to ensure that everything is right before they settle down. They want to be in the right kind of job and career situation, to have sorted themselves out money-wise, to have suitable housing and to be in the right relationship. Sometimes it seems that all these things are never right simultaneously (Hobcraft and Kiernan 1995). For over 30 years UK birthrates have been too low to maintain the population's size, and in the future this could become a far more serious issue for the country than the teenage pregnancies that the government wants to reduce (see Jones 2002).

Freedom and safety

This is another apparently contradictory pair of demands, in this case often voiced by the same individuals. Adults may often fail to understand that young people inhabit a dangerous world. Leisure places are particularly risky. Young people are the age group most likely to be convicted, but they are also the most common victims, of crime. Their property is at risk. Expensive bags, coats and mobile phones disappear if left unattended. Sometimes they disappear while attended! There is also the danger of physical assault from older or stronger young people, especially if they have been drinking. The most common reason young people give for carrying knives is self-protection. That said, their main defence mechanism is to keep their friends around them (Brown 1995).

Young people also feel threatened by adults, and there is a lot more fear and loathing from the old towards the young than vice-versa. Most young people report that they get on well (and even better as they grow older) with their own parents (Gillies et al 2001). Adults may trust the young people who they know personally but they are easily disturbed by groups who just hang about on the streets or in shopping centres. Adults may find young people's demeanour and dress disturbing. They are unlikely to appreciate the young people's music, especially if the volume is turned up. People aged over 40 are unlikely to be wise on the contemporary drug scene or to know exactly what happens in 'clubs'. Suspicion of the young is not new (see Eppel and Eppel 1966). It is among the constant research findings. Young people resent the suspicion that they attract. They feel unfairly victimised when residents complain to the police or to the local council about their presence on a neighbourhood's streets, or when they are asked to move on by police or security staff in shopping precincts.

Some adults are experienced as a more serious kind of threat. Being watched and even followed by an adult is quite a common teenage and childhood experience (Brown 1995). The adults about whom some young people feel most uneasy are relatives or neighbours (see Green et al 2000). This is part of the darker side of family and community life in present-day Britain (and no doubt elsewhere).

On the one hand, young people will say that they want simply to be left alone, to be accorded the same rights and respect as adults. At the same time, they want to live in safety from others. Don't we all! Simultaneously, young people want to take their own risks. Risk helps to keep life interesting. Nights out in city centres, with strangers all around, are exciting. Totally safe, hygienic leisure soon becomes boring (Rojek 2000). Young people know that there are risks attached to alcohol, tobacco, drugs and sex. They are not ignorant of, nor do they ignore, the risks. Rather, like most adults, they regard risk-taking as a normal part of present-day life (see Lupton and Tulloch 2002). Ideally, like adults, young people want to be able to control the risks. In other words, they want to be in control of their own lives. For this they need reliable information, not sermons. In practice, the messages that they receive are often confusing. Often it seems that friends are believed to be the most reliable informers.

Whose agenda?

Governments (central and local) spend a lot of money on leisure, including young people's leisure. The big problem is not the level of spending so much as how the money is spent. Government priorities do not match young people's issues, and neither wish list is wholly realistic.

Governments have incorporated their leisure spending on young people into the inclusion agenda, but who else wants to include the excluded? Ordinary youth are against it. They prefer to keep themselves apart. Their parents obviously want it this way. They do their best to ensure that their children do not attend 'sink schools' where they are likely to be contaminated by the wrong crowds (Willms 1996). There is a great deal of middle class duplicity: public support for inclusionary policies while in private engaging in exclusionary conduct.

Leisure is hardly the best place to begin to heal socio-economic divisions. People feel that they have the right to spend their free time where they want, doing what they want, with the people they choose to be with. In our highly commercialised times, 'good leisure' is the reward for 'good citizens' (and the children of good citizens) who have earned the money to pay for it (Ravenscroft 1993). There is a great deal of tokenism in the social inclusion agenda. Even targeted sport and arts projects may not attract truly disadvantaged young people. They are difficult to attract and retain (Kay 1987), and even when achieved this no longer includes those concerned in present-day, mainly commercial, mainstream youth leisure. The inclusionary efforts may work with some individuals, but if larger groups are attracted their own cultures are liable to overwhelm the provisions and repel ordinary working and middle class youth.

Young people's own priorities will be a better starting point for public and voluntary sector leisure provisions. What will this mean? First, providing activities and places for younger young people, the under-16s, who are betwixt and between the adult-led leisure of childhood and being able to access the commercial provisions and facilities which are intended for adults. Secondly, it will mean addressing young people's safety concerns. They do not want to be prevented from taking their own risks, but they do want protection from over-zealous, over-protective and paedophilic or otherwise exploitative adults, and from pilfering and violent age peers. Thirdly, there are the problems of the young adults who have become over-burdened by the demands of simultaneously earning and studying, then earning, saving and repaying debts while engaging in family and household formation (and enjoying leisure at the same time). Governments need to address these problems.

Social inclusion is a laudable aim, but young people's leisure is simply not the right place to begin. Exclusion is a product of late-twentieth century trends in the economy and labour markets, and these are the places where the search for genuine solutions must begin (and end).

References

Albermarle Report (1960) *The Youth Service in England and Wales*, London: HMSO.

Allatt, P. and Dixon, C. (2002) 'Dissolving boundaries between employment, education and the family', paper presented to the British Sociological Association Conference, Leicester.

Bennett, A. (1999) 'Subcultures or neo-tribes? Rethinking the relationship between youth style and musical taste', *Sociology*, 33: 599–617.

Brown, P. (1987) *Schooling Ordinary Kids: Inequality, unemployment and the new vocationalism*, London: Tavistock.

Brown, S. (1995) 'Crime and safety in whose community?', *Youth and Policy*, 48: 27–48.

Bugge, C. (2001) 'Reinventing subculture: forty years of marketing cool', paper presented to Conference on Global Youth, University of Plymouth.

Bynner, J., Elias, P., McKnight, A., *et al.* (2002) *Young People's Changing Routes to Independence*, York: Joseph Rowntree Foundation.

Carabine, E. and Longhurst, B. (2002) 'Consuming the car: anticipation, use and meaning in contemporary youth culture', *Sociological Review*, 50: 181–196.

Centre for Leisure and Sport Research (2002) *Count Me In: The dimensions of social inclusion through culture and sport*, Leeds: Leeds Metropolitan University.

Coalter, F., Allison, M. and Taylor, J. (2000) *The Role of Sport in Regenerating Deprived Urban Areas*, Edinburgh: HMSO.

Coleman, J. S. (1961) *The Adolescent Society*, New York: Glencoe Free Press.

Collins, M. (1999) *Sport and Social Exclusion*, Loughborough: Loughborough University.

Craine, S. and Coles, B. (1995) 'Youth transitions and young people's involvement in crime', *Youth and Policy*, 48: 6–26.

Department for Culture, Media and Sport, Policy Action Team 10 (1999) *Arts and Sport: A report to the Social Exclusion Unit*, London.

Department for Education (1995), *Young People's Participation in the Youth Service*, Statistical Bulletin 1/95, London.

Emler, N. and McNamara, S. (1996) 'The social contact patterns of young people: Effects of participation in the social institutions of the family, education and work', in H. Helve and J. Bynner (eds), *Youth and Life Management: Research perspectives*, Yliopistopaino: Helsinki University Press.

Eppel, E. M. and Eppel, M. (1966) *Adolescents and Morality*, London: Routledge.

Erikson, B. H. (1996) 'Culture, class and connections', *American Journal of Sociology*, 102: 217–251.

Fisher, K. (2002) *Chewing the Fat: The story time diaries tell about physical activity in the United Kingdom*, Working Paper 2002–13, University of Essex, Colchester: Institute for Social and Economic Research.

Gillies, V., McCarthy, J. R. and Holland, J. (2001) *Pulling Together, Pulling Apart: The family lives of young people*, London: Family Policy Studies Centre.

Green, E., Mitchell W. and Bunton, R. (2000) 'Contextualising risk and danger: An analysis of young people's perceptions of risk', *Journal of Youth Studies*, 3: 109–126.

Green, M. and Oakley, B. (2001) 'Elite sport development systems and playing to win: Uniformity and diversity in international approaches', *Leisure Studies*, 20: 247–267.

Hall, S. and Jefferson, T. (eds) (1976) *Resistance Through Rituals*, London: Hutchinson.

Hendry, L. B., Kloep, M., Espenes, G. A. *et al*, (2002a), 'Leisure transitions – a rural perspective', *Leisure Studies*, 21: 1–14.

Hendry, L. B., Kloep, M. and Wood, S. (2002b) 'Young people talking about adolescent rural crowds and social settings', *Journal of Youth Studies*, 5: 357–374.

Hendry, L. B., Raymond, M. and Stewart, C. (1984) 'Unemployment, school and leisure: an adolescent study', *Leisure Studies*, 3: 175–187.

Hendry, L. B., Shucksmith, J., Love, J. G. *et al.* (1993) *Young People's Leisure and Lifestyles*, London: Routledge.

Hobcraft, J. and Kiernan, K. (1995) *Becoming a Parent in Europe*, Welfare State Programme, London: London School of Economics.

Hollands, R. G. (1995) *Friday Night, Saturday Night*, Department of Social Policy, Newcastle: University of Newcastle.

Hollands, R. and Chatterton, P. (2002) 'Producing youth nightlife in the new urban entertainment economy: Corporatism, branding and market segmentation', paper presented to International Sociological Association Congress, Brisbane.

Jenkins, R. (1983) *Lads, Citizens and Ordinary Kids*, London: Routledge.

Jephcott, P. (1967) *Time of One's Own*, London: Oliver and Boyd.

Jones, G. (2002) *The Youth Divide*, York: Joseph Rowntree Foundation.

Karvonen, S., West, P., Sweeting, H., *et al.* (2001) 'Lifestyle, social class and health-related behaviour: a cross-national comparison of 15 year olds in Glasgow and Helsinki', *Journal of Youth Studies*, 4: 393–413.

Kay, T. A. (1987) *Leisure in the Lifestyles of Unemployed People: A case study in Leicester*, PhD thesis, Loughborough: Loughborough University of Technology.

Kenvyn, I. (2000) *The Ascribed Significance of Adolescent Free Time*, PhD thesis, Leeds: University of Leeds.

Leigh, J. (1971) *Young People and Leisure*, London: Routledge.

Lupton, D. and Tulloch, J. (2002) '"Risk is part of your life": risk epistemologies among a group of Australians', *Sociology*, 36: 317–334.

Malbon, B. (1999) *Clubbing, Dancing, Ecstasy and Vitality*, London: Routledge.

Miles, S. (2000) *Youth Lifestyles in a Changing World*, Milton Keynes, Buckingham: Open University Press.

Muggleton, D. (2000) *Inside Subculture: The postmodern meaning of style*, Oxford: Berg.

Murray, C. (1990) *The Emerging British Underclass*, London: Institute of Economic Affairs.

Murray, C. (1994) *Underclass: The crisis deepens*, London: Institute of Economic Affairs.

Organisation for Economic Co-operation and Development (2000) *From Initial Education to Working Life: Making transitions work*, Paris.

Parker, H., Williams, L. and Aldridge, J. (2002) 'The normalization of "sensible" recreational drug use: further evidence from the north-west England longitudinal study', *Sociology*, 36: 941–964.

Peterson, R. A. and Kern, R. M. (1996) 'Changing highbrow taste: From snob to omnivore', *American Sociological Review*, 61: 900–907.

Ravenscroft, N. (1993) 'Public leisure provision and the good citizen', *Leisure Studies*, 12: 33–44.

Roberts, K. (1996) 'Young people, schools, sport and government policies', *Sport, Education and Society*, 1: 47–57.

Roberts, K. and Brodie, D. (1992) *Inner-City Sport: Who plays and what are the benefits?* Culemborg: Giordano Bruno.

Roberts, K., Brodie, D. and Dench, S. (1987) 'Youth unemployment and out-of-home recreation', *Society and Leisure*, 10: 281–294.

Roberts, K., Campbell, R. and Furlong, A. (1990) 'Class and gender divisions among young adults at leisure', in C Wallace and M Cross (eds), *Youth in Transition*, London: Falmer Press.

Roberts, K. and Parsell, G. (1994) 'Youth cultures in Britain: The middle class take-over', *Leisure Studies*, 13: 33–48.

Rojek, C. (2000) *Leisure and Culture*, Basingstoke: Macmillan.

Roker, D. (1991) 'Gaining the edge: The education, training and employment of young people in private schools', paper presented to New Findings Workshop, ESRC 16–19 Initiative, Harrogate.

Shaw, P. (1999) *The Arts and Neighbourhood Renewal: A literature Review to inform the work of Policy Action Team 10*, Loughborough: Loughborough University.

Shildrick, T. (2002) 'Young people, illicit drug use and the question of normalization', *Journal of Youth Studies*, 5: 35–48.

Sugarman, B. (1967) 'Involvement in youth culture, academic achievement and conformity in school', *British Journal of Sociology*, 18: 151–164.

Thornton, S. (1995) *Club Cultures: Music, media and subcultural capital*, Cambridge: Polity Press.

Thurlow, C. (2001) 'The usual suspects? A comparative investigation of crowds and social-type labelling among young British Teenagers', *Journal of Youth Studies*, 4: 319–334.

Willms, J. D. (1996) 'School and community segregation: findings from Scotland', in A. C. Kerckhoff, (ed.) *Generating Social Stratification: Toward a new research agenda*, Boulder, Colorado: Westview Press.

Witt, P. A. and Crompton, J. L. (1996) *Recreation Programs that Work for At Risk Youth*, Pennsylvania: Venture Publishing.

Postscript on leisure

Carys Lovering

My name is Carys Lovering. I am 22 years old and live with my boyfriend in a village just outside Swansea, Wales. I grew up in a medium-sized village in South Wales where there was not very much for me to do when I was growing up. I am a full-time youth worker for the YWCA and I work with excluded young women – young mothers, young women who are not attending school who access our alternative curriculum scheme, young women who have experienced homelessness, young women who are bullied and the list goes on. I also volunteer with an integrated youth circus where young people of all abilities meet to learn circus skills. In the past I have worked with homeless people in a hostel in Swansea.

The problems young people face in leisure

As a young person I feel that not enough is available to me in my spare time. I graduated last year from Swansea University and decided to stay in the area because it is a good place for me to continue my long-term hobby – surfing. To be completely honest, the transition between university and working life has really had a large impact on my friends and I. When you've been in university for three years your social life is made so easy for you with things going on every night and posters everywhere letting you know about them. You've got countless amounts of clubs and societies to fill your spare time with and by the time you finish university and get on in the real world you think something's wrong. I found it such a big strain that I stayed in the place that I had attended university but all the friends that I had moved either back home or had gone travelling the world to 'discover themselves'! As there are so many people like myself who choose to work straight after university, I feel there should be something for us to do to keep up the busy social life that we experienced in university. I should imagine that there are groups like these that exist, but they are just not promoted enough in the right places. There should be boards in doctors' surgeries, in supermarkets and in other places that we have to go to. Something that has helped me meet and make new friends is volunteering, which is not promoted enough. Young people of all ages should be encouraged to volunteer and schemes like the Duke of Edinburgh award do this.

From my experience working with socially excluded young people, they do want somewhere to go and they are natural risk takers. I agree with Ken Roberts when he says that young people need/want better information on the risks of drugs or unsafe sex. However, in my experience, certainly in Wales, access to information is getting easier and drop-in information shops are springing up in areas of need. The wishes of some of the young women that I work with is for youth clubs to be open more hours, drop-in centres to find out what is going on and trips that are being organized, art projects such as building sculptures and gardens in the communities that they live in, computer courses, outdoor activities and more trips in holiday times. Outdoor activities seem to be very popular with so many young people, even those who don't like sports and even if a young person says that they won't take part, it's guaranteed at the end of the day they will be getting stuck in like everyone else in the group! Skateboard parks are another thing that young people are desperate for. Some young boys from our village were going round the village a few weeks ago with a petition for a skate park in the village. They are getting fed up with people moaning at them for skating in the street so they are taking action by using the only way they know how – a petition. The thing that all of these have in common is that they are all free! Ken Roberts says that some young people from disadvantaged backgrounds such as the unemployed cannot access leisure facilities that the government want them to because they cost money and therefore aren't being used by the people who 'most need them'. From working with young mothers I am aware that some of them only access our services because they are free and, if it wasn't for our service, they would not have any other means of socialising and meeting other people in the same situation. Young mothers also miss out on a variety of things due to lack of childcare facilities. A few young women from our young mums group have expressed to me that if it wasn't for the good childcare facilities in the project, they would not use the project.

What young people want

It's true from what Ken Roberts says that the government isn't entirely clear what it is that young people actually want. I know that youth work does have a positive impact on the lives of young people. I think the government should take note of what independent charities are doing in their work with young people. By providing specific groups where young people choose what they want to do and working with their ideas to deliver programmes that are best suited to the young people of that particular area and by working with young people and consulting with them in a participative and fun way, we can deliver what the young people themselves want in our groups. Young people are different from area to area, I have seen that by working with young women from three different areas in a relatively small area like South Wales. I think if there is a perfect answer to what young people really want, it is for youth organisations to consult with them about the projects or activities that they feel are most appropriate to them.

Part II

Specific issues

Chapter 8

Young people and unemployment: From welfare to workfare?

Peter A. Kemp

Introduction

The New Labour government has brought a renewed urgency and an enhanced commitment to tackling the problems of disadvantage and 'social exclusion' faced by large numbers of young people (Mizen 2003). Although a wide range of policies and initiatives for young people have been introduced – covering topics such as education and training, sexual health, drug misuse, homelessness and crime – employment is arguably the dominating theme of the government's social exclusion agenda (Levitas 1998). Economic and social changes over the past two decades have disproportionately affected disadvantaged young people and helped to make the school-to-work transition more protracted, more fractured and more risky (Furlong and Cartmel 1997, Coles 1995, Jones 2002). The New Labour government sees long-term youth unemployment as an important cause of social exclusion and has introduced the New Deal for Young People to tackle the problem.

In seeking to address social exclusion by helping young people into paid employment, the policy emphasis has been on the advice, training and other help that young people need to make them more 'employable'. In other words, policy has focused on the *supply* of youth labour and in particular on what are seen as the deficits and failings of unemployed young people as potential employees. Relatively little attention has been devoted to labour *demand*: that is, the number, type, quality and location of jobs available to young people. Or, to put it another way, the focus is on individual agency – young people's attributes, qualifications, decision-making and behaviour – rather than on the wider social and economic structures and the opportunities and choices that these offer to young people. While this approach is undoubtedly enabling many young people to move successfully from welfare to work, it is proving to be less successful at helping more socially excluded young people who have to cope with less resources and 'human capital' at their disposal.

The changing youth labour market

The past quarter century has seen a major restructuring – and some would say, collapse – of the youth labour market (Bynner *et al* 2002, Hasluck 1998, Maguire and Maguire 1997). This transformation has had profound implications for the school-to-work transition, which has become more complex and in some cases more fractured than in the past (Coles 1995, Furlong and Cartmel 1997). For much of the post-war period up to the mid 1970s, the majority of young people left school at 16 with relatively few qualifications and entered a restricted range of occupations. About a third of young men entered apprenticeships that enabled them to develop craft skills, which was often the route to relatively secure and well-paid skilled manual jobs. Meanwhile, a minority of school leavers entered higher education at age 18, which was generally a route into professional careers and better-paid employment opportunities (Ashton *et al* 1982).

By the time that New Labour came to power in 1997, that world had largely disappeared. As Fergusson *et al* (2000: 283) noted, 'By the 1990s these young workers were replaced by full-time students, trainees, part-time workers and the unemployed.' Over the past quarter of a century, there has been a sharp decline in craft jobs and a shift towards low-skilled occupations among young men. Meanwhile, there has been a shift from clerical and secretarial jobs to sales and personal service occupations among women. These new jobs are generally much less secure and offer relatively limited opportunities for advancement (Bynner *et al* 2002).

More generally, the demand for youth labour declined over the past quarter of a century. Many jobs that had previously been open to school leavers disappeared. By the 1990s, instead of apprenticeships, young people were more likely to be in youth training schemes, which were shorter, tended to have very low status and proved to be a far less certain route to a secure or well-paid job (Coles 2000). Some commentators even questioned whether a distinct youth labour market still existed (Maguire and Maguire 1997). Many more young people are now staying on in education in order to gain qualifications, which have become more important in the transition to full economic independence than was the case in the 1970s. With better-qualified young people staying on in education, the youth labour market has increasingly become a market for less well-qualified labour (Bynner *et al* 2002).

The net result is that fewer young people are in paid employment than was the case 20 or 30 years ago. Instead of typically entering the labour market at 16–19 years old, young people may not begin employment until their early 20s (Hasluck 1998, Millar 2000), leaving them financially dependent on their families or the state for much longer than before (Jones 1995, 2002). Analysis of the Youth Cohort Study by Dolton *et al* (1999) showed that the proportion of 19-year-old men in full-time employment declined from 60 per cent in 1987 to 38 per cent in 1994. Among 19 year-old women, the proportion declined from 58 per cent to 33 per cent. Meanwhile, the proportion in full-time education increased from 19 per cent to 40 per cent among men and from 18 per cent to 40 per cent among women at this age. The proportion of young people who were unemployed fell, but those in 'other' labour market states doubled among both women and men at age 19 between 1987 and 1994. The 'other' category comprises young people who are not in education, training or employment, such as the unemployed and those who are economically inactive (including people who are looking after the family home, are sick or disabled, or for some other reason are not looking for work). Bynner et al (2002) found that four times as many people born in 1970 compared with those born in 1958 who had been in the 'other' status at age 17, were unemployed at age 26.

Young people in general are better qualified educationally than previous generations. Bynner et al (2002) found that young people from poor and low-income backgrounds born in 1970 were more likely than those born in 1958 to gain academic qualifications. However, socio-economic differences continued to exist. Thus, young people from poor and low-income backgrounds in both cohorts were less likely than their better-off peers to still be in education after age 16. Compared with the earlier cohort, young people from poor backgrounds born in 1970 were more likely to be in training schemes, less likely to be in full-time employment, and had more experience of unemployment.

Young women are now less likely to stay at home and more likely to go out to work than was true of previous generations. Bynner et al (2002) found that young women aged 26 were much more likely to be in full-time employment, and less likely to be at home full time in the 1970 cohort compared with the 1958 cohort. Some 14 per cent of the later cohort, compared with 30 per cent of the earlier cohort, were at home full time. Meanwhile, 78 per cent of the 1970 cohort, compared with 58 per cent of the 1958 cohort, were in full-time employment. However, even among the 1970 cohort, young women from poor backgrounds were more likely than those from better-off backgrounds to be at home and less likely to be in full-time employment. Thus, 24 per cent of women from a poor background were at home full time at age 26 compared with 18 per cent of women from a low-income background and eight per cent from a higher-income background (Bynner et al 2002).

Although as a generation they are better off than their earlier counterparts, and despite their better qualifications, young people now earn less compared with adult workers than they did 25 years ago. Overlaying this trend, there has been an increase in earnings inequality among young people. Meanwhile, experience of substantial spells of unemployment appears to carry a significant 'wage penalty' for young people in terms of subsequent earnings (Bynner et al 2002). Unemployment thus has a 'scarring effect' among young people, as it does among people of working age more generally (Gregg 1998).

There also appears to be a trend towards increasing polarisation between those young people who stay on in education and gain higher qualifications, and subsequently move into 'career jobs' and better-paid occupations, and those who leave school with few or no qualifications, and move into insecure and low-paid jobs (Jones 2002, Bynner *et al* 2002). Moreover, Dolton *et al* (1999: 54) found that young people's success in the labour market is determined by 'factors beyond their control, such as where they live and when they were born'. In terms of both employment and earnings, young people from low-income backgrounds now face much greater relative disadvantage than their earlier counterparts (Bynner *et al* 2002). This structural disadvantage (Jones 2002) can create disaffection and social exclusion among young people (Coles 2000).

Although the overall employment outlook has improved over the last decade, with employment growing strongly and unemployment falling to relatively low levels, young people have not benefited from this to the same extent as older adults of working age. On the International Labour Organisation (ILO) definition, the unemployment rate for all adults halved between 1993 and 2003 (Office of National Statistics 2003). However, youth unemployment (ages 16–24) declined by only a third over this period. In April/June 2003 the unemployment rate for young people (12.5 per cent) was more than double that for people of working age as a whole (5.0 per cent). Table 8.1 shows that, in 2001/02, only about half (53 per cent) of people aged between 16 and 24 were in full-time employment, with a further 1 in 6 (17 per cent) in part-time work.

Young people on the margins of work

Thus, the youth labour market has been transformed in ways which have made it much more difficult for less well-qualified young people to make the transition from school to work. Instead of entering full-time and

Table 8.1 Employment status of young people aged 16–24

	Males (%)	Females (%)	All (%)
Full-time employment	60	45	53
Part-time employment	12	20	16
ILO unemployed	10	5	7
Student	12	13	13
Looking after family/home	–	10	5
Permanently sick/disabled	2	3	3
Temporarily sick/disabled	1	1	1
Other inactive	4	3	3
Total	100	100	100

Source: Department for Work and Pensions (2003a), Table 7.1.

permanent employment, perhaps after a period of apprenticeship, less well-qualified young people are more likely to experience a mix of training schemes, temporary and part-time jobs, and periods of unemployment. Meadows (2001) argues that while relatively few young people have no experience of paid employment, the difficulty is more about not being able to obtain a satisfactory long-term job.

In some respects, young men are less able than young women to compete successfully in this new and more insecure employment world. Stafford *et al* (1999) found that young men are proportionately more likely to be unemployed. However, young women are more likely to be looking after the home or family full time and not seeking paid work, which in some cases may be a response to not having a job. As well as being less likely than young men to be unemployed, young women are more likely to leave unemployment and have slightly shorter spells out of work.

Fergusson *et al* (2000) also found that young women 'outperformed men' in school and in their early work careers. Nevertheless, women also tended to have disrupted trajectories from school to work. The young people in their survey had unstable, complex and non-linear patterns of post-school experience. Indeed, they questioned whether these experiences could be said to resemble a 'career' or linear transition from school to work. Instead, young people experienced what Fergusson *et al* referred to as 'normalized dislocation' in which their lives were 'characterised by a *melange* of movement in and out of training courses, part-time, low-paid work. . . and unemployment' (Fergusson *et al* 2000: 286).

Further insights into the difficulties that young people can experience come from a study of a disadvantaged neighbourhood in Teesside in North East England (Johnston *et al* 2000a). The decline of manufacturing industry in the area since the 1970s had undermined local prosperity and economic security. The jobless rate was about 40 per cent in the area and employment opportunities for young people were very limited. Most young people saw getting a 'proper job' as an important aspect of adult status and one they wanted to attain, but only a minority had been able to secure long-term or rewarding employment in the area. Most crucially, their opportunities and decision-making were constrained by the limitations of living in a disadvantaged neighbourhood. Some young people had obtained secure, regular employment, but in many cases this was after repeated spells of unemployment. Many of the jobs that were available were short-term or part-time work or were low paid. Although young people's experiences varied widely, youth transitions were very complex and fast changing: 'The post-school "careers" that young people followed were unpredictable, insecure and largely lacking in regular employment' (Johnston *et al* 2000b: 2).

As well as living in areas of high unemployment, young people can be disadvantaged in other ways. Indeed, long-term unemployment can be a symptom of underlying disadvantages (Meadows 2001). Stafford *et al*

(1999) found that, for young men, shorter spells of unemployment and movements into employment were associated with living with a parent or relative (who was not a spouse or partner), having vocational qualifications, possessing a driving licence, having previous work experience and having no health problems affecting ability to work. Expressed differently, young men who did not have these characteristics had longer spells of unemployment and were less likely to move into employment than those who had them.

Young people with multiple disadvantages are especially vulnerable in the labour market and in need of support. A qualitative study by Lakey *et al* (2001a) examined the labour market experiences of young people who had multiple problems, including homelessness, disability, poor mental health, criminal records, family breakdown, drug and alcohol problems, or had been looked after by the local authority. Although the problems they faced varied, most of them had difficulty in obtaining or keeping paid employment. The majority had 'spent their working lives in and out of temporary, casual or part-time jobs' (Lakey *et al* 2001b: 2). Many referred to a lack of suitable jobs in their local areas and to employer discrimination.

Unemployed young people have only restricted entitlement to social security benefits. Those aged from 16 to 17 years old are not entitled to benefit at all, except in exceptional circumstances, single young people aged from 18 to 24 years old receive significantly less Jobseeker's Allowance than older claimants. Meanwhile, young claimants renting their accommodation privately are restricted to the 'single room rent', whereby the maximum housing benefit they receive is the average for shared accommodation in the locality (Kemp and Rugg 2001). Ostensibly, the rationale for paying young people aged from 18 to 24 years old lower rates of social security benefit is to maintain their incentive to work by ensuring that they are worse off on benefits than in paid employment. In general, young people are paid less than older adults and this is reflected in, and is reinforced by, the national minimum wage. Introduced by the New Labour government in April 1999, the national minimum wage has a lower rate for young people under the age of 22 years old. In addition, single people under the age of 25 years old are not entitled to the Working Tax Credit, an income-related wage supplement payable by the Inland Revenue to people in low-paid employment. In contrast to government concern about child and pensioner poverty, tackling income poverty among young people is scarcely mentioned in official documents.

New Deal for Young People

The Labour Party's manifesto for the 1997 general election included a promise to introduce a welfare-to-work programme for long-term unemployed young people. The new programme was to be paid for out of a windfall tax on the privatised public utility companies. The aim was to get a quarter of a million young people off benefit and into work (Labour Party 1997). Following the election, Gordon Brown, the new Chancellor of the Exchequer, confirmed New Labour's commitment to this New Deal for Young People (NDYP).

The NDYP was introduced in 12 'pathfinder areas' in January 1998 and rolled out nationally the following April. Initially, it was scheduled to last until 2002, but in 2001 it was announced that the policy would remain in place permanently (National Audit Office 2002). The new programme was widely viewed as the major plank of New Labour's strategy for tackling social exclusion among young people (Fergusson 2002). When it was introduced, almost 120,000 young people were long-term unemployed, of whom two-fifths had been out of work for one year or more (National Audit Office 2002).

The New Deal for Young People has often been described as one of New Labour's flagship policies (Bryson 2003, Ritchie 2000). It was devised in the wake of a series of youth training schemes that many participants viewed as failing them (Coles 2000). This new programme was to be a 'new deal' in the sense of being better funded and organised than previous youth training schemes. It sought to free itself of the negative image of previous training and employment programmes for young people 'by using real jobs, matched placements, market rates of pay, and certificated training linked to a life-long training strategy' (Fergusson 2002: 178). According to Ritchie (2000), an important feature of NDYP is that it provides advice, training and other support that is intended to match the specific needs of the individual participants. Hasluck (2001) argues that it is this feature that distinguishes the programme from previous youth training schemes.

The aim of the New Deal is to tackle long-term unemployment by helping young people get off benefits and into paid work. The theory is that getting them to compete for jobs would not only reduce social exclusion among young people but also, indirectly, increase the overall level of employment in the economy. According to one view, being out of work for a long time causes people to lose skills, thereby reducing their employability and undermining their confidence in being able to find work (see Hasluck 1998). The consequence is that young people risk becoming detached from the labour market and might give up searching for work. By re-engaging them with the labour market, young people's employability would increase and, by improving their job search, help the economy to run at a higher level of employment without causing inflation to rise (Layard 1997).

The NDYP offers young people a certain degree of choice (Bryson 2003), although not the option of non-participation. An important feature of the programme is that it is mandatory for all young people aged from 18 to 24 years old who have been unemployed and claiming Jobseeker's Allowance

(JSA) continuously for six months or more. The mandatory nature of NDYP has been criticised, but so has the fact that young people have to wait for six months before gaining access to the programme. All JSA clients are required to take steps to actively search for work, but otherwise are largely left to their own devices during the six-month qualifying period. For most young people, that might not be a problem, but for those facing significant barriers to employment who need support to find work, it delays the point at which their problems start to be addressed (Perkins-Cohen 2002). Young people who belong to certain disadvantaged groups can gain early access to the New Deal. This includes people with a health problem or impairment, people with literacy or numeracy difficulties, ex-offenders and recent leavers from local authority care (Ritchie 2000). However, relatively few young people enter NDYP under the early rules. Nationally, the figure is about seven or eight per cent of clients, but the figure is higher in areas of *low* unemployment and lower in areas of *high* unemployment. In other words, less use appears to be made of the early entry rules in areas where barriers to employment make it more difficult for vulnerable young people to get jobs (Perkins-Cohen 2002).

The New Deal has three main stages: the Gateway, Options and Follow-through. As the name implies, the *Gateway* is young people's point of entry into the New Deal. It is intended to be a period of intensive job search during which participants are expected to draw up an action plan with a New Deal personal adviser (Walker and Wiseman 2003). Those who are more distant from the labour market are given advice, counselling and support aimed at improving their employability. The aim is to address and resolve any immediate barriers to employment that young people may face. Although the Gateway was intended to last for up to four months, a significant minority of young people remain in this phase of the programme for longer than that owing to the severity of problems they face (Coles 2000). Young people who are unable to obtain a job during the Gateway period then move onto the Options phase of the programme.

The *Options* stage consists of four alternative types of programme:

1. In the *employment* option, the young person receives a wage and the employer gets a £60 per week subsidy for up to six months. In addition, up to £750 is available towards the cost of training for an approved qualification (such as an NVQ).
2. The *education and training* option lasts for up to 12 months for study towards an approved, work-related qualification. The young person continues to receive their JSA and any linked benefit during this period.
3. The *voluntary sector* option involves a placement of up to six months with a voluntary organisation, during which the young person receives their JSA and any linked benefits, together with a £400 grant payable

over the period, plus up to £750 towards the cost of training leading to an approved qualification.

4. The *Environmental Task Force* option lasts for up to six months, during which participants receive the same benefits and rights as in the voluntary sector. As the name suggests, the Environmental Task Force (ETF) involves projects that aim to improve the environment, such as reclaiming derelict land and tidying up green spaces in urban areas.

The particular option that young people participate in is determined by their preferences, the views of their personal adviser and the availability of placements (National Audit Office, 2002). However, young people participating in the New Deal tend to prefer the employment and the education and training options. The Environmental Task Force is generally viewed as the least attractive option (Hasluck 2000, Millar 2000).

Finally, the *Follow-through* is for people who have completed their New Deal option but have not been able to obtain unsubsidised employment during that period. It is intended to last for up to four months or more, during which participants' gains from the New Deal are supposed to be consolidated and further advice, counselling and support provided by their personal adviser. The evidence indicates that, by the time they have reached the Follow-through stage, some young people are 'clearly beginning to get disheartened about their future prospects of getting work' (Ritchie 2000: 310).

Following participation in the programme, young people who remain unable to find employment and claim JSA continuously for a further six months are required to re-enter the New Deal via the Gateway. By the end of October 2001, 18 per cent of New Deal participants had been through the programme more than once (National Audit Office 2002)[1].

The New Deal in practice

By September 2003, just over one million people had participated in NDYP, of whom 72 per cent were young men, 12 per cent were people with disabilities and 16 per cent were from minority ethnic groups. At that date, 89,000 young people were participating in the New Deal. Of these, 63 per cent were in the Gateway, 22 per cent were in one of the Options, and the remaining 15 per cent were in Follow-through. Almost half (47 per cent) of the young people in the Options stage were in education and training (Table 8.2).

There are significant gender and ethnic differences in Options participation. For example, as at September 2003, about one-third of young women in Options were working in the voluntary sector, compared with only one-sixth of young men. Around one-quarter of men were on the ETF compared with only one in every 18 women. Only one in 13 young people from minority ethnic groups were on the employment option compared with one

Table 8.2 Participation in the New Deal for Young People (as at September 2003)

	Number	% of total	% of options
Gateway	56,350	63	
Options:			
• Employment	2,770	3	14
• Education and training	9,340	10	47
• Voluntary sector	4,270	5	21
• Environment Task Force	3,700	4	18
Follow-through	13,000	15	
Total	89,420	100	100

Source: Department for Work and Pensions (2003b), Table 2.

in six whites (Department for Work and Pensions 2003b). In Scotland relatively fewer participants were in the education and training option, and more were on the employment option, compared with England and Wales (Lakey and Knight 2001).

Evaluations of NDYP highlight relatively high levels of satisfaction with the programme. For example, more than eight out of 10 participants interviewed in autumn 1998 said they were satisfied with their New Deal Option; indeed, two out of three were completely or very satisfied (Bryson *et al* 2000). It is clear therefore that the New Deal is offering something much better than the youth training schemes that preceded it (Millar 2000). Research indicates that the opportunity to undertake training and gain formal qualifications is one of the most highly valued features of NDYP, although in some cases the provision of training has been poor or badly organised. However, appreciation of on-the-job training is more mixed (Ritchie 2000). In general, the innovation of personal advisors is an aspect of the New Deal that young people particularly appreciated (Millar 2000).

Ministers have made clear that there is no fifth option. Failure to participate in New Deal and infringement of the rules of the programme can result in young people having their benefit sanctioned. There is a two-week sanction of benefit for a first infringement, four weeks for a second and 26 weeks for a third. Table 8.3 shows the number of sanctions imposed on young people in the Options phase of the programme in the first quarter of 2002 (separate figures are not available for sanctions imposed during the Gateway or Follow-through). It indicates that over 3000 young people – one in eight of the total number on Options – were sanctioned in that quarter. The proportion of young people sanctioned varied from only one in 20 of those on the employment option to one-third of those on the ETF. About half of the sanctions imposed on young people on the ETF option were for

Table 8.3 Sanctions on New Deal for Young People Options (first quarter 2002)

Number sanctioned	3,125
Proportion sanctioned	15.4%
Employer option	5.0%
Full-time educational training option	9.1%
Voluntary sector option	18.6%
Environmental Task Force	31.8%

Source: Bivand (2002), Table 1.

failure to attend. To some extent, these figures reflect the hierarchy in young people's perceptions of the four options (Bivand 2002).

Table 8.4 shows the stage at which leavers had departed the programme. About one in ten left *before* they had their first interview and just over one-half during the Gateway period. Adding these two together, means that two-thirds (66 per cent) of young people left New Deal before they got to one of the Options. One in five left during or at the end of the Follow-through stage (Department for Work and Pensions 2003b). Many of the young people who left NDYP before entering the Options stage did so because they were 'not particularly keen to be on an employment programme, even if it did come stamped with a "new" image. So they began to make much more concerted efforts to find work as soon as the programme began' (Ritchie 2000: 304).

Table 8.5 shows the immediate destinations of the NDYP leavers during the period from 1998 to September 2003. It is clear from this table that the programme has succeeded in meeting New Labour's target of getting 250,000 young people off benefit and into work. In total 371,000 young people, or two-fifths of all leavers, left New Deal to take up unsubsidised employment (Department for Work and Pensions 2003b). Although a significant minority (29 per cent) had left the programme for unknown destinations, research conducted for the Employment Service indicated that just over one-half of them had taken up paid employment (Hales and Collins 1999).

Table 8.4 Timing of departures from the New Deal for Young People (to September 2003)

Time of departure	Number	%
Left before having a first interview	102,510	11
Left during the Gateway	525,010	55
Left from Options	136,910	14
Left from Follow-through	192,110	20
All leavers	956,540	100

Source: Department for Work and Pensions (2003b), Table 4.

Table 8.5 Immediate destinations on leaving the New Deal for Young People (to September 2003)

Destination	Number	%
Unsubsidised employment	371,090	39
Other benefits	113,680	12
Other known	191,060	20
Not known	280,720	29
Total	956,540	100

Source: Department for Work and Pensions (2003b), Table 4.

Since NDYP was introduced, the incidence of long-term youth unemployment has fallen substantially. Between April 1997 and April 2002, the number of young people aged from 18 to 24 years old who were unemployed and claiming JSA for more than six months fell by more than one-half. The number out of work for one year or more fell by over 90 per cent (Finn 2003).

An important question for the New Deal is whether it has helped more people into unsubsidised work than would have been the case in the absence of the programme. Some young people who move off unemployment and into work would have done so without such help.

The National Institute for Economic and Social Research (Riley and Young 2000a) examined the difference that the NDYP has made, drawing on evidence up to March 2000. Their conclusion was that 'the NDYP programme is having a beneficial impact on the UK economy, although the magnitude of this impact cannot be quantified exactly' (Riley and Young 2000b: 1). They estimated that national income was roughly £0.5 billion higher as a result of the NDYP. About 200,000 young people had left unemployment *earlier* than they would otherwise have done during the first two years of the programme, of which 60,000 more moved directly into jobs than would have been the case. In total, youth unemployment was estimated to have been reduced by 40,000 and youth employment raised by 15,000 as a result of NDYP. The estimated cost of NDYP – after taking into account lower benefit payments and higher tax receipts – was £150 million, which was much lower than originally anticipated. This estimate takes no account of the wider social benefits that might have resulted from the programme (Riley and Young 2000a).

A further critical factor determining the success of the programme is the *sustainability* of the jobs into which leavers move. The government defines a sustainable job as being one that lasts for at least 13 weeks. Qualitative research on NDYP found that young people who entered employment at later stages of the programme appeared to have more potential stability than those obtained earlier. In addition, young people who had taken up employment largely as a response to features in the programme or its requirements were the most likely to have switched jobs. Young people who had completed their option or a substantial part of it were more likely to be stayers than those who had not (Woodfield *et al* 2000). Thus completion of Options appears to be critical to ensuring that young people move into sustained employment. The reasons for this reflect 'the acquisition of consolidated work experience and/or occupational skills; often, though not always, qualifications; and usually some aspect of self-development, like increased confidence or ease of communication' (Ritchie 2000: 307).

Whatever the stage at which people leave, the possibility exists that the New Deal may be facilitating 'churning' at the bottom end of the labour market, with young people repeatedly moving between unemployment and low-paid work and back again (Peck and Theodore 2000). This could deepen employment insecurity rather than lead to sustainable jobs that also provide some element of progression. Job retention and advancement is a relatively neglected aspect of the government's welfare to work strategy (Kellard 2002, Walker and Wiseman 2003). Instead, the main focus has been upon getting people into work (for at least 13 weeks).

A substantial number of young people who moved into paid employment after participation in the programme have subsequently become unemployed. Apart from churning, an important question is whether young people who complete NDYP are able to get other unsubsidised jobs and avoid returning to *long-term* unemployment. Government figures indicate that some young people who have left the programme do become long-term unemployed once again. Thus, by October 2001, 33,000 young people who had been on the New Deal more than once subsequently experienced spells of unemployment lasting six months or more (National Audit Office 2002). Thus, while the NDYP has reduced the extent of long-term unemployment among young people, it has by no means eliminated it. In 2001/02, a quarter of unemployed young people aged from 16 to 24 years old were long-term unemployed in that they had not worked for more than six months (Department for Work and Pensions 2003b).[2]

It is important to note that the programme has so far been operating during a period of strong employment growth and falling unemployment. It is not yet clear how successful the NDYP can be during an economic downturn (Coles 2000). There are also concerns about how successful the programme can be in localised areas of very high unemployment (Turok and Webster 1998). A survey of NDYP participants in Scotland found that 45 per cent had experienced job access problems such as lack of transport or no jobs nearby (Lakey and Knight 2001). In depressed local labour markets, the New Deal may initially raise young people's employability but without raising employment levels (Peck and Theodore 2000). The take-up of jobs as a result of the NDYP varies from one area to another and is affected by local labour market conditions. It is proving more difficult to get people into jobs and to retain them in structurally depressed areas than in more buoyant labour markets (Sunley and Martin, cited in Anon 2002).

Moreover, the changing circumstances of participants on the NDYP may also have implications for its future success. Many of the initial programme participants were job ready or almost job ready. But an increasing proportion of participants are 'hard to help' clients who face multiple or chronic barriers to employment. Indeed, according to a National Audit Office survey, only one-third of NDYP participants during 2000/01 had no barriers to employment (Table 8.6). A survey of NDYP participants in Scotland found that 16 per cent had experienced problems with drugs, alcohol, homelessness or the law (Lakey and Knight 2001). A national survey conducted in autumn 1998 found that participants from disadvantaged groups are less likely than other young people on the programme to find it useful and more likely to say that it has not improved their employability. They are also less likely to be satisfied with their personal advisor (Bryson *et al* 2000). A review by Hasluck (2000: 234) concluded that 'the scale of difficulties faced by some New Deal clients with multiple disadvantage were such that. . . [it could not] overcome their problems without other forms of support and assistance'.

Thus, the NDYP is less suitable for tackling the problems of young people who face multiple or entrenched barriers to employment, such as some homeless people and problem drug users, than it is for those who are not very distant from the labour market. A number of smaller-scale programmes have been introduced to tackle the difficulties faced by those young people and others who are hard to help. These include the New Futures Fund in Scotland, aimed at the most vulnerable, and Progress2Work, targeted at recovered and stable problem drug users. In addition, pilot schemes were introduced in April 2004 to provide intensive support to residents in neighbourhoods with very high concentrations of worklessness. But it remains unclear whether these small-scale initiatives can effectively tackle the chronic barriers to work faced by the most socially excluded young people.

Table 8.6 New Deal for Young People participants with barriers to employment in 2000/01

	% of participants
No barriers	33
One barrier	23
Two barriers	25
More than two barriers	19
Total	100

Source: National Audit Office (2002), Chart II.

Conclusions

Changes in the youth labour market and education in recent decades have helped to transform the school-to-work transition for many young people. It is possible to exaggerate the extent to which, in the so-called 'golden years' from the 1950s to the early 1970s, the school-to-work transition was smooth and unproblematic (Vickerstaff 2003). But there is little doubt that it is now more protracted, risky and fractured, especially for those from low-income backgrounds. This development has been accompanied by a trend towards increased polarisation among young people in relation to qualifications, occupations and earnings (Jones 2002). The most disadvantaged school leavers face the prospect of insecure, low-paying, dead-end jobs, interspersed with periods of unemployment or even long-term unemployment.

The New Deal and other welfare-to-work initiatives are focused not on this wider structure of opportunities and risks (Jones 2002) but on enhancing the employability of young people. In this deficit model, it is young people themselves who by implication are to blame for failing to find work, rather than wider structural forces over which they have little control (Davies 1986, Mizen 2003). Yet, as we have seen, structural factors including location are important determinants of success in the job market. Although NDYP has resulted in the creation of some new jobs, perhaps its main effect has been in 'redistributing available job chances in favour of the young long-term unemployed by bringing them closer to the front of the "queue" for work' (Mizen 2003: 464). It may also be facilitating churning between welfare and low-paid work, reinforcing young people's place within the low-wage economy (Byrne 1999), rather than promoting job retention and advancement.

Yet it is far too simple to describe the NDYP as merely a coercive regime to discipline the young unemployed and force them to take low-paid work, for the reality is much more complex than that (Finn 2003). Helping young people to improve their literacy skills, interview techniques and the effectiveness of their job search can enable them to better compete for jobs. Certainly, the evaluations of NDYP indicate that it has helped to get young people off welfare and into work and succeeded in reducing long-term unemployment among this age group. But for those who are most excluded or live in areas of relatively high unemployment and economic inactivity, existing welfare-to-work programmes may not be sufficient to overcome the barriers to work and lack of suitable job opportunities that they face. These wider problems may need to be addressed before they can realistically be expected to complete the New Deal and take up or retain paid employment. In that sense, it is not excluded young people who are 'failing' in the labour market, but rather the programmes that are designed to move them from welfare to work.

Endnotes

1 Immediate destinations on leaving the NDYP are discussed later in the chapter.
2 This excludes those that had never worked, who accounted for two-fifths of the total.

References

Anon (2002) 'New Deal for Young People', *Labour Market Trends* August, p 384.

Ashton, D., Maguire, M. and Garland, V. (1982) *Youth in the Labour Market*, Research Paper No.34, London: Department of Employment.

Bivand, P. (2002) 'Rights and duties in the New Deal', *Working Brief*, No.136, pp 15–17.

Bryson, A. (2003) 'From welfare to workfare', in J. Millar (ed.), *Understanding Social Security*, Bristol: The Policy Press.

Bryson, A., Knight, G. and White, M. (2000) *New Deal for Young People: National survey of participants: Stage 1*, Research report ESR44, Sheffield: Employment Service.

Bynner, J., Elias, P., McKnight, A., *et al.* (2002) *Young People's Changing Routes to Independence*, York: York Publishing Services.

Byrne, D. (1999) *Social Exclusion*, Buckingham: Open University Press.

Coles, B. (1995) *Youth and Social Policy*, London: UCL Press.

Coles, B. (2000) *Joined-up Youth Research, Policy and Practice*, Leicester: Youth Work Press/Barnardo's.

Davies, B. (1986) *Threatening Youth: Towards a national youth policy*, Buckingham: Open University Press.

Department for Work and Pensions (2003a) *Households Below Average Income: An analysis of the income distribution from 1994/5 – 2001/02*, Leeds: Corporate Document Services.

Department for Work and Pensions (2003b) *New Deal for Young People and Long-term Unemployed People Aged 25+. Statistics to end of September 2003*, London: Department for Work and Pensions.

Department of Social Security (1998) *New Ambitions for Our Country: A new contract for welfare*, London: The Stationery Office.

Dolton, P., Makepeace, G., Hutton, S. *et al.* (1999) *Making the Grade: Education, the labour market and young people*, York: York Publishing Services.

Fergusson, R (2002) 'Rethinking youth transitions: policy transfer and new exclusions in New Labour's New Deal', *Policy Studies*, 23: 173–190.

Fergusson, R., Pye, D., Esland, G., *et al.* (2000) 'Normalized dislocation and new subjectivities in post-16 markets for education and work', *Critical Social Policy*, 20(64): 283–305.

Finn, D. (2003) 'Employment policy', in N. Ellison and C. Pierson (eds), *Developments in British Social Policy 2*, Basingstoke: Palgrave Macmillan.

Furlong, A. and Cartmel, F. (1997) *Young People and Social Change*, Buckingham: Open University Press.

Gregg, P. (1998) 'The impact of unemployment and job loss on future earnings', in J. Hills (ed.) *Persistent Poverty and Lifetime Inequality*, London: HM Treasury and Centre for the Analysis of Social Exclusion.

Hales, J. and Collins, D. (1999) *New Deal for Young People: Leavers with unknown destinations*, Research Report No. ESR21, London: Employment Service.

Hasluck, C. (1998) *Employers, Young People and the Unemployed: A review of research*, Sheffield: Employment Service.

Hasluck, C. (2000) *The New Deal for Young People: Two years on*, Research and Development Report, Sheffield: Employment Service.

Hasluck, C. (2001) 'Lessons from the New Deal', *New Economy*, 8: 230–234.

Johnston, L., MacDonald, R., Mason, P., *et al.* (2000a) *Snakes and Ladders: Young people, transitions and social exclusion*, York: York Publishing Services.

Johnston, L., MacDonald, R., Mason, P., *et al.* (2000b) 'The impact of social exclusion on young people moving into adulthood', *Findings*, October, York: Joseph Rowntree Foundation.

Jones, G. (2002) *The Youth Divide: Diverging paths to adulthood*, York: York Publishing Services.

Kellard, K. (2002) 'Job retention and advancement in the UK: A developing agenda', *Benefits*, 10(34): 93–98.

Kemp, P.A. and Rugg, J. (2001) 'Young people, housing benefit and the risk society', *Social Policy and Administration*, 35: 688–700.

Labour Party (1997) *New Labour: Because Britain deserves better*, London: The Labour Party.

Lakey, J. and Knight, G. (2001) *New Deal for Young People in Scotland Phase 1*, Central Research Unit, Edinburgh: Scottish Executive.

Lakey, J., Barnes, H. and Parry, J. (2001a) *Getting a Chance: Employment support for young people with multiple disadvantages*, York: York Publishing Services.

Lakey, J., Barnes, H. and Parry, J. (2001b) 'Employment support for young people with multiple disadvantages', *Findings*, November, York: Joseph Rowntree Foundation.

Layard, R. (1997) *What Labour Can Do*, London: Warner.

Levitas, R. (1998) *The Inclusive Society?*, Basingstoke: Macmillan.

Maguire, M. and Maguire, S. (1997) 'Young people and the labour market', in R. MacDonald (ed.) *Youth, the 'Underclass' and Social Exclusion*, London: Routledge.

Meadows, P. (2001) *Young Men on the Margins of Work: An overview*, York: York Publishing Services.

Millar, J. (2000) *Keeping Track of Welfare Reform: The New Deal programmes*, York: York Publishing Services.

Mizen, P. (2003) 'The best days of your life? Youth, policy and Blair's New Labour', *Critical Social Policy*, 23: 453–476.

National Audit Office (2002) *The New Deal for Young People*. Report by the Comptroller and Auditor General, London: The Stationery Office.

Peck, J. and Theodore, N. (2000) 'Beyond "employability"', *Cambridge Journal of Economics*, 24: 729–749.

Perkins-Cohen, J. (2002) 'Extending New Deal to all young people', *Working Brief*, No.136: 18–20.

Riley, R. and Young, G. (2000a) *The New Deal for Young People: Implications for employment and the public finances*, Research & Development Report No. ESR62, Sheffield: Employment Service.

Riley, R. and Young, G. (2000b) *The New Deal for Young People: Implications for employment and the public finances*, Research & Development Summary, Sheffield: Employment Service.

Ritchie, J. (2000) 'New Deal for Young People: Participants' perspectives', *Policy Studies*, 24: 301–312.

Stafford, B., Heaver, C., Ashworth, K., *et al.* (1999) *Work and Young Men*, York: York Publishing Services.

Turok, I. and Webster, D. (1998) 'The New Deal: Jeopardised by the geography of unemployment?', *Local Economy*, February.

Vickerstaff, S. A. (2003) 'Apprenticeship in the "golden age": Were youth transitions really smooth and unproblematic back then?', *Work, Employment and Society*, 17: 269–287.

Walker, R. and Wiseman, M. (2003) 'Making welfare work: UK activation policies under *New* Labour', *International Social Security Review*, 56: 3–29.

Woodfield, K., Bruce, S. and Ritchie, J. (2000) *New Deal for Young People: National Options. Findings from a Qualitative Study among Individuals*, Research Report No. ESR37, London: DfEE.

Postscript on unemployment

Charlotte Ali

I am 22 years old and am currently living in Cardiff, where I work as a part-time youth worker in my local education centre. I have been receiving benefits since October 2003, and before this I was studying animal science for a six-year period since leaving school. Since finishing this and working part time, I have done various things to occupy my time, working with Cardiff young people's forum and 'Funky Dragon', the children and young people's Assembly for Wales, both working towards young people having their voice heard on issues that affect them. In April 2003, I represented young people from across Wales at a meeting at the House of Commons and appeared on the parliament channel. I class myself as a very active citizen on a local, national and international level. I recently returned from a Raleigh International Expedition to Ghana West Africa where I spent three months improving the community, doing environmental work and trekking and canoeing in the Lake Volta region.

I speak not just on my own behalf but on behalf of a lot of friends and family too. Young people I have met and attended the course with have a lot to say about the New Deal options and should be consulted about it as it affects them as well.

Working part time means I don't earn enough to live on and must claim Jobseeker's Allowance. After claiming benefits for a six-month period, I must attend the voluntary option with New Deal. The barrier that is holding me back is not being able to drive, and getting into a job that I enjoy and have been working towards. I have asked my New Deal advisor if I can have the driving lessons paid by New Deal, but was told that I need to have a letter saying that I will be employed full time if I have a driving licence, but I can't guarantee this. However, the cost to the government of me attending the voluntary option would cover my driving lessons and getting a job as a result would mean that I would not be claiming benefits for such a long period.

Personal advisers could be made more aware of the problems faced by disadvantaged young people and start advising them into the right training and jobs. They need to be able to liaise with a key worker for the young person to help with any additional problems with housing, etc.

I am now going into the third week of the voluntary option. My experience while attending the voluntary option has been very poor and I can't really understand what young people gain from it. The programme is not organised to a high standard. There is only one level of education and qualifications to work towards, the programme works with all levels of ability and it seems like they see all young people as the same. There is also no motivation or consistency amongst the staff who deliver these courses. The environment is very poor; the building is situated far from anywhere and is old and poorly equipped. Young people are being placed into charity shops as placements, but I don't see the point of this as young people should be attending placements where they will benefit from eventually being employed in relevant jobs that interest them. For example, there should be more trades such as carpentry and plumbing on the programme.

Before going onto the voluntary option, I attended the gateway to work course, which was worse. I didn't see the purpose of being there, talking about fantasy jobs and doing written exercises and having a day trip to the library. It was not entertaining at all. Young people are really not getting what they deserve and this should be investigated.

Young women are starting to have the same opportunities as young men but there are still some jobs young women cannot participate in, such as railway work. However, it is good that young women and men are doing the same type of training, such as carpentry, painting and decorating, and are working towards a career by attending courses and doing apprenticeships.

Some young people go through the New Deal several times, as Peter Kemp explained in his chapter, which shows it doesn't work for them and they are just repeating the work and not gaining anything at all. More work should be done after the period of the New Deal has finished, to get young people into employment or college courses. The government could create more jobs by making it compulsory for employers to take young people on, there should be no agencies that offer only factory production line work that is short term and recruitment agencies should not be paid by taking money directly out of young people's wages. Young people should be able to get into a job with less qualifications and more work-related experience.

Having a full-time job can help young people in the transition to adulthood as it gives them more responsibility and confidence. Working with all different ages and backgrounds will give young people more social skills and enable them to feel more of a citizen.

Young people are often blamed for their own unemployment, and this is not fair because in society today everything is qualifications: everything has changed from years ago. There should be more trades in school as young people are not being recognised by potential employers when they leave school and better training schemes apart from the New Deal should be in place for them. I feel strongly that the New Deal option is not being run properly. Are young people being consulted about these schemes and the skills needed to get the jobs they are interested in? I doubt it.

This chapter focuses on disadvantaged young people between the ages of 15 and 25 years old who face other problems, not just unemployment. Disadvantaged young people are worst off in the New Deal option as they are faced with other problems apart from unemployment, such as housing shortages, a lack of qualifications and poverty. Before going onto New Deal, it is important to make sure young people have good self-esteem, confidence and, in many cases, knowledge of their abilities. Many young people have very negative attitudes and perceptions of themselves, possibly perceiving formal training and employment as being way above their capabilities.

A lot of young people attending this programme have never attended any activity outside of school and, in some cases, literacy issues are the barrier. There is also a problem with the lack of availability in the school curriculum for relevant trades and skills. Young people could work towards a qualification to do with their chosen trade and attend a two-week work placement, leaving school qualified in a trade which would enable them to enter a job. This could work towards bringing the youth labour market back and cut the unemployment rate. Changing attitudes of others is important as young people think if they don't do well in school then they are not employable. Careers should work closely with employers to persuade them that school leavers are skilled and have the knowledge needed to do specific jobs.

In conclusion, young people should have their say on the whole of the New Deal as it affects them. There should, maybe, be an assessment to see if young people are ready to attend these courses, so that they do not see it as being like school or just going for their giro, but see what they will actually gain from it. So far, it is not benefiting me in any way. Young people in school and out of school should be asked what they think would work and what they would like to see available.

Chapter 9

Risk, social change and strategies of inclusion for young homeless people

Joan Smith

Homelessness can be a terrible experience for young people. In areas where there are few hostel, YMCA or foyer bed spaces, young people often 'sofa surf'; they sleep on a friend's sofa or floor, move to another friend, to another and also sleep rough for brief periods. Even in areas where there is provision for young homeless people, many will have difficulty finding that provision. On top of the insecurity, uncertainty and worry of homelessness there are also problems associated with why they became homeless. A minority may be homeless because they had spent some of their lives in institutions (care homes, or even custody), but others are homeless because they have been evicted from their family home, or chose to leave.

This chapter discusses youth homelessness in relation to a particular understanding of social exclusion, the family background of young homeless people and the different factors that put young people at risk of homelessness. The final part of this chapter looks at provision designed to offset the experience of exclusion through the work of one particular agency, the Foyer Federation, and changes in recent government policies designed to support the work of agencies in the field of youth homelessness.

Social exclusion and young homeless people

Ten years ago a group of British sociologists began to use the concept of social exclusion as a way of describing processes through which some UK households were becoming isolated from society, and living increasingly deprived lives at a time of extraordinary development of income inequality in the UK between 1979 and 1993. Room (1995) argued that previous theories of poverty had been concerned primarily with understanding the distribution of income and wealth in UK society and that the value of the theory of social exclusion was that it focused on issues of inadequate social participation, lack of social integration and lack of power. Therefore the concept of social exclusion provided an understanding of social justice that went beyond welfare theories of justice and welfare outcomes to relations between different social groups. As Wolfe argued: 'Exclusion is an active concept like exploitation. Someone or something bars out or drives out someone or something else, which reacts as best it can' (Wolfe 1995).

The concept of social exclusion provided an alternative perspective to that of the New Liberals or New Right, whose analysis was based on American theories of welfare dependency and the rise of an underclass of welfare dependents (Smith 1997, Anderson and Sims 2000). The origin of the term can be found in French debates over 'les exclus' in the early 1970s and the use of the concept of social exclusion during the French Presidency of the European Commission at the end of the 1980s[1]. Political scientists in the International Labour Office (ILO) initiated a research programme to explore the meaning of social exclusion in relation to the developing world.

For the purpose of this chapter it is Marshall Wolfe's contribution to the ILO programme that is important. He broke down the concept of social exclusion into six aspects:

- exclusion from gaining a livelihood;
- exclusion from social services, welfare and security networks;
- exclusion from consumer culture;
- exclusion from political choice;
- exclusion from bases of popular organisation and solidarity; and
- exclusion from understanding what is happening to society and to themselves.

Wolfe's understanding of social exclusion is more comprehensive than recent ones constructed in the UK: although from a current model, the additional dimension of exclusion from social interaction should be added to Wolfe's list (Burchardt *et al* 2001). The separate sections below consider each of Wolfe's six aspects of social exclusion in order to place in context the exclusion problems of young homeless people in the UK.

Exclusion from livelihood

From the late 1970s the Conservative government embarked on a financial and political experiment that, in the midst of a global recession, transformed both the lives of young people and the youth labour market. In 1977 the UK had levels of income inequality close to those of Scandinavia, and one in ten children lived in poverty; by 1997 UK levels of income inequality were close to those of Canada and the US and one in three children lived in poverty (Kumar 1993, Townsend and Gordon 2002).

The twin dogmas of non-interventionist support for manufacturing and the benefits of privatising all public utilities had enormous labour market consequences for young people who left school at 16 years in the early 1980s. In the 1970s a high proportion of young people had entered the labour market on wages that were a reasonable fraction of the adult wage, or entered apprenticeships that would lead to skilled employment. In the early 1980s, however, there was a huge leap in youth unemployment, and half of all apprenticeships disappeared. The government responded to youth unemployment by the establishment of a youth training labour market that paid benefit-level wages. By 1991 youth wages were 39 per cent of the adult wage (Kumar 1993).

During these years there was both a restructuring of the youth labour market into a youth training market and a deskilling of young people. The skills that young men could sell to private companies as electricians, carpenters or plumbers had often been learned as apprentices in the large nationalised industries that became private companies, in the direct labour departments of local authorities or in the large manufacturing companies that collapsed during the world recession of the 1980s that hit the UK doubly hard. As manufacturing declined, so too did the skilled and semi-skilled employment of young men's fathers and uncles, whilst guaranteed employment in publicly owned utilities and services changed into contract employment with newly privatised companies.

Youth unemployment and youth deskilling in the early 1980s had a long-term effect on whole neighbourhoods as well as individual young people, particularly young men. In all the surveys of young homeless people undertaken as part of the 'risk studies'[2] that are reported below, there is a huge gap between young people's aspirations for employment when they leave school and the employment that they are able to obtain – between aspiration and reality (Bruegel and Smith 1999, Smith *et al* 2000a, 2001, Smith 2003).

Exclusion from social services, welfare and security networks

Whilst the right to education and health remained universal rights in the UK, the right to welfare did not. By 1988 young people aged 16 and 17 years old were denied the right to claim income support. This was accompanied by an upsurge in youth homelessness, with destitute young people arriving at homeless shelters in London (Evans 1996). Henceforth, young people would have to prove estrangement from parents in order to claim benefits. In 1996 new rules on housing benefit also restricted young people's rights to shelter through restricting access to the private rental market. From January 1997 housing benefit for single people under 25 years was paid at the level of single room rent (i.e. not a flat) that was set for the local area. Rent levels had to be agreed with the landlord in advance and, not surprisingly, in areas of high demand for private rentals young people claiming housing benefit failed to find properties.

Exclusion from consumer culture

Compared with young people living at home, young people who become homeless and enter shared accommodation have few possessions. In a world of TVs, DVDs, CD players, computers and other household durables, they have very little and the little that they have can go missing or be stolen. One young woman who left care said:

> When you leave care you leave with your clothes . . . your black bags and that's it! . . . All of your life in black dustbin bags . . . !
>
> (care leaver, single parent, age 19, Smith *et al* 2000a)

Young people who were interviewed in foyers in 2002–3 were receiving Jobseeker's Allowance (JSA), paid fortnightly, or training allowances. Many were living on £42.70 per week, out of which they paid their personal rent costs, i.e. personal electricity and gas (£5–10 a week), bus fares to training, education or employment (£5–10 a week without a bus pass) and bought their food. They existed through living very cheaply, often at the cost of having too little food or living on frozen food. If they used a small amount of money to go to local clubs or pubs, they went without, but mostly they stayed in.

Exclusion from political choice

Democracy, of course, often depends on having an address as well as being over the age of 18 years old. Most young people do not stay in supported accommodation long enough to vote although there has been, in the past, campaigns by organisations such as CHAR (incorporated into the National Homeless Alliance and then Homeless Link) to encourage voting among homeless populations.

Exclusion from the bases for popular organisation and solidarity

Bases for popular organisation can be very different, including trade unions, credit unions, associations of those claiming welfare, or local community or neighbourhood associations[3]. Organisations working with young people go to great lengths to involve them in making decisions and encourage participation. However, although many young homeless people have common interests while they are homeless, such as income benefit levels, housing benefit rules and limited access to services, their time in supported accommodation is limited. Therefore, whilst young people are engaged in residents' groups or in some campaigns that are organised by service providers for brief periods, once they have moved on then other issues dominate their lives.

Exclusion from understanding what is happening

Young homeless people are most likely to explain their homelessness through their own history: they didn't get on with their mother, stepfather, brother or sister; they were living in care; or their parent had died. It is hard for them to understand that 30 or 40 years ago a young person to whom this happened would have been able to find affordable accommodation and a job that paid enough to live in that accommodation. For some, there is an element of self-blame and a loss of confidence or self-esteem:

JS: What are the differences you observe as young people stay with you?
R: Confidence . . . Self esteem . . . Trust . . . You get them into training or
    college or work and there is a stability in their lives, you replace the
    instability they have known.

(Foyer Assistant, Paines Mill Foyer: Smith 2004)

At the more practical level some are cut off from knowing anywhere beyond their immediate environment. On poverty-level benefits it is hard to move beyond even your immediate local area, although one of the benefits of some foyer placements was the opportunity to go abroad.

Social exclusions particular to homelessness

From research studies undertaken by the author it became apparent that two other areas of exclusion should be added to Wolfe's six-fold model. First, Wolfe places exclusion from shelter within exclusion from social welfare. However, although housing provision for the poorest can be part of welfare provision in some Western states, the attainment and maintenance of shelter is predominantly an individual struggle within a housing market, alongside of, and dependent on, the attainment of livelihood.

In the UK, housing has become an independent indicator of income, wealth and poverty. Using data from the National Child Development Study (NCDS), Hobcraft has argued that:

> Living in social housing at age 33 is associated with a wide range of other adverse outcomes in adulthood and might in some sense be regarded as the best single summary measure of social exclusion considered here.

(Hobcraft 2001: 64–67)

Living in social housing is a summary measure of pathways that include early parenting, extramarital births, multiple partnerships and poor qualifications. Hobcraft reports that one of the strongest links in the NCDS dataset is between adult homelessness and multiple cohabitations between

23 and 33 years old. In childhood, there is a strong relationship between remarriage of parents and homelessness (Hobcraft 2001: 78). Therefore, a seventh aspect of exclusion is *shelter exclusion,* in the sense of a shelter chosen by and suitable for the person. Living in some areas can be as excluding as being homeless for some young people. One young woman, recently re-housed in social housing, found herself harassed by her next-door neighbours and unable to buy food because they would walk in and eat it; she bought baby food and lived on takeaways herself. This young woman was isolated in this local area (Smith 2004).

The eighth aspect of social exclusion, apparent from interviews with young people and older homeless people, is *exclusion from personal social networks.* Three-quarters of all young homeless people are in touch with one or more members of their family. Many plan to go home at festivities such as Christmas. However, as managers of foyers report, the number who do go home range from three-quarters to almost none. Some go to return the same day. It is extremely difficult to overcome personal setbacks when the networks that should be holding one up are so frail. A research report into homelessness among single people has also reported on the loss of social networks and the fragility of these networks (Lemos 2000).

This discussion of different aspects of social exclusion in relation to youth homelessness raises the question of who is at risk of becoming so excluded in our society. The next part of this chapter summarises the work of the author and others on the 'risk factors' of youth homelessness, using insights from Beck's model of risk society.

Youth homelessness in the UK and the 'circle of risk' for young homeless people

In the mid 1990s it was estimated that large cities in the UK had five per cent of young people living in homeless circumstances – some in hostels, some with friends, some with overcrowded families (Evans 1996, Smith *et al* 1996). Up to one-third of young people had some background in local authority care – however, at 16 years old, only one in six were actually immediately from care. Obviously, being 'from care' could only explain between one-sixth and one-third of youth homelessness, whilst two-thirds of young people's homeless circumstances remained unexplained. Therefore, along with colleagues, I undertook a study of the family background of young homeless people in which 56 young people who became homeless from their family home were interviewed. In addition, in half of the cases, one or more of their parents were also interviewed.

The *Family Background of Young Homeless People* study identified a series of factors which contributed to the young person's homeless situation, including the young person's own behaviour (including the use of drugs, alcohol and criminal activity), the parent's behaviour (including violence towards the young person), and whether or not the family was reconstituted with a step-parent joining the family (Smith et al, 1998). Together, the factors could be described as a *Circle of Risk* for the young person (see Fig. 9.1), following Beck's theory of a 'risk society'.

Beck's Theory of Risk Society

Risk is such a common concept that it is possible to pour into it different layers of meaning. For the last 15 years the concept of 'risk' has carried a specific meaning in the social sciences, associated with Ulrich Beck (Beck 1992 translation). The impact of Beck's book can be compared with the impact of Esping–Anderson's theories of welfare regimes, or Bourdieu's theory of social capital or the development of the concept of social exclusion. All these theoretical developments were part of a strong resurgence in European social theory at the heart of which was the development of new concepts providing distinctive European ways of understanding society and social policy.

The core theory that Beck outlined in 1986 began with the premise that in advanced modernity the social production of wealth is accompanied by the social production of risks. Beck summarised his theory in a collection of writings by himself, Giddens and Lash (Beck *et al* 1994). His theory of reflexive modernisation proceeds from the analysis of a new process of change in industrial society that '. . . breaks up the premises and contours of industrial society and opens paths to another modernity' (Beck *et al* 1994: 3). There is no agency to this transformation except change itself and this makes it analytically distinct from earlier processes of social change and revolution. The specific result of this new modernity is the emergence of *Risk Society* and, as the old institutions of industrial society – family, community, social class – are undermined by the process of global modernisation, each individual must learn to navigate risk society for themselves:

> Opportunities, threats, ambivalences of the biography, which it was previously possible to overcome in a family, in the village community or by recourse to a social class or group, must increasingly be perceived, interpreted and handled by individuals themselves. To be sure, families are still to be found, but the nuclear family has become an even more rare institution.
>
> (Beck *et al* 1994: 8)

It could be argued that the individuals most threatened by these transformations in Western societies are both the old, who had supported the welfare of others (both through the state and privately) and had expected to be supported in turn, and the young. For the young the threat is intensified, having to navigate risk society while navigating their own 'ambivalent biographies' (Beck *et al* 1994) with the support of increasingly fragile social structures, including their own family, and in nation states that have restricted welfare provision for young people based either on their age or on their lack of employment history. Western states all have higher rates of youth unemployment than 20 years ago and have rising, some dramatically so, rates of family reconstruction. Figure 9.1 describes the 'Circle of Risk' found by our *Family Background* study.

One of the most important risks facing young people is a crisis arising in the *Fabric of the Family* in which they live (Fig. 1, Smith *et al* 1998). Whereas the majority of older young people (aged up to 29 years old) began to stay at home longer in the 1990s (the first reversal of the early leaving trend since the 1950s), some young people were forced out or left at an ever earlier age (Green *et al* 1996; Jones 1995). A study of young people in Scotland found that young people living with step-parents left home an average of two years younger (Jones 1995).

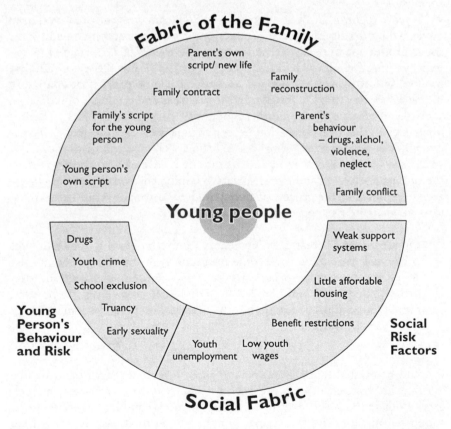

Figure 9.1 Circle of Risk for young homeless people (adapted from Smith *et al* 1998).

In our *Family Background* study (Smith *et al* 1998) the reconstitution of the family had an impact on the young person in several ways. Sometimes the new partner was abusive, or the birth parent became abusive, over conflict in the home. Sometimes there were arguments over the 'family contract', which included undertaking household chores or going to school/college or contributing to the household financially. Sometimes there was conflict between the script that the family had written for the young person – she is to go to college and achieve – and the script the young person wrote for herself. There could also be intense conflict with siblings, half-siblings or step-siblings and a belief by the young person that they were the unwanted child. Therefore, often, parental behaviour created the risk of homelessness for the young person:

> She kicked me sister out at 16, me brother first at 16 and me sister and then me . . . Me Dad [birth father, not stepfather] said 'You're next, don't worry about it'. I didn't believe him . . . just got kicked out. . . I was doing well at school . . . then when it started slipping and I stopped doing as well, that's when she started saying 'Look you've got to buck your ideas up, else you'll be out'. She always threatened to kick me out, and then when I left school . . . that's when they kicked me out.
>
> (young man, youngest of three, living in a hostel for homeless youth, father living in another city, Smith *et al* 1998)

The mother of this young man largely agreed with his account but said that he began taking drugs when she went away on her honeymoon with his new stepfather. She said:

> I mean if I hadn't married, I'd probably have my son back now. Probably ask him. And he'd probably come. Then my life would be on hold for how long? So I don't know if changing things works. I'd rather not think about it really.
>
> (mother of the young man above, Smith *et al* 1998)

Other young people described a history of violence that sometimes escalated before they finally moved out. In other families violence occurred against more than one family member. In one case a mother and daughter ran away when the husband and father, in this case the birth father, took a knife to his wife's throat. Because the daughter was over 16 years old, she and her mother were treated as separate cases of homelessness and were not housed together.

Sometimes, however, it was the behaviour of the young person that meant his or her parents could no longer cope. One couple lost all trust in their son after he sold their possessions when he needed money for drugs:

> We were just clearing out one day, we saw this empty case . . . some of
> my Wedgwood . . . jewellery . . . his father's medals . . . most of them
> we found in a second-hand shop. You can imagine . . . your child steal-
> ing from you . . . all, you know, your possessions that you've saved . . .
> that was the last thing really, the last straw . . . . I said, I've always been
> there for him but he's never, never appreciated it somehow . . . I'm ill
> now through, through all the stress over the years.
>
> (mother of young man living in a homeless hostel, Smith *et al* 1998)

Another mother was hospitalised for stress when her young daughter kept
staying out at night with her boyfriend who was 'twocing' (stealing cars to
joyride around town); she kept visualising her dead.

Included in the *Circle of Risk* for young people, therefore, are factors in
relation to the young person's behaviour that increased their risk of homelessness. Problems of substance misuse also caused tension in families. All
voluntary organisations have reported a rise in support needs among their
clients in relation to drug or alcohol use or mental or physical health needs,
and surveys of the needs of homeless people have found widespread problems of alcohol, drugs and mental health among homeless people (Craig
et al 1996, North *et al* 1996).

Being school excluded or being a truant also increased the risk of youth
homelessness, as did engaging in youth crime (young men) or early sexual
behaviour (young women). It surprised us how much parents still had different rules for their daughters than for their sons in relation to their behaviour. Young men were in trouble with their parents for violence (particularly
violence against the parent), drug-taking, stealing and truanting or being
excluded from school. Young women were in trouble with their parents for
the type of young man they went out with, because they were sexually
active at an early age or for truanting from school.

The other side of the *Circle of Risk* was the increasing likelihood that
young people could neither find employment, nor support themselves on
benefits, nor find housing outside of the family home. These are the risks
reported in the 'Social Fabric' part of Figure 9.1. Lower youth wages, youth
unemployment and numerous changes to their social security entitlements
have all affected young people's ability to support themselves outside of the
family home.

Above all, there is now a lack of affordable housing for any young person living outside their family home. This is not simply due to a decline in
the availability of social housing, and the very limited numbers of single
homeless people who qualify for social housing; it is also due to the decline
in supply of all forms of affordable accommodation. Young homeless people today could have found low-cost private rented accommodation in an
earlier period. The majority of people in the UK were housed in private
rented accommodation until the 1950s, and throughout the 1960s bedsitter

accommodation was particularly important in London as a source of cheap accommodation for single people. As in New York, one of the problems of London has been the decline of the old SROs (single room occupancy) buildings, as areas have become gentrified.

Identifying young people at risk of becoming homeless

Following the study of the *Family Background of Young Homeless People*, our research unit was commissioned, along with the Local Economy Policy Unit of South Bank University, to undertake a comparison of the social background of two groups of young Londoners aged 16–19 years old, in order to identify more precisely the particular risk factors in relation to becoming homeless. The study built on the 'Circle of Risk' findings and used a structured questionnaire to interview 200 young people living in homeless hostels, and compare their life experiences with 150 young people living in deprived areas, who were still living with their families.

The information collected from the two interview groups produced a measure of difference between those currently homeless and those not, in relation to an odds ratio (Table 9.1). It was found that the odds of being homeless were at their highest if the young person: did not get on with their mother, had moved house more than twice, had a younger mother, was badly off as a child, was not living with either one or two birth parents at age 12 years old, had been hit frequently during the course of an argument, had shared a bedroom, had lived in rented accommodation, had no car in household or had been school excluded.

There was a relationship between many of these variables, of course: for example, homeless young people not living with two or one birth parents

Table 9.1 Odds of being in the homeless sample: London 'Safe in the City' Survey 1998

Variable	Odds ratio
Didn't get on with mother/got on with mother	13:1
Moved house more than twice/less than twice	11:1
Mother aged below 25 years old at first child/mother older	6:1
Badly off as a child/not badly off as a child	5:1
Living with foster parent/care, step parent, or relative at 12 years old/ in two birth parent or one birth parent family at 12 years old	5:1
Hit frequently in course of argument/not hit, not hit frequently	4:1
Shared bedroom at 12 years old/not shared bedroom at 12 years old	3:1
In rented accommodation at 12 years old/in other tenure	3:1
No car in household/at least one car	3:1
Excluded from school/never excluded	2:1

Source: Bruegel and Smith (1999: 42).

but with a step-parent or other situation were more than twice as likely to have been school excluded. Therefore, we also ran a further analysis on all the young people to see which variables were independent. Living with a step-parent, foster-parent or other relative has an effect on the probability that a young person will be homeless that is independent of poverty, school exclusion, relationships with mother or violent arguments. Similarly, moving house more than twice has an independent effect.

It was also possible to map the areas of London where young people lived at age 12 years old and 16 years old through postcode information. Again, in nearly 90 per cent of the cases it would have been possible to predict these wards from the Ward Deprivation Index produced by the UK government, an indication of how the families of many young people who became homeless were themselves impoverished during the 1980s. The destructive impact of 'New Right' policies on poor neighbourhoods has been most graphically described in the reports produced by the Social Exclusion Unit (SEU 1998). A study of the areas of origins of the 200 young homeless people interviewed in London hostels in 1998 found that the borough probability of generating youth homelessness correlated with male registered unemployment at 0.9149 and the average index of deprivation for the borough at 0.7743 (Bruegel and Smith 1999).

The results of this comparative study have been important in targeting services in particular boroughs of London and the services provided also reflected the young homeless people's views on what services would be helpful to young people like themselves in the future. The most popular services were projects for runaways, more skills training and family respite services (a place for the young person to 'cool off'). Young people also reported preferring counsellors of their own age, and support for themselves in family disputes, i.e. young person advocacy rather than family mediation (Bruegel and Smith 1999: 105).[4]

Although the London risk study was not designed to quantify risk in relation to ethnic origins or gender, it was notable that our homeless sample from hostels was more often black African, black British or black African-Caribbean than the youth population of London, and more often male. The homeless were nearly four times more likely to be African-Caribbean than the London youth population although, in part, this may be due to our sampling procedures.

The risk of youth homelessness in other areas

The London risk study has been followed by three further studies in Birmingham, the Cotswolds and North Staffordshire. These studies show that the 210 young people interviewed in hostels in Birmingham, the 61 in the Cotswolds and the 52 in North Staffordshire (principally young people from Stoke-on-Trent) had similar risk profiles to young homeless people in

London. Each group of young homeless people reported that they came from more disrupted and poorer families, relationships within their family were much more frequently violent and they were much less likely to get on with their mother and had higher rates of school exclusion than the local reference sample in London of young people still living at home, despite the London local reference sample being drawn from similarly deprived areas.

One important difference between the homeless samples were that young homeless people in London and Birmingham reported that they were more liable to pick on others at school (be bullies), whereas young people in the Cotswolds and Stoke-on-Trent were more likely to be picked on (be the bullied). Overall, however, the risk factors that were identified in London were ones that young homeless people in other cities and a rural area shared.[5]

The Birmingham risk study proved to be particularly important because, unlike the London study, it was possible to quantify the risk factors of age, sex and ethnic group. Over a six-month period, any young person who reported as homeless to any agency, including the local authority and major housing associations, was included in a count of youth homelessness across the city. Over 6,000 records were collected and, after excluding young people who appeared twice in records, 5,374 individuals were included in the database. It was found that the majority of applicants were either homeless or potentially homeless – 3,287 over a six-month period (61 per cent). Comparing the homeless figure with the number of 16–25 year olds in Birmingham gave a rate of homelessness of five per cent, i.e. one in 20.

Among all applications, young white British applicants were under-represented (59 per cent of applicants compared with being 72 per cent of the local population), as were young Asian people from the Indian subcontinent (ten per cent of applicants compared with being 19 per cent of the local population). Young people of ethnic origins that they described as black British, or African-Caribbean or African were 20 per cent of applicants but only eight per cent of the local population. Half of applications were from men and half from women.

One of the most important differences between young men and young women was that one-third of young women applied as a single parent (34 per cent) and only just over one-half as a single person (54 per cent), whilst other young women applied as a part of a couple, with or without children. The vast majority of young men applied as single (88 per cent), three per cent as single parents and ten per cent as part of a couple (Smith *et al* 2000b).

Among the 210 young people living in Birmingham hostels, young women were more likely than young men to report parental behaviour that put them at risk of homelessness: six out of ten young women reported verbal abuse, or physical abuse, and parental problems such as drinking, drugs or mental health problems; by comparison, four out of ten young men reported such problems. Surprisingly, both young men and young women reported similar rates of school exclusion and, if anything, young white men and women had higher rates of school exclusion than young black men – this is an unusual finding and suggests either that school exclusion has an independent impact on becoming homeless, or that school exclusion is an outcome of extreme patterns of family disruption, violence and poverty that also lead to youth homelessness.

Developing social inclusion strategies for young homeless people

Given the risk of homelessness facing many young people in the 1980s, agencies began to address the issue of how young homeless people should be housed, providing separate supported housing for young homeless people. Nationally, YMCAs began to dedicate a large proportion of their beds to homeless young people, and in 1993 the first foyers were developed in the UK, in order to provide supported accommodation for young people who were prepared to enter into employment, training or education. In some cities local gold standard organisations developed extensive provision for homeless youth – Centrepoint in London and St Basils in Birmingham to name only two. As the problem of homelessness has grown across all regions, rural areas have also developed youth homeless provision.

Voluntary organisations offering supported accommodation to young people have also developed life skill training, basic skills training, counselling, support and other programmes. This has been particularly true of foyers accredited through the Foyer Federation. At the time of writing (March 2004), there are 129 foyers providing accommodation for approximately 7,000 young people. Their stated goal is simple, although hard to deliver:

> 'All young people need a home, support and a springboard into independent living, learning and work. Some don't get it. Foyers fill the gap.
> (www.foyer.net)

How can supported housing solutions offset the life risks that homeless young people face? How can they work to combat different aspects of social exclusion? Again, it is important to break down the different aspects of social exclusion, but this time in order to report on strategies of *social inclusion*. The next section and Table 9.2 summarise young homeless people's likely experiences of social exclusion, in its different aspects, and the possibilities of inclusion that can be offered by best practice in different foyers and other supported accommodation provided for young homeless people.

Providing supported accommodation

From a recent comparative study of 12 Foyers, and four floating support schemes, visited in 2002–3, it is possible to describe the social inclusion strategies pursued by Foyers. Group interviews with young people demonstrated that the support they received within their accommodation could help them turn their lives around. Inclusion of young people came about through the very positive relationships many had with housing staff, and, for some, the positive relationships they had with other residents. This support and these relationships addressed four aspects of social exclusion experienced by young people: exclusion from shelter; exclusion from social welfare; exclusion from social networks; and exclusion from understanding what is happening:

JS: What is the most important service you have got from the Foyer?
R: Support.
R: Yes support.
R: Someone to talk to.
R: Support.
R: I like (staff member). I can laugh and joke with her.
JS: What do you think they aim for you to get out of being here?
R: To get your life back on track!
R: Mm yes.
R: It's like being a stepping stone, until you are comfortable to do it on your own.
R: But when you move out of here they will still give you emotional support.
R: Anything else they could help you with really.

> (residents group interview, Salford Foyer, Smith 2004)

JS: What do you think is the most important service that you have been given?
R: It's a new start really, a new beginning.
R: Its like the Foyer gives you a step up.
R: They help you look after yourself, be independent.

> (residents group interview, Blackpool Foyer, Smith 2004)

Residents from other foyers also reported the importance of receiving staff support (Smith 2004).

For young people in South London, some of whom had experience of Social Service placements, or had been placed in a cold weather shelter, the fact that staff listened to them was a very important difference in their experience and one that allowed them to feel empowered:

R: Yeah, and they're (the staff) still pushing and they are going to try and do more and more.

R: And they're always asking your opinion in here. That's the thing that I like about it. They want to hear your views! What you got to say.

R: Like we, we mean something (All saying Yeah).

R: Like what we say might actually make a difference.

(residents group interview, ShortLife Foyer, South London, Smith 2004)

Foyers also provided other support that enabled young people to overcome other aspects of their exclusion. Some foyers had access to Family Mediation services, but even those that did not found that some young people's relationships with their family improved when they were living away from home. Other young people found that the friends they made within the foyer were very important to them. In both situations young people were helped to overcome social isolation. Scarborough Foyer residents (run by the charity Home and Dry, Scarborough) said that their three best experiences in the foyer were being housed, the support they received from Home and Dry staff and the friends that they had made. Residents of Blackpool Foyer also got a lot out of being together:

R: The best bit has been the new friends I have made.

R: Yes and we have had some good laughs.

R: The roof over my head (several agree).

R: They help you.

R: Yes they'll help you do what you need to do. Support you in what you want.

(residents group, Scarborough Foyer, Smith 2004)

JS: What has been the best experience for you?

R: Living together.

R: The practical jokes.

R: There is a lot of support from the others who are living here.

R: If you haven't got food, someone you know will help out.

(All agreeing)

R: If you need it you can get a bit of money from someone.

(residents interviews, Blackpool Foyer, Smith 2004)

Residents were also being offered opportunities that they might never have had. Several residents of Salford Foyer reported volunteering placements in Norway, Greece and Germany and language classes were offered in that foyer. In other foyers the favourite experience was often found through a Prince's Trust initiative or attending a regional meeting of foyer residents, a weekend course with staff and other residents.

The greatest limitation on addressing the social exclusion experienced by young people was presented by their entitlement to welfare benefits; although staff helped young people to claim welfare benefits, the entitlement to welfare for most young people was limited. Attempting to live on £42.70p (increased to £43.20p during the research project) paid at fortnightly interviews created great difficulties for all young people.

Table 9.2 Social exclusion and social inclusion strategies for young homeless people

Social exclusion	Young person experiences	Inclusion strategies
Exclusion from livelihood	Low wage, casual or part-time employment. Not the employment they wanted when they left school	Basic skills Independent living skills Modern apprenticeships and further education courses
Exclusion from social welfare Exclusion from consumer culture	Problems with claiming JSA or housing benefit Lack of own possessions	Training in benefits and anger management Collection of furniture and other goods before moving on
Exclusion from the bases of popular organisation and solidarity	Isolation from collective organisations	Possibility of joining organisations for young people
Exclusion from political understanding	Lack of knowledge or interest	Addressed through participation and volunteer skills
Exclusion from understanding what is happening	Individualised understanding of why they are homeless. Loss of self-esteem. At worse, self-blame and self-harm	Counselling and mental health support. Mixing with young people with similar experiences
Exclusion from shelter	From rough sleeping through to staying with relatives or friends	Safe supported accommodation and support in move-on accommodation and their own tenancies.
Exclusion from social networks	Majority of young people thrown out, asked to leave. Feel abandoned	Re-establish family networks, or contacts with an individual family member, or new friendships. Staff support

Employment and training strategies

In general, the policies of the Labour government between 1997 and 2001 sought to 'make work pay' through the development of a series of work-related benefits and also new procedures for attending job centres. The Jobseeker's Allowance and New Deal for Welfare were targeted at getting those on welfare benefits back into work. However, one of the issues facing young people was the conflict between what they wanted to do and what they were offered through New Deal:

JS: And so tell me about New Deal, what's that like in this area?
R: (Laughing) Sorry, didn't hear you . . . did you say Raw Deal! (All agreeing and finding it amusing). Well all right, they're going to sign me off after a year, and then telling me I couldn't do driving lessons any more! Oh yeah, and there was that business of saying to them that I actually had a 2-year course at College, and then they only paid for 1 year when they said in the beginning 'Oh yeah all the finance that's all fine', and then 'Oh no we can't pay for your second year'. I was like 'I can't leave then, I haven't done my two exams!'. So I sort of like complained to them, and sort of said well that's not fair and you know 'Help!', and they signed me back on again for another year. But they won't give me a third year. If I want to go to the Norwich School of Art I've got to find £1,000 for that year! From somewhere.
R: You're like a number to them basically.
     (Group Interview, HEART Dispersed Foyer, Norfolk, Smith 2004)

The current government has attempted to deal with different exclusionary issues as evidence has been presented. They have responded to concerns about the cut-off age for modern apprenticeships and raised that age to 25 years, to concerns about low wages by extending the minimum wage to all young people over the age of 16 years old, and now to concerns about young people being stopped from completing their course through the denial of benefits by creating a grant entitlement. A new Adult Learning Grant of £30 a week is being piloted which will help resolve this issue, but the payment is set at a level below benefit payments.

Outside of setting too low a benefit level for young homeless people, the government has instituted two programmes that are of enormous benefit to homeless youth. First, the development of Supporting People encouraged partnership between voluntary agencies, statutory authorities (Social Services and Probation) and local housing authorities, and gave the possibility of expanding provision prior to April 2003. Some local multi-agency partnerships used this opportunity very effectively, undertaking a rigorous local needs analysis that led to the creation of improved or new supported housing provision for different need groups, including the young homeless.

Secondly, the work of the Learning Skills Council in supporting post-school learning through its online courses, and the development of computer centres through UK Online, have allowed foyers and other supported housing providers to encourage many young people to retrace their steps and re-engage with learning. Given the basic skills deficit of many young homeless people, provision within their supported accommodation, or run by the providers of their supported accommodation, provides a safe learning environment. Such provision offers forms of training that are different from those previously experienced by residents: training in independent living, basic skills, gaining qualifications through college courses and training for employment. For some residents the certificates they received in the foyer were the first they ever had, and many received support from other foyer residents who did the course with them, as well as from the foyer training staff and the parent housing association (through small monetary rewards).

It is difficult for foyers to encourage young people into employment while they are living in the foyer; the wages that young people could earn would not allow them to pay their rent and the support costs. Under the new government policy of Supporting People, which separates payment of rent from payment of support charges, it was hoped that rent levels would be sufficiently low that young people could take up employment. However, only in some foyers are rents as low as privately rented rooms, and there are additional problems in the temporary nature of most employment now open to young people. A young person who takes a job and then loses it or gives it up can build up large housing benefit arrears that will eventually lead to them being evicted, or alternatively, having to stay in their accommodation for an additional period in order to pay off such arrears.

Conclusion

In the past 20 years there has been a dramatic rise in youth homelessness in the UK. This has been associated with the loss of a youth labour market, the loss of an affordable housing market (low-cost bedsitters) and a rise in rates of family dissolution and remarriage. This chapter has described the eight different aspects of social exclusion experienced by young homeless people, the risk factors that mean some young people are more likely to become homeless than others and the development of inclusionary strategies by providers of supported housing based on new government initiatives.

For young homeless people the way out of the poverty trap is two-fold: affordable accommodation and well-paying jobs. Labour government policies have concentrated on the latter part of the equation but for homeless young people the first priority, if they have no dependency issues to deal with in relation to drugs or alcohol, or no mental or physical health needs, is to find either independent housing or supported housing. Employment is secondary to finding secure accommodation; it is only in secure accommodation that young people can begin to reorientate themselves towards education, training and careers.

Although government policies are seeking to redress some of the worst aspects of the unequal society in relation to childhood poverty and have sought to support and reorganise supported housing through the specific provisions of Supporting People, there are other issues that have yet to be addressed. First, the low value of benefits paid in our society hampers young people in their attempts to live a less excluded life. Young people living on the basic amount of JSA are living below the poverty line and eating a poor diet. Benefit traps often mean they cannot live in supported accommodation and find work – the cost of supported housing or local housing is too high compared with local youth wages. Secondly, some benefit rights are restricted; young people under the age of 18 years old must prove estrangement from parents (which can be difficult) and housing benefits for single people aged under 25 years old are restricted to the average cost of a single room. Thirdly, young people attempting to continue in training and education face large hurdles if they are doing this without parental support.

The factors that exacerbate social exclusion among homeless young people are both individual and collective but their experience is that their exclusion is individual. Living in supported accommodation – receiving support from staff and other residents, participating in training and education and finding new opportunities – offers pathways out of social exclusion and addresses feelings of individual inadequacy. But supported housing providers cannot address the exclusions of low benefits or exclusion from livelihood without a change in the level of benefits paid to young people or changes to the rules under which housing benefit can be claimed.

Endnotes

1 The first time that the concept of social exclusion was used by the EC was in 1989: see CEC, 'Towards a Europe of solidarity: Intensifying the fight against society exclusion, fostering integration', Brussels, 12 December. (See also Wolfe 1995 and Anderson and Sims 2000.)

2 The 'risk studies' are four studies undertaken by individual interviews with young homeless people in four different districts. The earliest risk study was undertaken for Safe in the City, an action research programme working with young people at risk of youth homelessness. This study was followed by three others using a similar questionnaire in Birmingham, the Cotswolds and North Staffordshire. Two of the risk studies included group interviews – in Birmingham these were with young homeless people and in the Cotswolds these were with school students aged 14–15 years old.

3 Woolf (1995) argues that it is as these ties disappear that religious or ethnic associations become more important.

4 The full report of the original risk study in London and the report on the inclusionary strategies developed as part of the Safe in the City action research programme can be found on their website: www.safeinthecity.org.uk.

5 A brief summary of the risk studies and a guide for homeless agencies can be found on the Foyer Federation website at www.foyer.net. This organisation is taking forward the prevention package designed by Safe in the City, through its *Safe Moves* programme.

References

Anderson, I. (1993) *Access to Housing for Low Income Single People*, University of York and JRF: Centre for Housing Policy.

Anderson, I. and Sim, D. (2000) *Social Exclusion and Housing: Contexts and challenges*. Coventry: Chartered Institute of Housing.

Beck, U., Giddens, A., Lash, S. (1994) *Reflexive Modernization. Politics, Tradition and Aesthetics in the Modern Social Order*. Oxford: Blackwell.

Bruegel, I. and Smith, J. (1999) *Taking Risks. An Analysis of the Risks of Homelessness for Young People in London*. Peabody Trust/ Safe in the City. Available at *www.safeinthecity.org.uk*

Burchardt ,T., Le Grand, J. and Piachaud, D. (2001) 'Degrees of exclusion: Developing a dynamic, multidimensional measure' in J. Hills, J. Le Grand, and D. Piachaud (eds), *Understanding Social Exclusion*. Oxford: Oxford University Press.

Craig, T., Hodson S., Woodward S. and Richardson, S. (1996), *Off to a Bad Start, A Longitudinal Study of Homeless Young People in London*. Mental Health Foundation.

Drake, M. (1981) *Single Homeless People*, Department of the Environment.

Evans, A. (1996) National Inquiry Into Youth Homelessness, *We Don't Choose to be Homeless*, available from the National Homeless Alliance, London WC1H 8LS.

Green. H., Thomas, M. and Iles, N. (ONS), Down, D. (DoE) (1996) *Housing in England 1994/5*. London: HMSO.

Hills, J., Le Grand, J., and Piachaud, D., (2001) *Understanding Social Exclusion*, Oxford: Oxford University Press

Hobcraft, J. (2001) 'Social Exclusion and the Generations' in Hills J, Le Grand J, and Piachaud, D. (2001) *Understanding Social Exclusion*. Oxford University Press.

Jones G (1995) *Leaving Home*, Open University Press.

Lemos, G. (2000) *Homelessness and loneliness: The want of conviviality*. London: Crisis.

Lenoirs, R. 1989, *Les Exclus, un Francais sur dix*.4th Edition

Kumar, V. (1993) *Poverty and Inequality in the UK. The effects on children*. National Children Bureau.

Neal, J. (1996) *Supported Hostels for Homeless People: A Review*. York: Centre for Housing Policy Research, The University of York.

North, C., Moore, H. and Owens, C. (1996) *Go Home and Rest. The Use of an Accident and Emergency Department by Homeless People*. Shelter.

Pleace, N. (2000) 'The new consensus, the old consensus and the provision of services for people sleeping rough', *Housing Studies*, 15, 4.

Randall, G. and Brown, S. (1993) *The Rough Sleepers Initiative: An Evaluation*. London: The Department of the Environment, HMSO.

Randall, G. and Brown, S. (1995) *Outreach and Resettlement Work with People Sleeping Rough*, Department of the Environment, HMSO.

Rodgers, G., Gore, C. and Figuerido, J.B. (1995) *Social Exclusion: Rhetoric, Reality, Responses*. International Institute for Labour Studies, ILO, Geneva. Switzerland.

Room, G. (1995) (ed). *Beyond the Threshold: The measurement and analysis of social inclusion*. Bristol: The Policy Press.

Silver, H. (1995) 'Three Paradigms of Social Exclusion' , in Rodgers G, Gore C, and Figuerido J.B., (1995) *Social Exclusion: Rhetoric, Reality, Responses. International Institute for Labour Studies, ILO*, Geneva. Switzerland.

Social Exclusion Unit (SEU) (1998) *Bringing Britain together: A national strategy for neighbourhood renewal*, Cmnd 4045, London: HMSO.

Smith, J. (1997) 'Family and community: A new agenda for social democracy', London: Socialist Register.

Smith J. (2003) *Who is at Risk of Homelessness in North Staffordshire? A study of young homeless people and their pasts*. Staffordshire University. Centre for Housing and Community Research.

Smith, J. (2004) *Dispersed Foyers*, A report for the Foyer Federation. Available at: www.foyer.net.

Smith, J. and Simister, J. (2002) *Crisis Open Christmas: Housing 900 vulnerable single homeless people*. unpublished report, London: Crisis.

Smith, J., Gilford, S., Kirby, P., O'Reilly A. and Ing P. (1996) *Bright Lights and Homelessness: Family and single homelessness among young people in our cities*, London: YMCA.

Smith, J., Gilford, S. and O'Sullivan, A. (1998) *The Family Background of Young Homeless People*. London: Family Policy Studies Centre; York: Joseph Rowntree Foundation.

Smith, J. Ing, P. O'Sullivan, A. (2000a) *Routes In and Out of Homelessness: Informing a Youth Homeless Strategy for Birmingham*, Staffordshire University. Centre for Housing and Community Research,

Smith, J., Ing, P. and O'Sullivan, A. (2000b) *Towards a youth homeless strategy for Birmingham*. Staffordshire University: Centre for Housing and Community Research.

Smith, J., Ing, P. and Ing, M. (2001) *Making Youth Homelessness Visible*, Staffordshire University. Centre for Housing and Community Research.

Townsend, P. and Gordon, D. (2002) *World Poverty: New policies to defeat an old enemy*. Bristol: The Policy Press.

Wolfe, M. (1995) 'Globalization and social exclusion: Some paradoxes', in G. Rodgers, C. Gore, and J.B. Figuerido (eds), (1995) *Social Exclusion: Rhetoric, reality, responses*, Geneva: International Institute for Labour Studies, ILO, Switzerland.

Worley, C. and Smith, J. (2001), *Moving Out, Moving On . . . From Foyer accommodation to independent living*. England: YMCA.

Postscript on homelessness

Julie Johnson and Jon Paterson

My name is Julie Johnson. I am 22 years old and have lived at the Salford Foyer for most of the last six years. I now have my own home and I am currently employed. With the help and support of Salford Foyer and Salford Youth Service's Unwaged Project Salford (UPS), I have become an unqualified youth worker. This work has succeeded in building my self-confidence and self-esteem.

My name is Jon Paterson. I am 19 years old and I have been living at Salford Foyer for about two years. Currently, I am unable to work because I suffer chronic back pain and depression. I am classed by the state as being disadvantaged, disaffected and disassociated. This is not how I think of myself and these labels do little to help my self-esteem and self-confidence. The state also classes me as being homeless even though I reside at the Salford Foyer. I would prefer to describe myself as being a young 'independent liver'.

I (Jon) have had very negative experiences with social services. For example, when I was in the process of becoming homeless I approached them for help and support but they insisted that it was not their problem or policy to provide me with help and support because I was not officially homeless. The social services informed me that I would have to go away and come back to them when I had nowhere to live.

I (Julie) had a social worker before I moved in to Salford Foyer and when I became estranged from my family, social services did not provide the help and support that I needed. I had to support and provide help for myself. They only became interested when I approached them for references, which I needed to move into Salford Foyer. My social worker was concerned that I would find it difficult to cope on my own because I am a wheelchair user.

We both had extreme difficulties in finding support before we became officially 'homeless' (without a roof over our heads) and we were in 'crisis' before any support was offered in terms of accommodation. Professional support from social services and other relevant departments was fragile or non-existent. As Joan Smith has stated in her chapter, living on your own on a low income and being estranged from both family and friends was very hard and mentally draining. Equally, we agree with her statements in the chapter regarding reconstituted families being mainly negative due to our own past experiences with stepfathers being physically or mentally violent.

Fortunately, we were both, at different times, accepted for places in the Salford Foyer, where support was offered. If you needed, it extra support was provided by the UPS team.

Prior to leaving home I (Jon) was attending college but with the emotional turmoil and stress that I suffered it was difficult to keep up with the work and attend. I spoke to my tutors at the college but there was little or no understanding of what I was going through; they would not accept that a 17 year old could suffer from 'stress'. I continued and finished my course but in doing so received very low grades. When I had resolved some of my difficulties I tried to return to education, but was trapped in the benefit system. Being 19 years old whilst the course was still running meant that I had to either leave college or give up all entitlement to benefits.

Since becoming 'homeless' (an 'independent liver'), I have learned to become far more independent and assertive. I refuse to accept that my current situation excludes me from 'HAVING A VOICE' and taking my rightful place in the community. The current low level of benefit payments, as outlined in Joan Smith's chapter, is overwhelmingly correct. Young people from 'homeless' backgrounds have massive pressures placed on them to find suitable employment or monitory assisted education. Because they are living below the poverty line, they will continue to have poor diets and often suffer from mental health issues. Without proper intervention and support, young people will continue to feel socially excluded from today's society.

Since coming to the Salford Foyer over two years ago after leaving my family unit and friends, my life has been very different; I have experienced both good and bad times and attitudes. I am now a volunteer worker in the Foyer and work with City 2000 on a young persons' forum. I am also an active member of the UPS group and other voluntary sector placements. I feel that without the support I have been offered I would not have survived living alone, and although life is still very difficult at times, I feel I am making significant progress toward my goals.

Before moving into my own home I (Julie) lived at the Foyer for six years and received DLA (Disability Living Allowance) because of my disability. The Foyer and UPS helped me to receive the additional benefits that I was entitled to. I felt safe and stable in the foyer (although it was sometimes hard to adjust to the rules and regulations laid down by the staff), and I felt supported. It was at times difficult to live in an environment where there were so many young people in one building. The advantages were the friendships and social aspects (and the parties were good!!!). You were also encouraged to try new things with other groups such as the UPS; through this group I became a volunteer youth worker and have now secured paid employment. However, to get this job, I had to move out of the Foyer and lose the support and stability that was there. Both Jon and I agree with Joan Smith that it is difficult to find a job when you are living in a foyer because of not being able to pay rent on low wages. But, ideally, you need the support of the foyer in order to save money in the initial stages of receiving an income from employment.

Our immediate recommendations are as follows:

- The government should give more support, followed by money, to young people who are homeless.
- Young people should be asked their point of view more often regarding issues in their lives, including homelessness.
- Do not stereotype us into groups – we are all individuals with individual concerns and problems to deal with.
- Foyers should offer more support for young people who are working, as many young people who do find paid work have to pay a lot more rent. We think this should be reduced, and the whole issue of benefits reviewed.

Chapter 10

Young asylum seekers and refugees in the UK

Kate Stanley

Introduction

Asylum seeking and refugee young people[1] live extraordinary lives. Many will have experienced persecution or the persecution of their families, others will have experienced a terrifying journey across thousands of miles in the hands of people-smugglers or traffickers. When they arrive in the UK, their journey to safety and security will have only just begun, as they must then start the process of integration and seek inclusion in UK society. It would be fair to assume that policy and practice in the UK would be designed to ease this final journey. It would also be wrong.

Perhaps the greatest indictment of policy and practice relating to young refugees in the UK is evidence which shows that delays to asylum decisions may induce stress-related illness, causing further damage to mental health in a group that is already more likely to experience the negative effects to mental health of trauma and disruption (British Medical Association 2002). When we consider that the right of these young people to be here at all is the subject of intense scrutiny, it seems likely that deteriorating mental health is a result of insecurity as well as exclusion. They also face the very real possibility of what may be considered the ultimate exclusion from UK society – removal from the UK itself.

In this chapter, I will examine how much central government policy and practice[2] towards young asylum seekers and refugees[3] in the UK actively and explicitly seeks to exclude these young people from participation in social, economic and cultural life. The situation for young asylum seekers is particularly poor, partly because there is not even acknowledgement of the need to bring about their social inclusion. Young asylum seekers and refugees are treated as a threat and, whilst their resilience is often noted, their skills and talents are not encouraged to flourish as they might. I will consider the impact this has on young asylum seekers and refugees, and the direction policy must take to promote their inclusion. In order to do this, a fuller understanding of who these young people are and why they come to the UK is needed.

For those aged under 18 years old, the question of whether or not they are accompanied by a relative or carer is also crucial in determining how policy responds to them. Children in families and young people aged over 18 years old are supported through the provisions of immigration legislation by the National Asylum Support Service (NASS). Those aged under 18 years old and separated from both parents or carers (referred to as unaccompanied minors or separated children) are the responsibility of the local authority in which they presented and they are supported through the provisions of the Children Act (1989).

Asylum seekers and refugees coming to the UK

Much of debate that surrounds asylum in the UK centres around the notion that the UK takes more than its 'fair share' of asylum applicants and that most claimants are 'bogus' and do not deserve protection. Some facts are helpful in illuminating these issues.

Between 1999 and 2001, developing countries hosted almost three-quarters of the world's 12 million asylum seekers and only a small proportion came to the EU. In 2001, the UK received less than eight per cent of the world's asylum applications, ranking it the 32nd country in terms of numbers of applications relative to its size, population and wealth (IPPR 2003).

In 2002, the UK received the most asylum applications of any country in Europe but was still only eighth highest in Europe relative to population. The total number of applications was 110,700 (including dependants). One in three of all applicants were deemed to be in need of protection or leave to remain on humanitarian grounds and a further one in five were successful on appeal in 2002 (Home Office 2003a).

Statistics are not collected on the number of refugees in the UK, nor on the number of dependent children included in asylum applications. An estimate made in 1998 put the number of refugees in London at between 240,000 and 280,000 (IPPR 2003). In 2002, it was estimated that there were 82,000 asylum-seeking and refugee children in England[5] and 8500 unaccompanied minors with asylum seeker and refugee status (Save the Children 2003a). In 2001, the Home Office recorded 20,330 asylum seekers aged 18 to 24 years old in the UK (Home Office 2002).

In the decade from 1990, more than half of all asylum applications in the UK originated in ten countries characterised by repression and/or discrimination of minorities and/or ethnic conflict. The evidence strongly suggests that conflict is the primary underlying cause of asylum flows to the EU (Castles *et al* 2003). However, it is hard to separate out underdevelopment and conflict and 'the migration–asylum nexus' constitutes a major analytical and policy challenge not least because many migrants have multiple motivations (Castles *et al* 2003: iii).

The UK has placed an emphasis on reducing the numbers of asylum applications and this analysis suggests that a strategy of conflict prevention would have most potential to achieve this. Despite Home Office commissioned research (Zetter *et al* 2003) concurring with this, policy continues to be formulated instead to restrict entry into the UK and to proscribe the rights of those who do enter – e.g. through visa requirements, carriers' liability regulations and restricted access to welfare support. This is largely because there is a belief within government that the majority of asylum applicants are actually economic migrants. This strategy has begun to result in substantial reductions in the number of asylum applications. However, there are also indications that the focus on preventing the entry of asylum seekers has generated growth in illicit activities:

> [There is] strong circumstantial evidence, though little authoritative research, that restrictionism . . . led to growing trafficking and illegal entry of both bona fida asylum seekers and economic migrants.
>
> (Zetter *et al* 2003: 4)

NASS was established under the Immigration and Asylum Act (1999) to take over responsibility for the support of asylum seekers from local authority Social Services Departments. NASS was tasked with establishing a system of dispersal around the UK in order to reduce the concentration of asylum seekers in London and the South East. The dispersal system has distributed the asylum-seeking population around the UK[6] but asylum seekers, like refugees, continue to be concentrated in cluster areas in larger cities in England, Glasgow in Scotland and Cardiff in Wales. There are very small numbers of asylum seekers in Northern Ireland.

The majority of single asylum seekers are young males and approximately 60 per cent of unaccompanied minors are male (Home Office 2003a, Save the Children 2003c). There is no official source of data on the prevalence and type of disabilities amongst refugees. However, evidence suggests that there is a lack of consideration of the needs of disabled asylum seekers in the dispersal system (Roberts and Harris 2002). Evidence also indicates that the general health of asylum seekers is good when they arrive in the UK, although there may be a greater prevalence of certain illnesses, such as tuberculosis (Coker 2003). The deteriorating mental health of asylum seekers after arrival should, however, be an area of great concern.

I have sought to draw out some of the characteristics and motivations of asylum seekers and refugees in order to counter misapprehensions and establish some basic facts. However, this brief summary cannot begin to illustrate the heterogeneity of the refugee population in the UK. The only tie that binds young refugees together is the fact they have left their country of origin.

In the next section I will examine how the policies and practices that make up the asylum continuum impact on the lives of young refugees.

Policies underpinning the social exclusion of young asylum seekers and refugees

Policies should flow from the objective they are seeking to achieve. Currently, young asylum seekers and refugees are approached through a series of ad hoc arrangements with no underlying rationale or policy objective, partly because they are affected by at least three separate sets of policies with different objectives. There are policies which relate to their immigration status, through the asylum system; policies which relate to their youth, through the child protection and youth services; and policies which relate to their ethnicity through minority ethnic inclusion policies.

I cannot cover the vast range of these policies here, but examples follow from the above three areas, showing how policy and practice exacerbate the social exclusion of young asylum seekers and refugees. As we will see, the mantra of joined-up government is yet to be implemented in relation to young people who are asylum seekers or refugees.

Asylum policy

By the end of the 1990s, the government was compelled to respond to the massive backlog of unresolved claims and perceived crises in the asylum system. Wide-ranging measures were introduced, including major legislation in 1999, 2002 and 2003[7]. A new Home Office target was announced in 2002 to ensure that, by 2004, 75 per cent of substantive claims receive an initial decision within two months. The initial decision-making has sped up considerably as a result during the final quarter of 2003, with 80 per cent of claimants receiving an initial decision within two months (Home Office 2004). However, the quality of the decision-making and the integrity of the appeals system remain questionable.

While young people are awaiting an asylum decision, their lives are in limbo. It is extremely difficult for them to lay down roots both psychologically and in terms of accessing entitlements and gaining inclusion (Stanley 2001, Save the Children 2003b). Waiting for a decision is very stressful for many young people and it looms large in their everyday life. A study published in 2001 quoted a 17 year-old asylum seeker who epitomised this feeling:

> How long are they going to make us wait? How can we settle? How can we make plans? We can't without knowing our status. Our lives are always in the air . . . It is like they are killing us slowly.
>
> (Stanley 2001: 105)

He and his family had been waiting for four years for an asylum decision.

Whilst the appeals system has sped up, the quality and sustainability of initial decision-making remains questionable. For example, proportionately fewer young people who claim in their own right are granted asylum than those in older age groups. In 2000, just five per cent of unaccompanied asylum seekers aged under 18 years old were granted asylum compared to 27 per cent of applicants aged 25–29 years old. One possible explanation is that, up until very recently[8], under 18 year olds have not been required to have a substantive interview in which officials test and assess the veracity of their claim. Refugee and children's organisations argue that one reason for this may be that immigration officers do not have sufficient knowledge of child-specific forms of persecution upon which to base full assessments.

The complexities of returning unaccompanied minors to their country of origin mean the vast majority are awarded temporary leave to remain, which comes with a range of both entitlements and restrictions. For example, those with temporary leave can only access further education at the discretion of the institution to which they have applied, and can only access financial support for education after three years with leave to remain. Moreover, temporary leave provides no conclusion to the claim and will lead to an appeal, an application for an extension of leave to remain or possible removal. The uncertainty implicit in these possibilities is not conducive to integration and social inclusion. The possibility of being returned to their country of origin and/or the uncertainty can cause some asylum seekers to go 'underground', excluding themselves from all contact with authorities. They may seek work in the criminal or 'shadow' economy. The Home Office has no reliable estimates of how many people there are living illegally in this way.

While asylum seekers await a decision on their claim they may be detained at any stage, for any reason and for any length of time. Although the detention of asylum seekers is an administrative process rather than a criminal sanction, the regime in a detention centre (renamed removal centres) is the equivalent of a category B prison[9]. Detention has been increasingly used as a tool of asylum policy in the UK, and families with children can also now be detained, despite the United Nations High Commissioner for Refugees (UNHCR) describing the detention of asylum seekers as inherently undesirable. HM Inspector of Prisons (April 2003 recommendation 5 cited in Scottish Refugee Council 2003) recommended that 'detention of [asylum seeking] children should be avoided, and only take place for the shortest possible time, for no more than seven days'. The fulfilment of basic rights, such as educational provision in detention centres, is patchy and detained young asylum seekers are excluded from mainstream society in a very palpable way. The expressed need to detain them, despite the fact they have committed no crime, sends a very negative message to wider society about their supposed inherent danger.

Young people policy

The United Nations Convention on the Rights of the Child (UNCRC) is an international instrument[10] which sets out the rights necessary to ensure the survival and development of all children aged under 18 years old. Article 22 recognises that asylum-seeking and refugee children have special needs which must be provided in order for them to enjoy the rights set out in the UNCRC, making it clear that like-for-like treatment is not necessarily sufficient where children face particular disadvantage. However, when the UK government signed and ratified the UNCRC in 1991, it reserved the right not to apply the Convention to asylum-seeking and refugee children. Subsequent governments have refused to remove the Reservation, on the basis that it does not inhibit the discharge of obligations under Article 22 but is necessary in order to preserve the integrity of UK immigration laws.

However, this position has been challenged by legal opinion, which has pointed out the basic flaw in the government's insistence on the retention of the Reservation:

> [There is a] paradox at the heart of the UK Government's position, which is to maintain the Reservation whilst at the same time submitting that immigration laws are fully compatible with the CRC. If the latter were true there would be no need for the former.
>
> (Blake and Drew 2001: 1)

The Reservation reveals the primacy awarded to immigration legislation over welfare legislation. This is played out in many ways. One example is the location of the special grant for social services' support of unaccompanied minors with the Home Office, which has responsibility for matters relating to immigration, rather than the Department of Health, which has responsibility for matters relating to the welfare of all other children in public care. Another is the detention of asylum-seeking children, which violates the best interests principle and the duty of non-discrimination provided for in the UNCRC. The government is unapologetic that immigration and asylum are political issues. The consequence is that they respond to the issues with political measures in which considerations of welfare and social inclusion play only a minor role.

Minority ethnic inclusion policy

The government's analysis of social exclusion acknowledges the role race and ethnicity have in affecting outcomes for young people (Social Exclusion Unit 1998, 2000); immigration is also listed as a driver of social exclusion (Cabinet Office 2003). People from minority ethnic communities have been identified as more likely than others to live in deprived areas in unpopular and overcrowded housing, and more likely to be poor and unemployed, regardless of their age, sex, qualifications and place of residence. Racial harassment and racist crime are acknowledged to be widespread and under-reported and 'not always treated as seriously as they should be' (Social Exclusion Unit 2000: 7).

In recent years, considerable energy has been focused on reducing these indicators of social exclusion amongst minority ethnic groups and achieving community cohesion in areas of ethnic diversity. Strategies include early interventions (such as Sure Start[11]) and improving the accessibility of public services and employment opportunities in public bodies (for example, through the introduction of the Race Relations (Amendment) Act 2000). However, it could be argued that ambiguity remains in the experience of some children from minority ethnic communities: on the one hand, they receive the poorest and fewest services; on the other hand, they are labelled as being at fault over their quality of life in the community (Edwards 2002).

This ambiguity is exaggerated for young asylum seekers in particular. They receive even poorer and fewer services as part of an overt strategy to give them reduced rights and entitlements to deter future arrivals in the UK. This is done despite recognition of the particular risks of poor outcomes from social exclusion for young people.

Home Office commissioned research (Glover et al 2001: 3; 24–8) has identified policies which impact on the integration of young refugees and other migrants, including access to employment, benefits, opportunities for family reunion, citizenship policy and access to voting. If we assess the relevant policy areas, we find that they fall far short of supporting the integration of young refugees. For example, asylum seekers are not permitted to seek work and there is no policy to support the particular need of refugees in gaining employment. Asylum seekers have no access to mainstream welfare benefits (although they may be able to access other benefits via NASS provided they meet certain conditions). At present, there is no policy to encourage applications for citizenship and there is usually a requirement to have held ELR or HP for three years before having any rights to family reunification. Even full refugee status does not confer the right to vote[12].

The apparent contradiction between the approaches to asylum seekers compared to that of other minority ethnic communities is legitimised by the supposed necessity to give precedence to asylum policy over social inclusion, welfare and rights. It seems that a range of policies problematise young asylum seekers rather than seeking to develop their diverse skills and qualities.

The impact of policy on social exclusion and inclusion

Access to public services and housing

Approximately 85 million people arrived through UK ports during 2002; roughly one-third were overseas residents (International Passenger Survey 2003), and policy makers are tasked with identifying who of these belong to the 'community of legitimate receivers' of public services (Bommes 1999). If we try to ascertain what these judgements are and how they are made, we find that the rules about access to public services – though entirely necessary – are very complex. This means that service providers have little certainty as to which categories of migrants are entitled to what, and migrants themselves are uncertain of their entitlements.

Unquestionably, supporting diversity presents challenges to public services, particularly in London (Strategy Unit 2003), where people of 91 nationalities reside and 300 languages are spoken. Differing needs are not adequately reflected in the funding that service providers receive and national targets do not reflect changing priorities caused by the needs of refugees. These challenges are exacerbated by a lack of information about arrivals and departures, a significant issue given the high mobility of asylum seekers and refugees, and keeping count of those who arrive under one immigration and switch to another. Nonetheless, service providers often stress the contribution made by asylum seekers and refugees to community life (Stanley 2001).

Partly as a result of these challenges, young asylum seekers and refugees do not have full access to adequate public services. It has been estimated by the Refugee Council that approximately 2000 children in London were not in school in 2002. Despite these obstacles, asylum-seeking refugee children are often reported as having high ambitions for their education (Stanley 2001). However, obstacles exist at every stage. Universities have discretion whether or not they charge overseas students' fees or home student fees in relation to a student with only temporary leave to remain. Overseas student fees are frequently prohibitively expensive. Moreover, further education funding is based on completion rates, so institutions may be deterred from enrolling young asylum seekers with uncertain status.

Positive developments, such as the regionalisation of NASS which should make it more responsive to local circumstances, may be undermined by separate developments, for example, use of poor quality housing by NASS. Similarly, the Homelessness Act (2002) has had the unintended consequence of more 16 and 17 year-olds, including unaccompanied minors, being placed in bed and breakfast accommodation as homeless families are moved out. The use of poor-quality housing to accommodate young asylum seekers and refugees has been justified by some local service providers on the grounds that the accommodation is good compared to where they have come from. This justification reveals that young asylum seekers and refugees' rights are not judged against the same scale to those of the non-refugee population.

Poverty and worklessness

The Labour government has placed welfare-to-work initiatives and in-work benefits at the heart of strategies to meet its pledge to eradicate child poverty and increase social inclusion, but one policy runs entirely contrary to this approach. In July 2002, the provision for asylum seekers who had not received a final decision on their claim within six months to apply for permission to work was removed. This was justified on the grounds that no one would have to wait that long in future, as processing times were being substantially reduced. It was also based on the assumption that the ability to legally access the labour market acts as a 'pull' factor for economic migrants to use the asylum system to enter the UK. Young asylum seekers now have no means of supporting themselves in the UK and, for some, like those over compulsory school age, this might be a desirable option. They are also missing out on the important inclusionary benefits of work. Their worklessness does little to help reduce the negative impression of asylum seekers held by the wider public.

This means destitute asylum seekers must seek state support. Asylum seekers are excluded from access to mainstream welfare benefits, but if they meet certain conditions they are provided with accommodation and financial support by NASS. In 2003, a single asylum seeker aged 18–24 years old was entitled to £29.89 a week compared to £42.70 for British citizens of the same age (IPPR 2003). Income support is also a gateway to other benefits and other young people can access premium payments. It is widely accepted that the income support rates for young UK citizens are set at a level at which it is difficult to subsist, so young asylum seekers receiving 30 per cent less face severe poverty. A survey by Oxfam and the Refugee Council (Penrose 2002) found that 95 per cent of the surveyed adult asylum seekers could not afford to buy clothes or shoes and 80 per cent were not able to maintain good health. This will clearly impact on the children of asylum seekers as well as on single young asylum seekers.

Since the implementation of section 55 of the Immigration and Asylum Act in January 2003, some asylum seekers have also become ineligible even for NASS support. Section 55 requires that asylum seekers must make their asylum claim as soon as 'reasonably practicable' in order to be eligible for NASS support. This means that some asylum seekers who are assessed as destitute are not eligible for government financial support or accommodation. Families with children are exempt from this requirement but single young asylum seekers are not. This policy has been the subject of a failed judicial review and, it is argued by refugee organisations, is leading to overcrowding, homelessness and destitution.

If a young asylum seeker is granted leave to remain, he or she will be able to access welfare benefits and seek work and a way out of poverty. However, refugee unemployment is estimated at between 75 and 90 per cent, despite apparently high levels of qualifications (Glover *et al* 2001). The majority of refugees work in informal, short-term, menial, low-paid jobs with no job security. This is especially true for refugee women. Research suggests that barriers to employment include a lack of English language skills and knowledge about UK society, the labour market and support networks; lack of UK work experience; non-recognition of qualifications, and cultural barriers to effective job seeking (Glover *et al* 2001). There are also demand-side barriers such as employers' lack of knowledge about immigration status and racial discrimination.

The failure to promote the social inclusion of asylum seekers raises serious questions about social justice and our commitment to equality. But it also ignores the reality that many young asylum seekers will be granted leave to remain in the UK and that more still will remain here anyway because so few asylum seekers are actually removed from the UK. The Home Office does acknowledge that efforts should be made to integrate refugees, as illustrated in this statement:

> There is a need to invest early in integration to promote a quick move from dependency to self-value and sufficiency through work and inclusion in community and society.
> (Home Office 1999, quoted in Glover *et al* 2001: 48)

But despite low rates of return of those whose asylum applications have failed, the Home Office insists that the process of integration can only begin after a person has been granted leave to remain.

Public attitudes

Refugees in general tend to live in poor housing in poor areas, have a very high rate of unemployment, low incomes and can suffer poor health as a result. These indicators of social exclusion attract attention and their exclusion is reflected in and exacerbated by discrimination and public attitudes toward them. Public attitudes can be a powerful exclusionary force, and as race and immigration have moved up the political agenda, a mutually reinforcing rhetoric has developed between politicians and UK citizens that asylum seekers represent a threat that must be contained. This climate has created opportunities for far-right political organisations, such as the British National Party, to fuel such fears and misapprehensions. In turn, this has caused mainstream politicians to call for still tougher approaches to immigration in order to prevent this kind of capital being made by the Far-Right. The European Commission Against Racism and Intolerance has laid considerable blame at the door of UK politicians:

> Many politicians have contributed to, or at least not adequately prevented, public debate taking on an increasingly intolerant line, with at times racist and xenophobic overtones. Public statements have tended to depict asylum seekers. . . as a threat.
>
> (ECRI 2000: II.58)

Of all the polls that have revealed negative public attitudes toward asylum seekers and/or refugees, one of the most worrying found highly intolerant attitudes amongst young UK citizens. It found that six in ten young people aged 15–24 years old thought that refugees do not make a positive contribution to the UK, and 23 per cent believed Britain should not offer a safe haven to people fleeing war and persecution (MORI 2003a). Far from supporting any efforts towards inclusion, almost one-third believed that rights to education, liberty and work should not apply to asylum seekers. Much public concern centres on numbers, with nine out of ten voters in 2003 believing the number of asylum seekers in Britain is a serious problem (IPPR 2003). Nonetheless, 78 per cent in this poll did think it is right that Britain should continue to let in people seeking asylum if their claim is genuine. Public attitudes are important in shaping public policy. More immediately, these attitudes, reflected in racist attitudes more generally, are experienced through discrimination against refugees.

There are indications that greater familiarity with refugees creates a greater level of tolerance. One survey found that Londoners tend to think that asylum seekers and refugees come to the UK for 'a better life for themselves and their family' (MORI 2003b), whereas more than half of people asked elsewhere believed they came to the UK because it was a 'soft touch' (MORI 2001). This belief that the UK is a 'soft touch' is partly founded on the misapprehension that asylum seekers receive generous welfare support. A poll in 2000 (Bouquet and Moller 2001) found that people thought asylum seekers received an average of £113 per week. At the time asylum seekers were entitled to just £36.54 per week.

Future policy directions

> At a time of great population movements we must have clear policies for immigration and asylum. We are committed to fostering social inclusion and respect for ethnic, cultural and religious diversity, because they make our societies strong, our economies more flexible and promote exchange of ideas and knowledge.
>
> (Berlin Communique 2000)

It seems that little progress has been achieved towards the inclusion and respect described in the above quotation. This ambition must be renewed with a clear strategy for its achievement. The first step must be a new kind of dialogue between policy makers and the wider public which acknowledges the positive impact asylum seekers and refugees – including young asylum seekers and refugees – can and do have on the UK.

Secondly, a correlation has been identified between the economic success of migrants and their method of entry into UK (Glover *et al* 2001), with those entering through the asylum system having most restrictions upon them and, as a consequence, least success. This suggests that joining up entry policy with wider social and economic objectives would be beneficial for all. This means reformulating the asylum continuum so that it runs from entry through to settlement and social inclusion.

A successful and joined-up asylum policy will deliver both an asylum policy that has integrity and a welfare policy that delivers opportunities for young asylum seekers and refugees to achieve social inclusion. There have been some suggestions of better things to come for young refugees through initiatives such as the Home Office (2000) strategy for the inclusion of refugees. The strategy aimed to help refugees develop their potential and contribute to cultural and economic life, to set out a clear framework to support the integration process and to facilitate access to support for the integration of refugees. However, resources were not allocated for the implementation of such an ambitious strategy and it applies only to refugees.

Conclusion

The UK has a duty to ensure that when young asylum seekers and refugees reach this country their rights and entitlements are such that those who are granted leave to remain have the opportunity to grow and develop as members of British society, and those who are not are not damaged by their experiences here. If the UK is to deliver human rights, including those enshrined in the UNCRC, the UN Convention on the Status of Refugees and the Human Rights Act (1998), we need to reconsider policy and practice towards asylum seekers and refugees. This needs to begin with a change in the language we use to talk about asylum, and with raising awareness of the circumstances of refugees and the UK's role in refugee protection. We then need to acknowledge that many young asylum seekers and refugees will spend much of their lives in this country and we should take pains to ensure their social inclusion from the time they arrive.

Endnotes

1 In this chapter young people refers to those aged 15 to 25 years old.
2 There is good practice amongst many voluntary organisations and some local authorities but we concentrate our attention largely on central government policy and practice.
3 Policy and practice varies considerably between asylum seekers and refugees. Throughout this chapter I indicate where I am referring specifically to policy and practice in relation to asylum seekers; at other times I refer to both asylum seekers and refugees.
4 HP replaced Exceptional Leave to Remain in April 2003.
5 Stephen Twigg MP in a speech, 5 March 2003.
6 Only those who require or choose to live in accommodation provided by NASS are dispersed.
7 The Immigration and Asylum Act (1999), the Nationality, Immigration and Asylum Act (2002) and the Immigration and Asylum (Treatment of Claimants etc.) Bill (2003). There was also major immigration legislation in 1995 and 1997. More legislation is planned in 2004.
8 Substantive asylum interviews are due to begin with some under 18 year olds in 2004.
9 Category B prisoners are defined by the prison service as 'prisoners for whom the highest conditions of security are not necessary, but for whom escape must be made very difficult' (www.hmprisonservice.gov.uk).
10 The UNCRC is not legally binding.
11 Sure Start was launched in 1998 to support children and families from pregnancy until the child is aged 14 years old. Sure Start seeks to achieve better outcomes for children by increasing childcare; improving children's health, education and emotional development; and supporting parents' employment aspirations (www.surestart.gov.uk).
12 Some refugees may have the right to vote, but this is due to their nationality not their status as refugees; for example, citizens of commonwealth countries may vote in the UK.

References

Berlin Communique (2000) 'Progressive governance for the 21st century', issued on 2nd/3rd June 2000 by Heads of Government on President Clinton's visit to Germany. Available:
www.usembassy.de/events/clinton2000/final.htm (accessed 22 March, 2004).
Blake, N. and Drew, S. (2001) *In the Matter of the United Kingdom Reservation to the UN Convention on the Rights of the Child:* Opinion, London: Matrix Chambers and Tooks Court Chambers.
Bommes, M. (1999) 'Migration, belonging and the shrinking inclusive capacity of the national welfare state', presented at HUGG Berlin Conference, October 1999.
Bouquet, T. and Moller, D. (2001) 'Are we a tolerant nation?' in *Reader's Digest – British Edition*, London: Reader's Digest – British Edition. Available: *www.readersdigest.co.uk/magazine/tolerant.htm* (accessed 30 July 2003).
British Medical Association Board of Science and Education (2002) *Asylum Seekers: Meeting their healthcare needs*, London: British Medical Association.

Available: *www.bma.org.uk/ap.nsf/Content/Asylumseekers?OpenDocument&High light=2,refugees*

Bynner, J. (2003) 'The Future of social exclusion: Patterns and trends', paper delivered at Strategy Unit seminar, 7 May 2003.

Cabinet Office (2003) *The Future of Social Exclusion: Drivers, patterns and policy challenges*, London: Social Exclusion Unit, Office of the Deputy Prime Minister and the Strategy Unit.

Castles, S., Crawley, H. and Loughna, S. (2003) *States of Conflict*, London: Institute for Public Policy Research.

Coker, R. (2003) 'Migration, public health and compulsory screening for TB and HIV', Asylum and Migration Working Paper 1, London: Institute for Public Policy Research.

Cole, E. (2003) *A Few Families Too Many: The detention of asylum-seeking families in the UK*, London: Bail for Immigration Detainees.

Dustmann, C., Casanova, M., Fertig, M., *et al.* (2003) *The Impact of EU Enlargement on Migration Flows*, Home Office Online Report 25/03, London: Home Office. Available:
www.homeoffice.gov.uk/rds/pdfs2/rdsolr2503.pdf (accessed 30 July 2003)

Edwards, R. (2002) 'Children and the local economy: another way to achieve social inclusion', presented at a conference in November 2002.

European Commission Against Racism and Intolerance (ECRI), *Second Report on the United Kingdom* (adopted 16 June 2000) Strasbourg: Directorate General of Human Rights. Available:
press.coe.int/dossiers/105/E/e-uk.htm

Fitzpatrick, P. (2003) 'Poor, excluded and forgotten: asylum seekers and the welfare state', *Poverty* No. 115: 12–17.

Garvie, D. (2001) *Far from Home: The housing of asylum seekers in private rented accommodation*, London: Shelter.

Glover, S., Gott, C., Loizillon, A., *et al.* (2001) *Migration: An economic and social analysis*, London: Home Office.

HM Prison Service, 'Factsheet'. Available:
www.hmprisonservice.gov.uk/faq.asp (accessed 3 March 2004)

Home Office (1999) *A consultation paper on the integration of recognised refugees in the UK*, London: Home Office.

Home Office (2000) *Full and Equal Citizens: A strategy for the integration of refugees into the United Kingdom*, London: Home Office.

Home Office (2002) *Asylum Statistics United Kingdom 2001*, London: Home Office.

Home Office (2003a) *Asylum Statistics United Kingdom: 4th Quarter 2002*, London: Home Office.

Home Office (2003b) *HM Inspector of Prisons Report*, London: Home Office.

Home Office (2004) *Asylum Statistics: 4th Quarter 2003*, London: HMSO.

IPPR (2003) *Asylum in the UK: A fact file*, London: Institute for Public Policy Research.

MORI (2001) *The Mail on Sunday Asylum Poll*, London: MORI. Available:
http://www.mori.com/2001/ms010106.shtml (accessed 8 March 2003)

MORI (2003a) *Young People and Asylum*, London: MORI. Available:
www.mori.com/polls/2003/asylumseekers.shtml (accessed 8 March 2004)

MORI (2003b) *British Views on Immigration*, London: MORI. Available:
www.mori.com/polls/2003/migration.shtml (accessed 8 March 2004)

Office for National Statistics (2003) *Travel Trends 2002*, London: TSO.
Available:
www.statistics.gov.uk/downloads/theme_transport/TTrends02.pdf

Penrose, J. (2002) *Poverty and Asylum in the UK*, London: Oxfam and Refugee
Council.

Refugee Council, 'UK asylum law and process: latest changes to the asylum system'.
Available:
www.refugeecouncil.org.uk/infocentre/asylumlaw/latest.htm (accessed 8 March
2004)

Refugee Council (2002) 'The Nationality, Immigration and Asylum Act 2002:
Changes to the asylum system in the UK', Refugee Council Briefing, December
2002, London: The Refugee Council.

Roberts, K. and Harris, J. (2002) *Findings: Disabled people in refugee and asylum-
seeking communities*, York: Joseph Rowntree Foundation.

Save the Children (2003a) *Young Refugees: A guide to the rights and entitlements
of separated refugee children*, London: Save the Children.

Save the Children (2003b) *Young Refugees: Providing emotional support to young
separated refugees in the UK*, London: Save the Children.

Save the Children (2003c) *Young Refugees: Working with unaccompanied asylum-
seeking children at ports*, London: Save the Children.

Save the Children and UNHCR (2000) *Separated Children in Europe Programme.
Statement of Good Practice*, London: Save the Children and UNHCR.

Scottish Refugee Council (2003) *Briefing: Detention*. Glasgow: Scottish Refugee
Council, available:
www.scottishrefugeecouncil.org.uk/Document/detention.pdf (accessed 8 March
2004)

Social Exclusion Unit (1998) *Bringing Britain Together: A national strategy for
neighbourhood renewal*, London: Social Exclusion Unit.

Social Exclusion Unit (2000) *Minority Ethnic Issues in Social Exclusion and
Neighbourhood Renewal*, London: Social Exclusion Unit.

Stanley, K. (2001) *Cold Comfort: The experiences of young separated refugees in
England*, London: Save the Children.

Strategy Unit (2003) *London Analytical Report*, London: Strategy Unit.

Sure Start, 'About Sure Start'. Available:
www.surestart.gov.uk (accessed 3 March 2004).

Taylor, D. (2003) 'Desperately seeking safety' in *The Guardian*, 27 June 2003,
London: The Guardian. Available:
society.guardian.co.uk/asylumseekers/comment/0,8005,986151,00.html
(accessed 30 July 2003)

Travis, A. (2003) 'Outcry as asylum 'whitelist' extended' in *The Guardian*, 18 June
2003, London: The Guardian. Available:
www.guardian.co.uk/Refugees_in_Britain/Story/0,2763,979619,00.html
(accessed 30 July 2003).

Zetter, R., Griffiths, D., Ferretti S. and Pearl, M. (2003) *An Assessment of the
Impact of Asylum Policies in Europe 1990–2000, Findings*, London: Home
Office.

Postscript on asylum seekers and refugees

Kh. Mustajab Malikzada and Ahmad Qadri

My name is Kh. Mustajab Malikzada. As a young asylum seeker myself from Afghanistan, now aged 21, I found the whole process of asylum complicated with great obstacles to find a way into the mainstream society and form a relation with the host community. I was committed and passionate about working in the community, so I had to struggle extremely hard to participate in local youth activities and other local affairs. I also experienced a lack of information and apprehension about local and national services for refugees and asylum seekers and was not advised on how to go about applying to college or for a doctor. I even had to find my own solicitor to deal with my immigration case. If I had to rely on the government structural procedures I would not have been able to learn the language, attend mainstream education courses and eventually go to university. I have lived in this country for over four years now and I am doing a three-year degree course in Politics and International Relations at the University of Essex. However, at the age of 21, my future is in limbo because I have to wait for the extension of my ELR to remain in this country.

My name is Ahmad Qadri. I am 19 years old and I was born in Afghanistan where I lived most of my life. I moved to the United Kingdom as an asylum seeker in 2000 and have been living here since then. Today I am a British citizen as well as an Afghan and I feel I have duties in life towards these two nations. I started school from year 10 here in England and I am now in sixth form studying A Level Maths and Sciences, aiming to get into medical school. Since I started living independently from such an early life, studying towards my goals has never been easy and I always had to work extremely hard to succeed. However I have never felt any lack of motivation in myself because in everyday life I can still see people who are in need of help.

Young asylum seekers and refugees have different experiences as they come from various countries of the world with diverse religious, cultural and linguistic backgrounds, but stigmatisation as asylum seekers or refugees brings them together. Also they travel in the same boat once they have arrived in the UK, by going through a similar process of immigration, settling down among others, learning the language and integrating in the society by participating in the local communities' activities. But there are obstacles in doing so, created by government policies and procedures. The journey that brings a young asylum seeker to safety is one harsh reality and then the legal process that this requires is another harsh reality, as illustrated more comprehensively by Kate Stanley, author of this chapter. The first is short term with long effects and the destination is uncertain sometimes. However, the latter is long term, and, in most cases, the effects are perpetual without recognition by authorities and one's future destination is also uncertain – where you will end up, either in a detention centre, hostel, dispersed from one place to another or left on your own to survive and make your way in a strange and unfamiliar country. Life becomes like a complicated puzzle sometimes with no way out and one question remains unanswered: what is going to happen next?

Once arrived in the UK, young asylum seekers confront issues such as legal information on their process of asylum; services for asylum seekers; health and well-being; discrimination and prejudices by a number of groups of people in society; education; welfare; and accommodation. Moreover, they are not considered and treated by statutory organisations as 'young people' but as 'asylum seekers' or 'refugees'. The fundamental problem at the initial stage for young asylum seekers is the decision of their asylum cases, which cause great tension and worries as the uncertainty about the decision increases and the length of time it takes. Also in some instances they have to provide evidence of their age as the basis of which their cases are said to be decided, which seems sometimes impossible as most of these young asylum seekers come from war-torn countries with no culture of birth registration. Most young asylum seekers do not have the knowledge of the asylum continuum, which is described in detail by Stanley, and they have differing levels of knowledge of their rights and entitlements depending on the stage of their cases. Until, or if, their cases have been decided, their lives are in limbo and they cannot make any decision about their future or even if they do (e.g. education, a job or settling down in the community), there is always the worry of whether they would be able to continue to stay or not. This all adds to the psychological stress and disconsolation of young asylum seekers, which weakens their prospects of integrating in the society.

However, Kate Stanley seems not to have recognised or acknowledged a crucial issue surrounding young asylum seekers and refugees: the discriminatory immigration policies and the different policies for different age groups and the implications of these on both young people and on the government. Yes, the destiny of young asylum seekers pretty much depends on their age when they arrive in this country and who is eligible for particular services during various stages. For instance, those who are under the age of 18 years old are looked after by Social Services or foster families with adequate and decent services which enable them to access education and other mainstream services for young people. This can eventually lead to better integration in the society and play an active role in most cases. On the other hand, however, those asylum seekers who enter the UK after their 18th birthday confront a dissimilar situation. They immediately confront the other challenge of their lives, which sometimes can be as damaging to their mental health as the persecution that they had run away from in their home countries. When one turns 18 years old, rights and entitlements of young asylum seekers change and one is no longer a young person anymore, as Kate Stanley shows. Moreover, the significance of this discriminatory policy is that it does not just result in, or drive young asylum seekers to, exclusion but it also sends a negative message to their home countries, encouraging the ones who are on their way to lie about their age so as to escape the unwelcome reception that they would have received if they had given their real ages when arriving in the UK. As a matter of fact these young people do benefit from an easier start in life by lying about their age but later on they all experience even more severe social problems as they are introduced to a new society which is unique in its own distinct way, with lots of opportunities but dependence on others for some time, accommodated with the wrong age group or in incorrect classes at schools or colleges. In most cases all these factors would result in extreme social exclusion as they drop out of school or college and their future becomes even more insecure. So all of this happens because of the way the UK government's immigration policies treat asylum seekers who are under and over 18 years old in ineffective and contradictory ways.

Kate Stanley argues that, once their cases are refused and they are told they will be deported or that there is uncertainty about their cases, some asylum seekers will go 'underground' and exclude themselves from all contact with authorities and seek to work in a criminal or 'shadow' economy. But she seems to forget the impact or effects of the decisions taken as a result of unfair policies of government. First of all, those who go 'underground' are young people with not much experience of working in dodgy systems with no precautions to protect them from exploitation and, more importantly, ill health. They would not be able to approach the NHS services but they nevertheless accept that risk.

The issue of health and well-being is important for young asylum seekers and refugees. As they go through difficult circumstances both at home and on their journeys, they suffer from psychological or mental and physical illnesses. But because of the legal process with their asylum case, their main priority remains the legal case rather then their health. Also with a lack of information and understanding of how the system works – e.g. how to register with a GP or dentist – problems of communication lead to such young people forgetting their health, resulting in deterioration rather than improvement. All this contributes to the further isolation of young asylum seekers in society.

Although there are numerous voluntary and statutory organisations working to support asylum seekers and refugees in general but young asylum seekers in particular, these young people are not provided information about their rights to those services and are therefore left in the dark. Also as a result of immigration rules or not being given enough information about local mainstream services that are widely available for young people more generally, young asylum seekers and refugees are excluded from the community. As a result, there is a further gap created between the local community and asylum seekers and refugees as a consequence of a lack of information.

Young asylum seekers are discriminated against in all stages of their asylum life by officials: i.e. they are not treated as young people and there is always the culture of constant interrogation either by Social Services or other departments. There is also widespread prejudice generally about asylum seekers in the country, which is obviously a by-product of the immigration policies that are designed and implemented by policy makers and propagated by mass media. These all contribute to the misunderstanding caused between both groups in this society which highlights the contradictory policies of the UK government, e.g. immigration versus social policies.

Education is also important but that also depends on one's legal status. In some cases young people are refused places in schools or colleges. This happens in two forms: first, the young person is not the right age to enter school because of the age considered appropriate by the Home Office; and secondly, colleges will not accept a young person because he or she is too young. So there is always a barrier or obstacle to make a difference. These young people are determined to learn the English language and proceed to further mainstream education but they are mostly barred because of unrealistic government policies.

Young refugees and asylum seekers are in essence locked in the legal procedure's cage which prevents them from understanding and socialising in British culture, systems and way of life. And these abstract and uncohesive government policies prevent them from integrating in society and encourage them to disintegrate further and make their life parlous. The government should consider young refugees and asylum seekers as young people first, and then as asylum seekers. Then the tangible immigration policies would be inconsistent with pragmatic social inclusion policies and definitely should not be precarious. The government should also realise the potential of these young people by giving them the opportunity to explore and improve their skills by attending either college, school or other educational institutions, instead of locking them up in the legal system.

The UK government in the last few years has put great emphasis on the participation of minorities and inclusion of excluded groups in society, asylum seekers and refugees among them. It also seeks to promote multiculturalism by reconciliation and accommodation of asylum seekers, and especially refugees with legal status, with other minority groups in the society. But if young refugees and asylum seekers face the dilemmas or issues mentioned above, how can they integrate or understand the importance of integration or participation in the community and society? All these policies of immigration and social inclusion embody ideas of segregation and conflict.

Chapter 11

Contemporary youth justice systems: Continuities and contradictions

David Smith

There has been a good deal of academic commentary on the youth justice policies of the New Labour government, and nearly all of it has been highly critical, notably of the policies that have been introduced in England and Wales. In this chapter I will describe the main lines of criticism and assess how far they are justified. I then compare youth justice policies south of the border with those in Scotland, and discuss the extent and import of the differences. I will argue that both north and south of the border policies are often contradictory and incoherent, and that some positive initiatives in support for families, for example, and in trying to improve the experiences of looked after children, are liable to be undermined by youth justice policies – and their accompanying rhetoric – that are overwhelmingly punitive and stigmatising, and are apparently based on the assumption that children in need and young offenders are two quite distinct categories. Finally, I explore alternative approaches to youthful offending that may have the potential to be more effective in the short term and less damaging to young people's lifelong prospects.

Labour and youth justice in England and Wales

When New Labour came to power in 1997, government policy on young offenders had been overtly punitive for at least four years (Goldson 1999), and Labour in opposition, anxious about appearing soft on law and order, had essentially acquiesced in the Conservatives' ratcheting up of the rhetoric of penal toughness. So it is not surprising that, in government, New Labour should have pursued policies on youth justice whose resemblance to those of its predecessor is more striking than its difference from them. Jones (2002) stresses the sheer amount of work that went into New Labour policies in this field in the five years before the election, and it was this that enabled the then Home Secretary, Jack Straw, to produce the first White Paper on youth justice only months after the election (Home Office 1997). This paper announced what it claimed to be a radically new approach in which the 'culture of excuse' – in which young people's offending was supposedly excused rather than condemned, their parents were allowed to evade their responsibilities, and professionals in the system were habituated to delay, avoidance of effective action and lack of public scrutiny – was to be swept away and replaced by a culture of responsibility. Since then, a rhetoric of innovation and radical rejection of the policies of the past has been maintained, especially in the pronouncements of the Youth Justice Board, whose 'Year Zero' style explicitly treats as irrelevant all policy, practice and research preceding its own creation in 1998 (Jones 2002, Pitts 2001).

But the actual content of the legislation tells a different story. The first new Act, the Crime and Disorder Act of 1998, did indeed introduce a wide range of new measures, but it is not difficult to imagine that, if the Conservatives had remained in power, they would have done something similar. Conservative criminal justice legislation in 1993, 1994 and 1997 had increased the scope of custodial sentencing (in a sharp reversal of the previous Conservative government's policies, as expressed in the 1991 Criminal Justice Act), and this pattern was followed in the 1998 Act, with the Detention and Training Order. Arguably, however, Labour broke new ground by presenting custody as a positive option not only for the law-abiding public but also for young offenders. Similarly, the replacement of police cautions by a much less discretionary system of reprimands and final warnings continued a process of restricting the scope of diversion from prosecution begun by the Conservatives in 1993 (again reversing their own previous policy). None of the Act's other measures – Action Plan Orders, Anti-Social Behaviour Orders, Reparation Orders, Parenting Orders, Child Safety Orders and child curfews – represents a clear departure from the punitive orientation of Conservative policy after 1993.

Pitts (2003: 88) cites Jack Straw as claiming that the Crime and Disorder Act represented 'the most radical shake-up of youth justice in 30 years', but what the Act changed was not the ends of youth justice but the means by which they were to be pursued. In particular, Youth Offending Teams were established with the aim of increasing efficiency through improved inter-agency cooperation. In identifying what is new about 'the new youth justice' (Goldson 2000a), one feature that deserves notice is a revival of a policy commitment to what John Pratt (1989) called the third model of youth justice – neither justice nor welfare but 'corporatism'. Greater inter-agency and inter-professional cooperation in criminal justice had been high on the government's agenda in the late 1980s and early 1990s, only to be abandoned after 1993, when a punitive populist approach swept all before it. Labour's commitment to joined-up solutions to 'joined-up' problems (Social Exclusion Unit 2001) produced a more rigorous version of inter-agency cooperation than the Conservatives had aspired to, and the 1998 Act provided it with a statutory basis for the first time, not only in Youth Offending Teams but in crime and disorder partnerships and the Youth Justice Board itself.

More substantive innovation of a kind that might be seen as reflecting a strand in New Labour thinking that is distinct from mere punitiveness came in two subsequent pieces of legislation: the 1999 Youth Justice and Criminal Evidence Act and the 2000 Criminal Justice and Court Services Act. Both include elements of restorative justice, the former in the shape of the Referral Order, the latter in the idea of 'restorative cautioning' (Holdaway *et al* 2001). Interest in restorative justice is not the preserve of New Labour, but it is consistent with the communitarian concerns of 'Third Way' thinking (Muncie 2000) and with the commitment that follows from these to encourage public participation in resolving crime problems and to promote dialogue and social reintegration. Referral Orders are meant to replace conditional discharges and to be the normal response to offending that brings young people to court for the first time. The referral is to a Youth Offender Panel, which includes a representative of the local community, and provides a setting for informal dialogue and exchange about the reasons for and effects of the offending, and what can be done to put matters right. The Panel's work is to be informed by considerations of 'restoration, reintegration and responsibility' (Home Office 1997: 32). The Youth Court itself has been encouraged to develop a less legalistic style of conducting its business, to allow more opportunities for dialogue (Home Office 1998), though how far it has done so seems to be unknown; and research on the introduction of Referral Orders suggests that in most cases it is not meaningful to speak of anything having been restored to victims (Earle and Newburn 2002). The Referral Order has been criticised by those who are unhappy about all forms of restorative justice on the grounds that it threatens to abuse the rights of (alleged) offenders (e.g. Haines 2000) and, more persuasively, by those who are unhappy about the abandonment of diversion or minimum intervention as policy aims in favour of an explicit commitment to early intervention (e.g. Goldson 2000b); this follows, of course, from the starting point 'no more excuses'. These measures may therefore be failing to realise their communitarian and restorative aims, but the aims are present nevertheless, and I will return to the positive potential of restorative and participative approaches at the end of this chapter.

New Labour and its critics

Newburn (2002) and Smith (2003a) are among the very few academic voices that have suggested there might be anything positive about New Labour's reforms; the great majority of academic comment has been exclusively hostile, both towards what is taken to be the punitive, authoritarian orientation of policy overall and towards specific measures. So, in addition to the criticisms of Referral Orders, writers have attacked the abolition of the presumption of *doli incapax* (incapable of crime) for 10–13 year olds (Bandalli 2000), the blaming and stigmatisation of parents (Drakeford and

McCarthy 2000), the continuing over-reliance on custody (Moore, 2000), the infringement of children's rights in Child Safety Orders and curfews (Bell 1999) and the potential for such infringement in Anti-Social Behaviour Orders (Jones 2002). The very name of Youth Offending Teams is taken as an ominous sign that young people's needs are being made secondary to their offending, as is their organisational separation from child and family social work (Goldson 2002). Their inter-agency constitution is also held to be likely to promote more punitive reactions to young people's offending. Jones (2002) lists these criticisms and summarises the main lines of the overall critique as follows: New Labour's youth justice policies erode children's rights, are in contradiction with policies on child care and protection, blame and punish parents (in reality, mothers) and have discarded everything that is known about effective practice. They will inevitably lead to the further social exclusion of vulnerable children and young people, through widening the scope of criminalisation and increasing the use of custody.

It would be wrong not to attend seriously to such critics, or to treat them simply as disappointed Labour supporters who misguidedly hoped for better things when the party finally came into power. The writers cited are by no means all radical academics professionally committed to perpetual dissatisfaction with whatever government does; they include people with long and distinguished experience of youth justice as social work or legal practitioners, and with a demonstrable commitment to the welfare of young people. They deserve to be taken seriously, and there is no doubt that there is much force in their criticisms. But there is also a sense, certainly from the earlier critiques, of minds made up in advance: even if New Labour could not realistically have been expected to move youth justice policy in a direction that could lead to accusations of being soft on crime, there is still a sense of disappointment, of having been let down. (The sheer volume of published work, starting very shortly after the 1997 election, is testimony to this strength of feeling.) The criticisms tend to predict failure, or worse, rather than to demonstrate it; they assume that political rhetoric accurately describes what is actually happening; they tend to be abstract rather than informed by data from research; and they rely heavily on rights-based arguments rather than on considerations of young people's needs and problems. The abstract and general nature of these criticisms is inevitable, given that they appeared before research data became available, but it is a limitation, as is their focus on rights without specification of what human goods the rights are meant to safeguard: rights are liable to become 'vacuous' (Braithwaite 2002: 167) if they remain abstracted from moral purpose, and have often been invoked in the cause of self-interested professional legalism.

However, research has begun to appear that will allow for the critics' predictions to be tested (and it is surely to the government's credit that it has devoted substantial resources to the evaluation of its new measures). For example, Ghate and Ramalla (2002) evaluated Parenting Orders and parenting programmes, and found that, contrary to predictions, over 90 per cent of parents (in line with predictions, over 80 per cent were mothers) found the programmes helpful and would recommend them to other parents in difficulties. Earle and Newburn (2002) evaluated the introduction of Referral Orders, and found that the Youth Offender Panels introduced to implement such orders had been successfully established, managed to recruit lay members, and worked in a way that allowed young people and their parents to state their position in an atmosphere that conveyed hope and respect. The great majority of young people who attended meetings signed a contract, which in most cases contained some element of reparative action. Victims, however, were involved in only six per cent of all cases: this is hardly a story of overwhelming success, and it is still open to critics to dismiss the idea of Referral Orders on principle, but it does show that a radical and risky new measure was implemented as intended, with a genuine element of lay participation. Holdaway et al (2001) evaluated the pilot Youth Offending Teams and concluded that despite some organisational problems – such as uneven levels of commitment from different agencies and lack of clarity about responsibilities in central government – the new teams had 'added value' to youth justice practice and demonstrated a model of cooperative inter-agency working that could be useful in other fields, such as child protection and community safety. These emerging research findings, while certainly not telling a story of unalloyed success, still suggest that the new measures may not prove as disastrous as the critics have tended to claim.

The available statistics on the number of juveniles entering the criminal justice system also fail to support the claims made by the fiercest critics of 'the new youth justice'. The Home Office (2001a) shows that the number of juveniles cautioned or convicted for indictable offences in 2000 was substantially lower than in 1990 – at the end of the decade when what are generally regarded as successful forms of practice with young offenders had developed. It is difficult to infer from this the massive extension of surveillance and control that critics have suggested is entailed by the government's youth justice strategy since 1997. The authors of the Criminal Statistics (Home Office 2001a: 100) note the decline in the number of younger (10–14 year olds) males entering the system and suggest that it may reflect widespread use by the police of informal warnings. This would presumably not be a practice Jack Straw or his successor David Blunkett would approve of, redolent as it is of the culture of excuse, so it may be that as the police are brought into line under the new culture of responsibility the scope for this informal method of diversion will decrease. To date, though, the figures do not suggest that the net of disciplinary control has been widened so as to catch more young people in its punitive mesh.

The statistics on young people in custody provide stronger support for the critics' arguments. Newburn (2002) notes that the trend towards a greater use of custody for young people continued after 1997. The Home

Office (2001b: 52) analysis of trends over time shows that the number of sentenced young offenders in custody dropped by one-half between 1980 and 1993, but then began rising steadily, so that by 2000 it was two-thirds higher than seven years before. Elkins and Olangundoye (2001) give the average number of sentenced young male prisoners in 2000 as 8070, and of sentenced young females as 380; at the June census date in 2001 the figures were 8320 and 390, respectively (Home Office 2003: 49); 23 per cent of this population were 17 years old or under, representing an increase of six per cent over the previous year. The authors of the latest *Prison Statistics* (Home Office 2003: 50) comment that there have been annual increases in the number of sentenced young offenders since 1993, with the exception of 1999. It is clear that the long-term upward trend was maintained after the 1998 Act, though the rate of increase is not as dramatic as some critics have suggested (Pitts 2001). Since fewer juveniles were being criminalised in the years immediately following the Crime and Disorder Act than ten years previously, a far higher proportion of those who did enter the system must have received custodial sentences. It is not clear how far this change is a result specifically of the reform of youth justice, but it is hard not to read it as a result of the continuation under Labour of the kind of rhetoric that characterised the last of the Conservative governments – a rhetoric that presented youth crime as a problem spiralling out of control, and made clear to sentencers that there was no reason why they should seek to avoid the use of imprisonment; indeed, in Labour's version of this, custody could actually benefit young offenders. Given this 'down-tariffing' of imprisonment, it is inevitable that the increased use of community penalties for young offenders from 1990–2000 (before Referral Orders came on stream) should have brought under statutory supervision young people whose offending was at a level that would previously have attracted less intrusive sentences. While it would be irrational to regard community supervision as inherently damaging, or even as more likely to do harm than good, it seems clear that young people who offend are more likely than in the early 1990s to receive sentences that not only entail some intrusion into their personal and family lives but also may, in the event of a subsequent conviction, increase the risk of a custodial sentence later on.

Thus, while some of the criticism of Labour's youth justice strategy has been exaggerated and polemical, and not well supported by what is actually known about the effects of the innovations, there are good grounds for thinking that under Labour the proportionate use of custody has increased. It seems unlikely that the government will take the electoral risk, as it sees it, of listening to those in the judiciary and the prison and probation services who warn that the prison system is under severe stress and that many who receive prison sentences would be better dealt with in another way. The case of Scotland, discussed below, presents some instructive differences as well as some worrying similarities.

Youth justice in Scotland

The differences between the Scottish youth justice system and that of England and Wales provide perhaps the best known and most obvious contrast between the two jurisdictions. The Scottish Children's Hearings System (CHS) was established following the Social Work (Scotland) Act of 1968, and represents a thoroughgoing commitment to treating children who offend (under the age of 16 years old) as children in need and not as young offenders. The CHS has survived largely intact despite occasional political scepticism and repeated criticism from advocates of rights-based approaches (Lockyer and Stone 1998) for its insistence that needs, not rights, are the focus of its work. Legal representation at hearings is specifically prohibited by the legislation, though a solicitor can attend as a 'friend' of the child or family; proceedings are deliberately informal, with a minimum of legalistic jargon and ritual; the adversarial model of a criminal court has no place in a hearing; and the aim is to promote open discussion of problems and possibilities with a view to reaching agreement among all present on what would be a helpful and appropriate response to the offence (conceived as one among several 'grounds of referral'). Considering the agitation of some commentators south of the border about the supposed lack of attention to children's formal legal rights in the introduction of the Referral Order, for example, it is hard to imagine what their reaction would be to the CHS – whose existence is surprisingly little noticed in England and Wales, and has rarely entered debates about possible reforms of the system there.

In Scotland, the anti-custodial agenda survived after 1993, and in general law and order issues, among them youth crime, had for a long time a lower profile than south of the border (McIvor 1996). Whether this is still the case is doubtful. The main contribution of the Labour government to the development of youth justice in Scotland was not any criminal justice legislation but the devolution of political power. The creation of the Scottish Parliament has allowed law and order issues to become more overtly politicised, and introduced policy uncertainties where previously the main lines of policy were based on a broad consensus. The CHS, in particular, was seen (rightly) as a distinctively Scottish achievement, which enjoyed the support of those who worked within it, of the police and social workers, and of the majority of politicians. Since devolution it has become the target of more hostile criticism. There is no reason to suppose that youth crime is an increasing problem in Scotland – rather the opposite (Smith 2003b). Crime rates in Scotland have overall been persistently lower than in England and Wales, and the crime survey evidence is that they have fallen over the past 20 years (MVA 2000); and, importantly, this fall has occurred without an increase in the prison population of anything approaching the proportion by which it has increased south of the border. But it would be impossible to

infer this from the pronouncements of the main political parties. This politicisation of youth crime helps to explain an apparent loss of confidence in
the CHS. In November 1999, the Scottish Executive commissioned a review
of youth crime, and the report of the group that undertook the review was
published in June 2000 (Scottish Executive 2000). It was strongly in favour
of maintaining the established approach to young offenders, based on the
principle that their welfare should be the paramount consideration in deciding how to respond to an offence. More, it proposed an experimental extension of the welfare principle to 16 and 17 year-olds, through a 'bridging
pilot scheme' that would take young offenders of this age out of the Sheriff
Courts and into the CHS. This clear recommendation was, however, not
quickly taken up (it was found to require new legislation) and the Scottish
Executive began to sound much more cautious about the virtues of the
CHS, let alone about its extension to an older group of offenders.

The main opposition party in the Scottish Parliament, the Scottish
National Party (SNP), has – rather surprisingly – been sceptical about
whether the CHS is the right forum in which to deal with (older) young
offenders. Despite the evidence of the Scottish Crime Survey, the SNP's pronouncements on youth crime have (rather like New Labour's when in opposition) suggested that the problem is worsening and that no adequate policy
exists to deal with it. A press release on 2 October 2002, for instance (see
www.snp.org.uk) claimed that the party had found a 'secret spin plan' by
the Scottish Executive that showed the 'truth about youth crime', and that
the relevant ministers, worried about appearing 'soft', were covering up an
'absolute disaster' in their youth crime policies. In a speech in the previous
month, the SNP's spokesperson on youth justice told her audience that the
CHS was 'overburdened', and that it was wrong to 'treat 16 and 17 year-
olds as if they were just children'. (There are echoes of 'No more excuses'
here, although the SNP presumably arrived at its position independently.)
The Scottish Executive (2001) in its action plan for 2002 did make a commitment to legislating for the pilot scheme recommended by the advisory
group, but its tone was much less confidently pro-welfare than the earlier
report had been. Subsequently, and no doubt partly in response to the SNP's
claims, the Executive became still less confident; a press release of June
2002 praised the CHS and said there was 'little evidence to support its radical replacement' (Scottish Executive 2002). Someone, then, had been talking about radically replacing it. There was also a U-turn on the issue of
youth courts. Whyte (2000: 124) cites the then deputy minister for children
as saying in 1999 that Scotland 'will not go down the youth court route',
but in 2002 the Executive announced a project to assess the feasibility of
youth courts for persistent offenders aged 16–17 years old, with enough
flexibility to include some 15 year-olds. Rather than extending the welfare
principle to an older age group, this would extend the punitive principle to
a younger one.

There is no doubt that the CHS has allowed for forms of practice with young offenders, even those whose offending was persistent and serious, that are virtually unimaginable south of the border. The Freagarrach project, for example, worked with most of the serious and persistent juvenile offenders (as judged by the number of times they were charged by the police) in central Scotland on a completely voluntary basis, and produced very promising results in terms of known reoffending (Lobley *et al* 2001). Hardly anyone contacted by the researchers about the project thought that its work needed in some way to be tightened up or made more rigorous and demanding, or that there should be some punitive sanction for young people who reoffended or failed to respond to what the project offered. All of this is in dramatic contrast with practice with persistent young offenders south of the border, for whom the Youth Justice Board has demanded intensive surveillance (involving electronic monitoring and voice recognition technologies) and almost full-time attendance at programmes, under the aptly named Intensive Supervision and Surveillance Programme – which uses a criterion of persistence in offending which is less stringent than that used by Freagarrach. The ideological climate is sufficiently different in Scotland for a project like Freagarrach to receive government support, to develop its work and to survive (though, despite favourable publicity, no project quite like Freagarrach has appeared elsewhere). Anybody interested in more inclusive, responsive and supportive work with young offenders must hope that the different Scottish climate persists – and can dream that it might be exported south of the border. It is as well to recognise, however, that the political pressures that led to New Labour's determination not to be outflanked on law and order issues also exist in Scotland, and that the CHS itself, the keystone of Scottish juvenile justice, is no longer regarded as inviolable.

Doing good by stealth

The welfare approach to young offenders, then, has been ostensibly abandoned in England and Wales and is under pressure even in Scotland. But there is a contradiction within government policy that was foreshadowed in the famous slogan used by Tony Blair when he was shadow Home Secretary: 'tough on crime, tough on the causes of crime'. Toughness on crime has been amply and proudly demonstrated since 1997; toughness on the causes of crime has been much less visible. Toynbee and Walker (2001), reviewing the performance of the first New Labour government, write of the twin-track approach of policy: while loudly announcing that there would be 'no more excuses' for youth crime, the government defined poverty as the essential cause of crime, and embarked on a range of measures to alleviate it and to support the poorest families and communities, but – with a few exceptions such as the New Deal for the young unemployed, which could be presented as involving a bracing element of coercion – it did so almost in secret. Committed to avoiding any rise in income tax during its first term, the government was keen to keep a low profile for the various redistributive initiatives it undertook. Not all of New Labour's policies on children and families have been punitive and stigmatising, though one has to look behind the headlines to find this out.

The Sure Start programme, for example, works with children and their families in the poorest electoral wards in the country. It provides pre-school education, family counselling and support from social workers, and intensive advice and help from health visitors. It was influenced by research on the long-term outcomes of these forms of early intervention that found positive results in adolescence and adulthood for children from disadvantaged areas (and for their parents) in terms of lower levels of criminal involvement, better mental health, better educational and employment records and greater stability in family relationships (Karoly *et al* 1998). Involvement with Sure Start is voluntary; it has no connections with the criminal justice system; and its interventions are designed to be supportive, not stigmatising. It represents a very different approach to disadvantaged children and families from that of most of the criminal justice legislation. The same is true of the work of the Children and Young Persons Unit, established in 2000 to coordinate government initiatives on child and family poverty and given the task of managing the Children's Fund, through which the main voluntary organisations for children and families receive resources for preventative work with vulnerable children. The Children and Young Persons Unit (2001) declared a commitment to reducing the need for custodial sentences for young people at the same time as the Home Office produced another White Paper that announced a further expansion of the prison system.

The government has also taken action to improve the situation of looked-after children, a social group particularly at risk of long-term disadvantage and of criminal involvement (Taylor 2002). The Quality Protects programme (Department of Health 1998) is meant to transform social services for children by improving the quality of their care, and to improve their life chances by supporting them at school and on leaving care, and reducing their involvement in offending. The Children (Leaving Care) Act of 2000, implemented in October 2001, gives local authorities new responsibilities for young people leaving care: they must keep in touch with formerly looked after young people until they reach the age of 21 years old, and each young person must have a personal advisor who will help in drawing up and seeing through a 'Pathway Plan'. It is too early to assess how much of an improvement this will bring about, and Taylor (2002) identifies a number of potential problems (for instance, what will happen to young people whose relationship with the local authority has broken down?); but it is clearly positive that the government should have shown such interest in the experiences of looked-after children both during and, importantly, after their time in care.

Government policy in this field recognises that rates of offending among young people who are or have been looked-after are higher than for the young population as a whole, and aims to reduce the various disadvantages that contribute to this. But government policy also entails that if a looked after young person does become involved in offending, he or she is at once liable to be defined as something quite other than a child (or young person) with needs and problems. The same is true of a young person from a poor neighbourhood with high levels of unemployment, low levels of educational achievement, high levels of crime and disorder, and so on. Toynbee and Walker (2001) wrote of a 'twin-track' approach, but this image implies that the tracks are close to each other and lead in the same direction. We need an image instead that conveys that once a young person offends (or is offi- cially known to have offended) he or she is meant immediately to cease to have any claim on our sympathy or understanding (Goldson 2002). The child in need, deserving supportive attention, becomes the young offender, deserving only just deserts.

Even though the punishments that have actually been imposed on young people who offend have, so far, been less drastic than much critical com- mentary has implied, it is easy and tempting to conclude that there is little anyone can do to change the direction of current policy. New Labour is, arguably, inherently so anxious about the possibility of being thought soft on crime that it will never take the risk of sounding anything other than harshly punitive. It has evidence, after all, that people are much more likely to think that young offenders are treated too leniently than that they are treated too harshly (Mattinson and Mirrlees-Black 2000). To be outflanked by the Conservatives on law and order issues, as the Labour/Liberal Democrat coalition risks being by the SNP north of the border, would represent a return to Labour's worst electoral nightmare of long-term unelectability.

There may well be force in such an argument. But we should remember that in the fairly recent past a strongly punitive official line from govern- ment was accompanied by the development of practice with young people in trouble that reduced the numbers entering the criminal justice system and going into custody (Smith 1999). The 1980s was the decade of the triumph of Thatcherism and the radical erosion of the welfare state. But it was also a decade that, in England and Wales, saw practitioners in youth justice gradually reversing the punitiveness of the late 1970s through intelligent, informed approaches to their work based on a sophisticated recognition of the connections between decisions on individual cases and longer-term out- comes within the system (for example, that well-intentioned early interven- tion could increase the chances of repressive interventions later on). It may be that social work and probation practitioners have less freedom of manoeuvre now than they did in the 1980s: the Youth Justice Board and the

National Probation Service were established partly to ensure that this became the case. But it is certain that workers in other parts of the system – in the judiciary and the prisons, for example – are unhappy with the prospect of a drift into a response to young people's offending that offers nothing but coercion, surveillance and punishment. Social workers concerned to work for change would not lack allies. And, as we have seen, there are contradictions within the government's own range of policies that may provide opportunities for alternatives to punitiveness to be developed.

Conclusion: Towards more inclusive practice?

I will conclude with hopes and possibilities rather than with certainties about how policy might be influenced in more socially inclusive directions. Sure Start and similar programmes have the potential to produce a base of knowledge and understanding of good practice that could expose the limitations of a purely repressive response to young people who offend. Certainly, they should make it more difficult to ignore the complex causes of youth crime, and attribute it solely to wickedness or indiscipline. Goldson (2002: 693) cites the American penal reformer, Jerome Miller, on the advantages of policies that 'save us from the messiness of knowing too much about delinquents, their families, their lives, their opportunities, their backgrounds or their experiences'. Social programmes like Sure Start make such comforting ignorance less easy to maintain.

There are also, as noted above, restorative, communitarian strands in New Labour policy that could, if developed, help to promote a more inclusive approach. At present there is – and for some time there has been – a gap between aspiration and achievement in restorative justice in Britain: the high promise of the approach as persuasively described by Braithwaite (2002) seems remote from the modest realities of practice in the context of Referral Orders, for example (Earle and Newburn 2002). But a restorative response to young people's offending has proved feasible elsewhere, and there are elements in recent policy that at least allow for its feasibility to be explored in England and Wales, along with the potential for greater public participation in resolving crime-related problems. (The CHS could have been specifically designed for a restorative approach, though Whyte (2000) suggests that its potential in this regard has been less, not more, exploited in recent years.) Allen (2002) argues that public attitudes to crime and punishment are not as straightforwardly punitive as is generally believed, and that there is much scope for marketing alternatives to prison (see also Hastings *et al* 2002). The British Crime Survey evidence is that much of the public's impression of crime and the criminal justice system is based on ignorance and unnecessary fear: many people believe both that crime is increasing and that lenient sentencing is partly to blame (Mattinson and Mirrlees-Black 2000). Opportunities for active participation in dealing with crime problems could be a means of enabling people to discover a sense of control instead of a sense of powerlessness, and they would become better informed about the realities of crime and criminal justice in the process (the commercial media cannot be relied on to give this information). What is often regarded as a New Labour think-tank, the Institute for Public Policy Research, has a Criminal Justice Forum that has worked on exactly these ideas, so there is interest in circles from which the government draws its ideas in ways of engaging the public in responses to crime, as is envisaged by advocates of restorative justice (Edwards 2002). None of this guarantees that positive and effective alternatives to exclusionary policies will develop, but there are enough signs of interest in them for despair to be premature on the part of criminal justice practitioners or troubled young people and those who care about them.

References

Allen, R. (2002) 'What does the public really think about prison?', *Criminal Justice Matters*, 49: 6–7.

Bandalli, S. (2000) 'Children, responsibility and the new youth justice', in Goldson, B. (ed.), *The New Youth Justice*, Lyme Regis: Russell House.

Bell, C. (1999) 'Appealing for justice for children and young people: A critical analysis of the Crime and Disorder Bill 1998', in B. Goldson, (ed.), *Youth Justice: Contemporary policy and practice*, Aldershot: Ashgate.

Braithwaite, J. (2002) *Restorative Justice and Responsive Regulation*, Oxford: Oxford University Press.

Children and Young Persons Unit (2001) *Tomorrow's Future: Building a strategy for children and young people*, London: Children and Young Persons Unit.

Department of Health (1998) *Quality Protects: Transforming children's services*, London: Department of Health.

Drakeford, M. and McCarthy, K. (2000) 'Parents, responsibility and the new youth justice', in Goldson, B. (ed.), *The New Youth Justice*, Lyme Regis: Russell House.

Earle, R. and Newburn, T. (2002) 'Creative tensions? Young offenders, restorative justice and the introduction of referral orders', *Youth Justice*, 1 (3): 3–13.

Edwards, L. (2002) 'Public involvement in the criminal justice system', *Criminal Justice Matters*, 49: 16–17.

Elkins, M. and Olagundoye, J. (2001) *The Prison Population in 2000: A statistical review* (Home Office Research Findings 154), London: Home Office.

Ghate, D. and Ramalla, M. (2002) *National Evaluation of the Youth Justice Board's Parenting Programme*, London: Youth Justice Board.

Goldson, B. (1999) 'Youth (in)justice: Contemporary developments in policy and practice', in B. Goldson, (ed.), *Youth Justice: Contemporary policy and practice*, Aldershot: Ashgate.

Goldson, B. (ed.) (2000a) *The New Youth Justice*, Lyme Regis: Russell House.

Goldson, B. (2000b) 'Wither diversion? Interventionism and the new youth justice', in Goldson, B. (ed.), *The New Youth Justice*, Lyme Regis: Russell House.

Goldson, B. (2002) 'New Labour, social justice and children: Political calculation and the deserving–undeserving schism', *British Journal of Social Work*, 32(6): 683–695.

Haines, K. (2000) 'Referral Orders and Youth Offender Panels: Restorative approaches and the new youth justice', in B. Goldson (ed.), *The New Youth Justice*, Lyme Regis: Russell House.

Hastings, G., Stead, M. and MacFadyean, L. (2002) 'Reducing prison numbers: Does marketing hold the key?', *Criminal Justice Matters*, 49: 20–21.

Holdaway, S., Davidson, N., Dignan, J., *et al* (2001) *New Strategies to Address Youth Offending: The national evaluation of pilot Youth Offending Teams* (Home Office Occasional Paper 69), London: Home Office.

Home Office (1997) *No More Excuses: A new approach to tackling youth crime in England and Wales* (Cm 3809), London: Home Office.

Home Office (1998) *Opening up Youth Court Proceedings*, London: Home Office.

Home Office (2001a) *Criminal Statistics England and Wales 2000* (Cm 5312), London: The Stationery Office.

Home Office (2001b) *Prison Statistics England and Wales 2000* (Cm 5250), London: The Stationery Office.

Home Office (2003) *Prison Statistics England and Wales 2001* (Cm 5743), London: The Stationery Office.

Jones, D.W. (2002) 'Questioning New Labour's youth justice strategy: A review article', *Youth Justice*, 1(3): 14–26.

Lobley, D., Smith, D. and Stern, C. (2001) *Freagarrach: An evaluation of a project for persistent juvenile offenders*, Edinburgh: Scottish Executive.

Lockyer, A. and Stone, F.H. (eds) (1998) *Juvenile Justice in Scotland: Twenty-five years of the welfare approach*, Edinburgh: T. and T. Clark.

McIvor, G. (1996) 'Recent developments in Scotland', in McIvor, G. (ed.), *Working with Offenders*, London: Jessica Kingsley.

Mattinson, J. and Mirrlees-Black, C. (2000) *Attitudes to Crime and Justice: Findings from the 1998 British Crime Survey*, London: Home Office.

Muncie, J. (2000) 'Pragmatic realism? Searching for criminology in the new youth justice', in Goldson, B. (ed.), *The New Youth Justice*, Lyme Regis: Russell House.

MVA (2000) *The 2000 Scottish Crime Survey: First results* (Crime and Criminal Justice Research Findings 51), Edinburgh: Scottish Executive.

Newburn, T. (2002) 'Young people, crime and youth justice', in M. Maguire, R. Morgan, R. Reiner, (eds) *The Oxford Handbook of Criminology*, 3rd edn, Oxford: Clarendon Press.

Pitts, J. (2001) 'Korrectional Karaoke: New Labour and the zombification of youth justice', *Youth Justice*, 1(2):3–16.

Pitts, J. (2003) 'Youth justice in England and Wales', in R. Matthews, and J. Young, (eds) *The New Politics of Crime and Punishment*, Cullompton: Willan.

Pratt, J. (1989) 'Corporatism: The third model of juvenile justice', *British Journal of Criminology*, 29(2): 236–254.

Scottish Executive (2000) *Report of the Advisory Group on Youth Crime*, Edinburgh: Scottish Executive.

Scottish Executive (2001) *Scotland's Action Programme to Reduce Youth Crime 2002*, Edinburgh: Scottish Executive.

Scottish Executive (2002) *Executive's Youth Crime Review: Report and statement on recommendations*, Edinburgh: Scottish Executive.

Smith, D. (1999) 'Social work with young people in trouble: memory and prospect', in Goldson, B. (ed.), *The New Youth Justice*, Aldershot: Ashgate.

Smith, D. (2003a) 'New Labour and youth justice', *Children and Society*, 17: 226–235.

Smith, D. (2003b) 'Comparative criminal justice: North and south of the border', *Vista: Perspectives on Probation*, 8(1): 2–8.

Social Exclusion Unit (2001) *Preventing Social Exclusion*, London: Social Exclusion Unit.

Taylor, C. (2002) 'The relationship between care and criminal careers', unpublished PhD thesis, Lancaster University.

Toynbee, P. and Walker, D. (2001) *Did Things Get Better? An Audit of Labour's Successes and Failures*, London: Penguin.

Whyte, B. (2000) 'Between two stools: Youth justice in Scotland', *Probation Journal*, 47(2): 119–125.

Postscript on youth justice

Michael Fadipe and Lance Gittens-Bernard

Michael Fadipe

> My name is Michael Fadipe, I am aged 15 and of African origin. I live and was brought up in West London. Ever since the age of 13 I was wise enough to know what was going on in the streets and from there I entered into the criminal justice system. I'm not a known offender. I see myself as number one, not a criminal. I am sitting my GCSEs at an early stage and from there want to take my education further, as I see it as a key to many opportunities in life. In this book I just wanted to get my personal views across on how I see road [street culture] and the bias of the government. My dream is to be an entrepreneur, make money work for me and study law, business and psychology.

I think young people offend because of lack of education, things to do, places to go and peer pressure. For example, if a young person bumps into a bunch of boys and they force him to steal: if he refuses he gets beaten up; if he does it, he's free to go (so it's also about the young person's safety). Another example is the local youth club closes early for the night (in most cases), then shift us onto the streets when for one reason or another the young people don't choose to go home, leaving them searching for something to do. Having money problems is another example: in the society we're living in, youths want the latest Nike trainers or the latest camera mobile phones. Even members of the public looking down on youths, and peer pressure. At home young people may feel it's their responsibility to put food on the table because the parent may not be able to afford it, or to look after their siblings, or buy things for the family, and they may think the only way they can do these things is through crime.

I think extra help is needed for young offenders who come from disadvantaged family backgrounds, such as help with schooling, family support, money every six months for clothing or short breaks for the ones who aren't so fortunate. There should be more projects to help the young offender get an opportunity to get things which he/she maybe thinks are unattainable without resorting to crime: e.g. if young people wanted to go to Wales rock climbing or canoeing, etc., they would have to commit themselves to participate in all the other things that the project's doing. There should also be support for the young offender's family so that the young offender doesn't return to the same environment and go back to square one, like if there's something wrong in the family or in the local area. I'd like to see politicians living with a disadvantaged family for a week and see what it's like, so that they experience what youths and their families feel. They're not working with us; they don't consult us about anything.

I think good ways of dealing with youth crime are more community work, more offence-related work, victim awareness, more projects for young people to use their time constructively (not just the one-off Summer Splash, which only offers leisure activities and education during the summer months), more apprenticeships, jobs/professions, for example. If a young person was to use all his time graffitying and was to get caught and forced to clean it, it would then help the young person to realise the time and effort needed to clean it and the effect of what the young person did. On the other hand, the government should channel that interest because the young person could be the next best artist, so an art course/apprenticeship can also be an option: whilst the young person is serving their punishment they could do the art course at the same time (buy two for the price of one!).

I think the bad ways of dealing with crime is just automatically locking a youth up or sending him straight to the crown court. I think youth courts should have more power because the surroundings are a bit more laid-back, and they should be able to deal with an offence that would otherwise go to the crown court. Youth courts look more at your background and if they see an opportunity for you to change, they'll help you, whereas the crown court is not as laid-back, it's tense.

Putting a youth in the environment of an adult offender (like throwing them in Securicor vans alongside murderers and drunks) is very uncomfortable and has a psychological effect on the youth; also shifting them around different places (like from one prison to another) is bad. Also being constantly reminded of your offence by the police (getting stopped on the street and 'we know you, you're that one that did this', etc.) has a negative effect on a young person and reinforces negative labels. The police should have better training in dealing with young people and how not to discriminate against young black males. I don't see white young people getting stopped so much. The police are just always on your case if you're black; white young people don't get so much hassle.

In short, criminal justice agencies are nosey and I believe there should be a barrier in how much they know; it's like an invasion into our private lives (*we* don't know what goes on behind *their* doors). I personally think it's wrong. At least leave it down to the youth and his family to tell them how much they want the agencies to know. Right now with the increase of surveillance (and all the rest of it) it seems a youth cannot walk down the street without being stopped by police or being told where you can and cannot go. Whatever happened to human rights? It doesn't count for us. It seems youths of today have already been penalised. The other question is how would it reflect on the parents with those agencies breathing down their necks, saying they're failures, and all the hassle on them. I think the agencies need to step back.

I honestly don't think the government is soft on crime. In actual fact I think being placed in custody is harsh enough: away from family and those you love and care for. Especially if you're placed far away from home, where a phone call is the only thing you look forward to. And in most cases a visit is out of the question. If it was years ago, we might have got away with crime, but nowadays it's a slim chance you'd get away with it, what with the increasing level of police on the streets, the YOT offices, three appointments a week, even down to being followed around like a dog with its owner. You can't play on the streets any more, what with the police and the community patrols and everything.

I think the right way to go about reducing crime is by offering youths a second chance, e.g. offering them education, help, accommodation and youth projects. If the youth doesn't take hold of it, it's down to him/her. But I believe it will help the youth become steadfast and disciplined in the long run, e.g. the Intensive Supervision and Surveillance Programme (ISSP) which is an alternative to custody. Not putting on lots of pressure but making them learn there's more to life than crime. Maybe bringing in past criminals/non-criminals or somebody in a profession who has come from a bad background, etc., and has succeeded in life, to show youths.

It is true that the government is increasingly talking about punishing rather than helping young offenders because the government doesn't want to seem soft on crime. Instead they should be looking at the background of youths, their culture and the community/society the young person is living in. I would like to see politicians seeing the streets through our eyes, the dangers (fights and gangs) and good times (chilling, relaxing with friends) on the streets. I think their main concern is about what other people think of them. Instead they should be looking at the bigger picture, which is not just locking young people up.

Lance Gittens-Bernard

> My name is Lance Gittens-Bernard and I was brought up in Hammersmith, West London. I'm 16 years of age and I attend a local school where I'm taking nine GCSEs and am expected to get A–C grades for eight of them. The area in which I was brought up has been labelled as producing many criminals but fortunately I have been able to take the straight and narrow path by keeping myself occupied with music and sports and also having the right type of friends around me who are not

afraid to tell someone when they've done wrong. I wanted to write this postscript because I would like to find out how politicians have decided what is the best way to deal with young offenders. I think I'm able to argue my point, and I won't stop until my point is heard!

From what I have read in this chapter, I think the British government believes that putting young people down by labelling and incarcerating them is the right thing to do, but deep down they know that there are other ways of dealing with the problem. For instance, you could sit the young person down and talk to him/her and try to find out why they offended and what ways you could help them to not re-offend. Youth Offending Teams are good because you can talk to the workers and know it won't be relayed back to the police – it's like a trust between them and you.

Sending young people to prison for minor offences is stupid because all the government is doing is paving a path for the young person to consistently re-offend because the government has robbed them of the chance of having a proper education. And whilst they are inside, their minds become corrupted by criminals who are inside for more serious offences.

I think that the government is too tough on crime, although with serious crimes they are correct in what they do. I'm not being hypocritical. I think they should review ways they deal with less serious young offenders instead of jumping straight to a decision to imprison them. The government doesn't want to use different ways of dealing with youth offending because they would rather get it over and done with than deal with the problem in a more effective way.

David Smith talks about schemes where young offenders meet with the victim. I'm not sure that would be successful all the time due to the fact that the young person would inevitably feel uncomfortable around the victim. But in some cases if this was to happen, the offender might show sympathy for the victim if they met them face to face and could apologise. The victim most probably gains more self-esteem and it shows the offender has respect for them by apologising face to face and in a letter. I agree with the Scottish system which helps offenders as well as victims.

Politically, the politicians are trying to protect the older generation rather than trying to put straight the young offenders. Instead of helping the offender, who may come from a disadvantaged family, to gain education opportunities and teaching them awareness, politicians feel that they should help the adults/victims due to the fact that they are taxpayers. Society treats young people as a lower class. They don't really take our views into account, only if it is vitally needed like how to improve a youth project, but never when it's into politics, because older people believe that young people don't have the right views and understanding about politics.

If politicians consulted young people, it would make it easier, but their views of solving crime are to automatically put young people in prison, and if you look at the latest prison figures, many young people are inside for minor offences, whereas this could have been avoided if the government showed more interest in helping young people.

Overall, this chapter is very interesting, although many of the words (like 'rhetoric') are hard to understand.

Chapter 12

'There's helping and there's hindering': Young mothers, support and control

Alison Rolfe

Teenage motherhood is commonly viewed as a problem for young women, families and societies. The focus for concern and for intervention by policy makers is the sexual behaviour, actions and decision-making of individual young women. However, this focus detracts from the real site of difficulty, which lies in the social context within which marginalised young people live, negotiate social conditions and form relationships.

There is also widespread ambivalence about teenage mothers. Sexuality, mothering and caring form central elements to what it means to be a woman, yet young women are liable to be punished by society if they become mothers under the 'wrong' circumstances. The unspoken question running through both policy debates and media discourses is whether young women should be supported or controlled. This ambivalence has led to a policy focus on the reduction of teenage pregnancy, but a relative neglect of support for young women who become mothers.

There are differences between 'insider' and 'outsider' accounts of teenage motherhood (Phoenix 1991a), yet young women's own views of mother-hood and mothering are rarely considered. This is part of a wider tendency for young women's voices not to be heard (Taylor *et al* 1995). Listening to young women's own accounts of pregnancy and motherhood can provide a different perspective on their experiences and on how best to support them and their families and unless young women's accounts are taken into con-sideration, policy is unlikely to succeed. The young mothers whose views are presented in this chapter were mainly attenders of projects run by NCH, a national children's charity. They took part in interviews across England, in groups and individually[1], as part of a qualitative research project on the views and experiences of young women who become mothers below the age of 21 (Rolfe 2002).

The chapter begins with a review of the policy framework. This is then compared and contrasted with the views of young mothers themselves. Most of the young women see teenage motherhood as far from ideal, and consider their lives to be constrained. Ideally, they would have postponed having children until they were more settled. However, motherhood can also be a much more positive experience than is frequently thought. The young women consider this to be largely unrecognised by health and welfare professionals with whom they come into contact and who they view as having low expectations of their ability to succeed. Their accounts suggest that a shift is required, in policy and practice, towards an approach based on the strength and resilience of young people, and on the recognition that young mothers and their children can do well.

The 'problem' of teenage motherhood

The stated aim of current policy is to provide more choice, information and opportunities to young women. At the same time, this is set within a wider discursive framework in which teenage motherhood is viewed as a problem spiralling out of control. The main target of recent policy initiatives around teenage motherhood is, therefore, young people's sexual activity. In this section the research evidence on the extent and pattern of teenage motherhood is briefly reviewed. This is followed by a critical review of the current policies aimed at tackling it.

One of the key reasons given for concerns over teenage motherhood is that Britain currently has the highest teenage pregnancy rate in Western Europe[2] (Social Exclusion Unit [SEU] 1999). Since the 1960s, there has also been a marked rise in the proportion of British teenage mothers who are unmarried. However, the rate of teenage births reached its post-war peak in 1971 (Selman 1996). Furthermore, the vast majority of births to teenage women are to young women between the ages of 16 and 19. In 1999, there were 92,400 pregnancies to women under 20, of which 7400 were to under-16s (Department of Health, 2003). Recent figures show a ten per cent reduction in pregnancies amongst under-18s between 1998 and 2003 (Teenage Pregnancy Unit 2003).

Previous research indicates a number of 'risk factors' for becoming a teenage mother (SEU 1999), and suggests that pregnancy and motherhood are considerably higher amongst groups of young people who are socially excluded. For example, young mothers are much more likely to come from economically disadvantaged families (Babb 1994, Kiernan 1997, Hobcraft and Kiernan 2001). Other groups of young women 'at risk' of teenage pregnancy include those of Bangladeshi, Pakistani and African Caribbean origin (SEU 1999), and those who have been in public care. Between one in four (Biehal *et al* 1992, 1994) and one in seven (Garnett 1992) care leavers become teenage parents. However, the picture is considerably more complex than is suggested by these bare statistics. The term 'risk factors' is negatively loaded, and the presentation of such factors masks the different circumstances and experiences of individual young people.

The current policy framework

Support for teenage mothers in England is subsumed under the government's Teenage Pregnancy Strategy, which aims to halve the rate of pregnancy among under-18 year olds by 2010. In Wales and Northern Ireland, the national assemblies have similarly developed action plans on teenage pregnancy (National Assembly for Wales 2000, Department of Health, Social Services and Public Safety 2002). The Scottish Executive has established a Sexual Health Reference Group with a view to drawing up a sexual health strategy (to include teenage pregnancy) in 2003[3].

The Teenage Pregnancy Unit (TPU) was established in 1999 to implement the teenage pregnancy strategy for England, and is now part of the Directorate for Children and Families within the Department for Education and Skills (DfES). Every English top-tier local authority now has a ten-year strategy in place, agreed with health and other partners. Local coordinators are supported by a network of regional coordinators, who have the task of ensuring that the teenage pregnancy strategy is joined up with other initiatives, such as Connexions, National Healthy School Standard and Sure Start. The strategy includes measures to provide more advice and information on sex and contraception to young people.

Twenty 'Sure Start Plus' pilot projects have also been established across England. These provide each pregnant young woman with a personal adviser to help her decide whether to continue with the pregnancy or have a termination, and whether or not to consider adoption. Advisers also coordinate a support package for young parents, including childcare provision to enable them to return to education, training or employment. The aim is to increase the rate of participation by teenage mothers in education, training and work to 60 per cent by 2010. From September 2002, new national entitlement arrangements have been piloted in four areas, providing childcare support of up to £5,000 per year per child to young parents aged 16–19 years old in education. This childcare is funded by the DfES, employing registered childminders. Under the banner, 'Caring to Learn', this scheme will be extended into a universal scheme for all parents under 19 years old in education from August 2004. In addition, the Education Maintenance Allowance initiative provides young people living on a low income £30–40 a week if they stay in education. From 2003–4 local authorities in areas of social deprivation will be able to use a Vulnerable Children's Grant to improve educational support and attendance at school for mothers of school age. Finally, six semi-independent supported housing schemes are currently being run as pilot projects. These are intended for 16 and 17 year-old lone parents who are unable to live with their birth family. The aim is to provide supported housing by the end of 2003 for all teenage parents unable to live with their birth family or partner (Teenage Pregnancy Unit 2003).

Support or control?

Current policy measures are intended to provide more information to young people to enable them to make informed choices around sexual health, and should enable some young mothers to continue with education and training. However, current efforts being put into the prevention of teenage pregnancy are not being matched by support for teenage mothers. As the government-appointed Independent Advisory Group on Teenage Pregnancy points out, 'Many young parents still have very low incomes, face many obstacles in returning to education and work, and do not live in appropriate housing' (Teenage Pregnancy Unit, 2003: 39). The group advises that the government should prioritise the provision of financial incentives for young parents to return to education. They also argue the need for adequate and affordable childcare, and suitable, affordable housing.

These recommendations are important in continuing the push towards improved conditions and opportunities for young parents. However, in order to see why support for teenage mothers is still not adequate, debates over policy initiatives also need to be considered in a wider context of power relations, structures of disadvantage and oppression. It is no coincidence that fears over 'threatening youth' have become increasingly prevalent since the 1970s (Davies 1986, Scraton 1997). During this time, there has been a major shift in the terms of the debate concerning the ways in which welfare has been provided and working-class young people have become the target of increasing social control. Fears around escalating rates of teenage mothers living on benefits are part of an increasingly punitive climate in relation to vulnerable young people. There are also clear moral undertones to the debate over teenage pregnancy. In a newspaper article on teenage pregnancy in the *Times*, Tony Blair remarked, 'I believe now that it is the decent majority, who play by the rules, who want us to take a lead in defining a new moral purpose' (Blair 1999: 6). This implicitly marked out an 'indecent' minority, containing teenage mothers and their families, who do not 'play by the rules'. There is, therefore, a tension running through debates on teenage motherhood between support and social control. In this climate, it is perhaps unsurprising that young mothers' accounts are rarely sought, yet where they are, they may reveal a rather different picture.

Young mothers' accounts

During 1999 and 2000, 33 young mothers took part in research interviews, individually and in groups[4], and the following discussion draws on their accounts. All of the participants were in their teens or early 20s and had become mothers between the ages of 14 and 20, with an average age of giving birth for the first time of 17. They were living in socially deprived areas on low incomes. Around a quarter were from minority ethnic groups. Just

over two-thirds had been in care, and only one was living with both her
birth parents[5].

The main messages to emerge from these interviews are that, for most of
these young women, pregnancy was unplanned, yet by the time they
became mothers they had adjusted to their new role and 'grown up' as a
result of motherhood. They stressed that motherhood was hard work, but
that they also gained a great deal from it. However, they had to struggle
with poverty, unstable housing and with the low expectations of adults
towards them. Their accounts suggest that the experiences and meanings of
motherhood need to be socially located, and teenage motherhood understood as a means of negotiating personal and social worlds.

Teenage pregnancy and motherhood in social context

Young women living in deprived communities may not deliberately choose
pregnancy, but may view it positively if it occurs (Davies *et al* 2001).
Almost all of the pregnancies were unplanned[6] so, for most, pregnancy led
to altered plans and expectations. However, some women may not make a
definite 'plan' of pregnancy, yet may not take measures to prevent it. For
example, Trish (19 years old) remarked, 'It was like a case of, if I did, I did.
If I didn't, I didn't'. Around a third of participants said that pregnancy had
been greeted immediately with happiness, and this included many
'unplanned' pregnancies. Several young women considered termination but
decided against it. Public perceptions sometimes led young women to feel
they are in a no-win situation, of condemnation for abortion and equally
for childbirth. As Emma stated: 'You get a lot of digging. But if you was to
have an abortion, or if you was to adopt them out, "Oh, you know so-and-
so, she gave her kids away. She got rid of it" . . . . So you can't win'. Several
young women decided that, on balance, motherhood would be a positive
choice. As Ebele (17 years old) stated, 'In the end I decided to keep the baby.
You know, effectively, there was nothing to lose, and everything to gain'.

Young women who have very few prospects of training or work can find
motherhood a source of pride and satisfaction and a means of constructing
an identity when other options are limited (McRobbie 1991, Phoenix
1991b, Craine 1997). Opportunities for young women have apparently
expanded in unprecedented ways in recent years, with young women over-
taking young men in 'A' level results and the 'feminisation of labour'
enabling women to take more of a role in the workplace. However, such
shifts are extremely patchy and have been accompanied by a contraction of
opportunities for working-class young people and the 'feminisation of
poverty'. Putting off motherhood may make little sense to young working-
class women with limited opportunities (Phoenix 1991b). Young women's
traditional (and socially sanctioned) identification with the home, family

and with a caring role may be further accentuated by the lack of alternative sources of identity.

For care leavers, there may be additional considerations. Previous research suggests that they are likely to face particular difficulties in personal and social identity, stemming from trauma before going into care, instability of placements, institutionalisation and sometimes abuse in care (Department of Health 1997). On leaving care, a lack of support and stability can further compound a sense of not belonging, at least temporarily (Biehal *et al* 1995). This, added to the lack of opportunities for education, training and work for care leavers (Stein and Wade 2000), can mean that pregnancy is more of a gain than a loss. As Linda (a care leaver) stated, 'Some people want to have their babies when they're young, because they want to grow up and settle down'.

It is sometimes assumed that black young women become pregnant for different reasons than white young women, with studies of black teenagers focusing on cultural explanations (Phoenix 1992). However, there were no notable differences between the meanings of motherhood for black and white young women in this study[7]. Moreover, a focus on culture is often based on a mistaken notion of homogeneity amongst black young women, and places black young people outside of British culture (Phoenix 1992). The young women in this study described themselves variously as Black African, Black Caribbean, British Asian, Pakistani and of mixed heritage, and their experiences and cultural identities differed, though they are likely to have had a shared experience of racism. Material deprivation and social marginalisation, rather than shared culture, may be more important factors in attempting to explain early motherhood amongst young women from minority ethnic groups.

Being a 'young mum': The gains and the losses

The meanings and experiences of motherhood for the young women were, in many ways, strikingly similar to those of older women. Teenage mothers are frequently associated with an 'underclass' (Murray 1996) which rejects mainstream norms and values, but the young women who took part in the research generally subscribed to mainstream values of femininity. They wanted to be married, have good careers and be part of a traditional two-parent family. However, they differed in the specific ways in which motherhood intersected with youth, class and biography.

The young women were proud of their children and of their own mothering abilities. They all saw advantages, as well as disadvantages, to being a young mother. They felt that they would have more patience and understanding for their children, compared with older parents. Those who had become mothers over the age of 16 years old tended to feel that it would be more difficult to be a mother under 16 years old. However, most participants felt that age did not affect their mothering abilities, and they stressed that a far more important factor was the willingness to accept responsibility. For example, Sam (20 years old) stated:

> Somebody who's had their kid young, they could turn out brilliant, but you see, like, 32 year olds that don't give a crap about their kids . . . . It's not on age, it's all on responsibility.

A few young women had a history of offending or substance abuse. However, they stressed the personal and lifestyle changes that they underwent during pregnancy and the early days of motherhood. Some who had been 'in with the wrong crowd' had made a fresh start. This was seen as a key part of growing up and becoming responsible:

> You're a mum, aren't you? It's different to being a teenager and running around. You have responsibility . . . . I needed to get out of the crowd that I was in, because I would have ended up in trouble, and there were drugs floating about and the like. I needed to make a fresh start.
>
> (Jan, 21 years old)

The young women generally saw themselves as having changed, made sacrifices and 'grown up' as a result of becoming mothers. They also felt more determined to succeed now that they had children to care for, and wanted to give their children a better start in life than they had had. Whilst politicians speak of young mothers being part of a 'cycle of deprivation' (Social Exclusion Unit, 1999: 4), many were actively engaged in improving their own skills and qualifications, and others planned to do so once their children were older. One had 'A' levels and was at university. Three other young women had NVQ or BTEC qualifications, and two more were working towards 'A' levels. Several had recently enrolled for GCSE and nursing courses at college, including two who had missed a considerable time from school. Many who had previously not been particularly interested or motivated in their education suggested they had a new determination to gain qualifications and a 'decent job' once they had their child. Many identified with a caring role, reflected in the common wish for jobs in nursing or care work.

Some young women took motherhood in their stride. For example, Trish described herself as initially frightened to find herself pregnant at the age of 17 years old. However, she 'talked to lots of people' about it, and by the time her son was born, the fear had gone. She stated, 'he was just there and I loved him . . . . I'd baby-sat for babies and everything before. I'd a load of experience there'. Thus, for some, the adjustment to motherhood is relatively unproblematic, and considerably easier than they had previously anticipated or been told to expect by others.

In spite of the gains, the young women were also almost unanimous in saying that they wished they had waited. Most felt that if they were older, they would be better off financially, have a career and be married. There was also considerable diversity in experiences of motherhood, with some young women finding the adjustment much more difficult than others. This seemed to depend on a variety of factors, including the level of social support, the behaviour of the baby and the mother's response to this, past experience of childcare, professional support, material resources (including money and housing), emotional resources and resilience.

Not all of the difficulties faced by the young women were about motherhood or their age per se. They were also about the social context in which they were caring for their children, including poverty, poor housing, social stigma and low expectations by professionals of their ability to succeed. A key disadvantage to being a young mother was having to struggle financially. Many of the mothers went without to ensure that their children could be fed and clothed. Care leavers were likely to face particular financial challenges in equipping their new homes, particularly if this involved acquiring equipment for a baby. They all received a grant, but the amount varied from £720 to £1,800, depending on the local authority. This sometimes barely covered the essentials involved in setting up a home for themselves and their children. Many ended up taking Social Fund loans for essentials, which meant that they were under even more pressure.

Many young women also experienced unstable housing during pregnancy and beyond. Seven young women were homeless during pregnancy, five staying in hostels and two with friends. Moves were particularly numerous for care leavers, but were not restricted to this group. Of the eight young women who were not care leavers, only two had not moved by the time of childbirth. Housing moves amongst the young mothers were influenced by both 'pull' and 'push' factors. 'Pull' factors included wanting to leave care or the parental home and set up independently. For those living with one or both parents, 'push' factors included overcrowding, arguments, being 'thrown out' of home by parents, and fleeing violence. For those in care, they included the breakdown of foster placements, residential placements being considered unsuitable for pregnant young women and having to leave because of 'causing trouble'.

'You're expected to fail: End of story'

In addition to financial and housing worries, the young women felt that others had low expectations of their abilities to both cope with parenting and to achieve anything with their lives. As Lucy (who was 22 years old and at university) commented, 'They just expect me to be a failure because I've had a baby so young'. There is some support for Lucy's suspicions. For example, Jack Straw (the then Home Secretary), stated: 'If you get a situation where young mothers feel happy about adoption that's so much the better. It is better if these adoptions are done voluntarily than if the children are later taken into care' (The *Times*, 26/01/99). The assumption here seems to be that young mothers cannot provide adequate care for their children.

For the care leavers, the stigma of being a teenage mother tended to be magnified. They often felt that their past actions were interpreted by professionals as indicative of individual disturbance, pathology or deviance. In other words, they were seen as 'trouble' or 'troubled'. When they became pregnant, it was sometimes assumed that they did not have the capacity to break out of chaotic lifestyles and patterns of behaviour that would be likely to impact negatively upon a child. As Ebele remarked:

> People automatically think, because you've been in care, you're going to be a bit messed up in your head, and if you have a child, you won't be able to cope. That's the automatic stereotype, like a game of dominoes, you do this, this will happen, this will happen, this will happen.

Rather than viewing past trauma as a reason to set in place additional support mechanisms that are sensitive to the needs of individual young women and their children, the young mothers felt that services tended to focus on child protection. They felt that having been in care was taken as evidence of their risk to their own child. Furthermore, as young people from ethnic minorities are over-represented in the care system (Biehal *et al* 1995, Ince 1998), the increased surveillance of their behaviour, and particularly of their parenting, can add to a wider tendency for black young people to be pathologised.

Such fears were significantly lower amongst mothers who had not been in care. Interestingly, only two participants felt that they had received insufficient contact with social services as young mothers. One of these had been in care and had a child with severe disabilities. The second had no care history and felt that she needed more support and advocacy as a young mother. A third reported that her own mother felt that her grandson, who was registered as a child 'in need', had received insufficient input from social services. In contrast, many of the young women themselves felt that they had received sufficient contact, but insufficient support.

The participants clearly recognised that parenting can be difficult and that some people may be unable to manage. They recognised the importance of child protection, and some also recognised and appreciated the concern of professionals for the welfare of *their* child. However, in many cases they felt that if they asked for help, they were unlikely to receive it unless there was a clear risk to their child. Moreover, many feared that they must keep out of the spotlight of professional surveillance or else run the risk of losing their child. Jan stated:

If you've been in care, you're expected to fail. End of story (. . .) Social services and all that support, don't just stop there. They have to pass that line. You end up with more crap than what you started with.(. . .) There's helping, and there's hindering.

Thus, there may be little help available to young women unless it is in relation to their mothering. Women who have the least resources are frequently those to whom the least is offered.

Implications for policy and practice

Policy should start from the young woman's experience of herself as resourceful and resilient and on the whole, able to manage. Some young mothers were already experienced in childcare and found motherhood straightforward and very rewarding. The young women felt that they had changed and had had to grow up through motherhood, and argued that responsibility is more important than age in mothering. However, not all young women can cope with motherhood with equanimity. Like mothers of all ages, the young women considered motherhood to be a very demanding job, and this may be compounded for some mothers under 16 years old, lone mothers and for care leavers. This is not helped where there is a lack of financial, practical and emotional support available.

There are many positive steps currently being taken to improve sex and relationship education offered to young people. There are also steps to improve the situation of young mothers. However, despite a raft of recent measures in this area, there are still gaps in services for young mothers, and in opportunities available to them and their children. This is, at least in part, due to ambivalent views on teenage motherhood. This translates into policies that focus on the prevention of teenage motherhood and on child protection, but put less emphasis on enabling young people to succeed, both as mothers and in their own right.

It is sometimes argued that improving the material conditions of young parents will act as an incentive to pregnancy, but this argument cannot be sustained. No research to date has found evidence of the provision of social housing and extra money to be a motivation to teenage pregnancy (Allen and Bourke-Dowling 1998), and this argument does not fit with young women's accounts of pregnancy as almost always unplanned. Neither can it be argued that poverty is simply an outcome of teenage pregnancy. Poverty commonly predates motherhood for teenagers (Phoenix 1991b) and care leavers face huge obstacles to employment and prosperity (Biehal et al 1995, Stein and Wade 2000). The situation of young mothers could be improved by a number of specific measures, including the reinstatement of equitable benefit levels for young people under 25 years old. In order for this to happen, the financial circumstances of young people living away from their birth family, unemployed young people, young parents and care leavers need to be fully recognised and addressed.

The need of special financial provision for care leavers has been recognised in the Children (Leaving Care) Act 2000[8]. This Act makes financial support available from social services, instead of from social security funds. It is a positive move that the financial needs of care leavers have been recognised. However, the income level for care leavers has been set at the basic Income Support level. Care leavers are likely to have additional needs, which are not taken into account by this arrangement. Maintaining the poverty of young mothers through low levels of financial support ultimately punishes both young people and their children.

There needs to be a variety of options in housing for young people, to suit different needs and preferences. This applies to all care leavers, but the issue is thrown into particularly sharp relief in the case of young women leaving care pregnant or with a baby. The pilot housing schemes which are being developed under the Teenage Pregnancy Strategy may provide more adequate supported housing for young mothers who have been in care. However, such schemes are not likely to suit every individual. For some young women, this kind of housing may feel too institutionalised, and may feel too much like residential care. For some, a formalised extension of fostering may be more appropriate. For others, supported lodgings may offer the best option. The main criticisms made by the young women are that they were not able to stay in the same placement when pregnant and that they were not given any real choices. Sometimes, the options given to them did not feel like options at all, because they involved living in a hostel, living with their birth family or living in a different geographical location. The most important factor, then, is the availability of a variety of housing options, offering varied levels of support.

Conclusions

Where alternative routes to adulthood are blocked, motherhood can be a route into adulthood. However, young mothers' attempts at social inclusion are rejected by adults and they are pushed further into social exclusion. This is partly due to poverty, inadequate housing and limited life chances amongst marginalised young people, but is also due to the consequences upon young parents of the ways in which teenage motherhood is viewed by adult society.

If young families are to be socially included, more services need to be developed which provide advice and support for young mothers in a non-judgmental manner. There is a particularly urgent need for more services for young care leavers who have children. Expectations of young people, and particularly of young people who have been in care, also need to be raised. Where the mother is young, and particularly if she has been in care, low expectations of her may precede her and may result in a regulatory and sometimes punitive focus upon her mothering. However, parents and children do not always have the same interests and needs, and it is important that such services are kept separate, as far as possible, from child protection work, so that young mothers have sufficient trust to enable them to access appropriate services. The best and most cost-effective form of child protection, in the long run, may well be supporting and protecting mothers.

Young women require support in their own right, as potentially vulnerable young people. Such support should be available to a young mother whether or not child protection concerns exist, and should be provided separately from services in relation to the child. Also, young women who have been in care may require ongoing support at various points in their lives, on the basis of individual need. Young women's own accounts and views on motherhood provide a powerful case for a move to a more strengths-led model in relation to services for young people and for young mothers particularly.

Endnotes

1 Five group interviews and 28 individual interviews were conducted.
2 Scotland, Northern Ireland and England have similar rates, whilst the rate in Wales is slightly higher (SEU 1999).
3 The main focus here is on the strategy for England, since the research interviews were conducted with young women living in England.
4 Interviews were semi-structured. This means that an interview guide was used, but that this was more flexible and conversational than a questionnaire approach.
5 Six had two children. The children were aged between four weeks and five years. At the time of childbirth, of the 28 participants in individual interviews, eight were living alone with their baby, ten were with the baby's father or a new partner and the remaining ten were living either with their parents or in care.
6 Four pregnancies were planned. Two were first pregnancies, and two second.
7 It is important to note that I am a white researcher, and that different findings may have emerged had the interviewer been black.
8 This Act covers England and Wales. Section 6, on social security benefits also applies in Scotland. Scotland is covered by the Children (Scotland) Act 1995, the Regulation of Care (Scotland) Act 2001 and the Support and the Assistance of Young People Leaving Care (Scotland) Regulations 2004. For Northern Ireland, see the Children (Leaving Care) Act (Northern Ireland) 2002.

References

Allen, I. and Bourke-Dowling, S. (1998) *Teenage Mothers: Decisions and outcomes.* London: Policy Studies Institute.
Babb, P. (1994) 'Teenage conceptions and fertility in England and Wales, 1971–1991', *Population Trends,* 74: 12–17.
Biehal, N., Clayden, J., Stein, M. *et al.* (1992) *Prepared for Living? A Survey of Young People Leaving the Care of Three Local Authorities,* University of Leeds.

Biehal, N., Clayden, J., Stein. M. *et al.* (1994) 'Leaving care in England: A research perspective', *Children and Youth Services Review,* 16: 231–254.

Biehal, N., Clayden, J., Stein. M. *et al.* (1995) *Moving On: Young people and leaving care schemes,* London: HMSO.

Blair, T. (1999) 'Teenage mums are all our business', *The Times,* 8 September.

Craine, S. (1997) 'The 'black magic' roundabout', in R. MacDonald (ed.), *Youth, The 'Underclass' and Social Exclusion;* London: Routledge, pp130–152

Davies, B. (1986) *Threatening Youth,* Milton Keynes: OU Press.

Davies, L., McKinnon, M. and Rains, P. (2001) 'Creating a family: perspectives from teen mothers', *Journal of Progressive Human Services,* 12: 83–101.

Department of Health (1997) *People Like Us: The Report of the Review of the Safeguards for Children Living Away from Home* (The Utting Report), London: HMSO.

Department of Health (2003) *Health and Personal Social Services Statistics, Table A13, Conceptions, ONS* http://www.doh.gov.uk/HPSSS (accessed 26/07/03).

Department of Health, Social Services and Public Safety (2002) *Teenage Pregnancy and Parenthood: Strategy and action plan,* Belfast.

Garnett, L. (1992) *Leaving Care and After,* London: NCB.

Hobcraft, J. and Kiernan, K. (2001) 'Childhood poverty, early motherhood and adult social exclusion', *British Journal of Sociology,* 52(3): 495–517.

Ince, L (1998) *Making it Alone. A Study of the Care Experiences of Black Young People,* London: British Agencies for Adoption and Fostering.

Kiernan, K. (1997) 'Becoming a young parent: A longitudinal study of associated factors', *The British Journal of Sociology,* 48(3): 406–428.

McRobbie, A. (1991) *Feminism and Youth Culture: From Jackie to Just 17,* Hampshire: MacMillan.

Murray, C. (1996) *Charles Murray and the Underclass: The Developing Debate,* London: I.E.A.

National Assembly for Wales (2000) *A Strategic Framework for Promoting Sexual Health in Wales: Post-consultation action plan,* National Assembly for Wales.

Phoenix, A. (1991a) 'Mothers under 20, outsider and insider views', in A. Phoenix, Woollett and Lloyd (eds), *Motherhood, Meanings, Practices and Ideologies,* London: Sage.

Phoenix, A. (1991b) *Young Mothers,* Cambridge: Polity.

Phoenix, A. (1992) 'Narrow definitions of culture: The case of early motherhood', in L. McDowell and R. Pringle (eds). *Defining Women,* Milton Keynes: OU Press.

Rolfe, A. (2002) 'Young Mothers on the Margins: The meanings and experiences of early motherhood in and out of care', Unpublished PhD thesis, University of Warwick.

Scraton, P. (ed.) (1997) *'Childhood' in 'Crisis'?* London: UCL Press.

Selman, P. (1996) 'Teenage motherhood then and now: A comparison of the pattern and outcomes of teenage pregnancy in England and Wales in the 1960s and 1980s', H. Jones and J. Millar (eds), *The Politics of the Family,* Aldershot: Avebury.

Social Exclusion Unit (SEU) (1999) *Teenage Pregnancy,* London: HMSO.

Stein, M. and Wade, J. (2000) *Helping Care Leavers: Problems and strategic responses,* London, Department of Health.

Straw, J. (1999) ''Give babies for adoption call' by Straw', The *Times*, 26 January.

Taylor, J.M., Gilligan, C. and Sullivan, A.M. (1995) *Between Voice and Silence: Women and girls, race and relationship*, Cambridge, Mass: Harvard University Press.

Teenage Pregnancy Unit (2003) *The Independent Advisory Group on Teenage Pregnancy, Second Annual Report*, London: Department of Health.

Postscript on young mothers

Annmarie Fraser and Stephanie George

Annmarie Fraser

My name is Annmarie Fraser, I live in Aberdeen and am 18 years old. I have a 21-month-old daughter called Megan. I fell pregnant with Megan when I was 16 years old and still at school doing my Highers. Although I found it quite tiring I was determined to stick at it and get my exams done to enable me to have a better future for myself and my daughter, and to prove to all the people out there that being a teenage parent doesn't need to ruin your life. I am currently working full time as a Trainee Project Worker for Save the Children, and Megan goes to a childminder through the day.

At the start of my pregnancy I got very little support from the school, well not so much the school but one teacher in particular – who was the head of my year – so I found this very disappointing. It took me ages to get a meeting with my midwife, health visitor and social worker just to get things sorted out for my exams, etc. There is no support whatsoever for teenage parents staying in education in Aberdeen. I have to disagree with Alison Rolfe when she states that most teenage mothers come from disadvantaged families or have just left care. Being a young parent and a community worker myself, I see young mothers every day and most of them actually come from 'normal' families.

In general, I think the chapter is quite well written. It has a lot of useful information, although I feel that it reflects England more than Scotland, so not much of the information is of use to me. However, the Sure Start Plus scheme seems like a brilliant idea – it just seems a shame that it's only available in England. What about young parents in Scotland? In Aberdeen there is only one parent support group that I am aware of and you must stay in the area in order to join it, so what is the point in that? And as far as social workers are concerned, as long as your children are not at risk then you don't get any support unless you have had a social worker yourself in the past, e.g. if you were in care or you had other problems.

I have to agree with Sam (20 years old) who was quoted in the chapter as saying that being a young mum isn't just about age, but about responsibility. If you are 16 years old and a parent, it does not mean you are less capable of being responsible for a child than someone of 32 years old. At the end of the day, everybody is an individual and we all grow up at our own pace. I feel that a lot of people put downers on young parents, but then I also feel a lot of young parents can put downers on themselves. You do get the young parents that stay on benefits and feel that they can't return to work, education, etc., and this is because it has always been drummed into their heads that they can't do any better.

Stephanie George

> I'm Stephanie George, I'm 22 years old and I have a son who will soon be six years old. We've lived by ourselves in a two-bedroom council flat in Aberdeen since he was two months old. I'd never lived on my own before this and it hasn't been easy. I had few possessions when I moved into my flat – only the contents of my teenage bedroom – so I had to build up our home from scratch. I spent the first four years of my son's life on benefits (income support). During my time on benefits, I did some part-time work in a teen mums' creche and applied for some college courses, but I wasn't able to start these due to lack of child care. In January, 2003 I took up the post of Trainee Project Worker with Save the Children, on their Saying Power Scheme. It gives young people aged 16–21 years old the chance to run an 18-month project that will benefit other disadvantaged or discriminated young people. My project is a young mums' project: I wanted to offer help and support to other young mums in my area.

Due to my job and my own personal circumstances, I was very interested in the topic of this chapter. I think that Alison Rolfe has managed to get across the majority of the issues that face young mums in Britain, although the focus is on England; being a young mum in Scotland, I could not really relate to some things she mentioned, like policies, as these don't often apply in Scotland. There is very little reference to other areas in Britain. For example, as far as I know, Scotland does not have a strategy in place for teenage pregnancy, and if they do, it is not publicised very well.

The support that is available in Scotland is quite difficult to access. When I had my son I didn't know who to contact for support. I knew very little about benefits or housing and there is no specific organisation in my area to direct you to such organisations or support. I think the Sure Start Plus pilot schemes running in England are a great idea, and it should be rolled out to cover Scotland as well.

If you fall pregnant at 16 or over in Scotland and do not have a social worker already, it is difficult to access services. I had to find and contact local charities myself for help with things like furnishing my house, whereas friends of mine who were slightly younger and had social work involvement received a lot of help.

Alison Rolfe talks about certain risk factors that can lead to a young woman becoming pregnant. I do not agree with this. I think that if a young woman becomes pregnant, she becomes pregnant. I do not think that her parents separating at an early age or living in a deprived area causes this. However, Alison Rolfe comments on young mothers being part of a 'cycle of deprivation'. This will remain the case unless support and encouragement are offered to young mums to break the cycle.

Alison Rolfe doesn't really discuss the actual amount of benefits young mums receive. I think this needs to be looked at by government as just now the benefit amount rises by the mother's age and not the child's. I can see how this is useful for an 18 year old who has the extra financial burden of council tax, but I think it should also rise by the child's age: a six month-old baby can sometimes cost a lot less than a three year-old attending nursery five mornings a week.

In the conclusion to the chapter, Rolfe states: 'Where alternative routes to adulthood are blocked, motherhood can be a route into adulthood.' This comment seems to suggest that motherhood is an easy option to becoming an adult. This is by no means the case. Equally, being on benefits seems to be seen as an easy ride for young mums, which it is not. Most young mums are struggling to get by financially and often get further and further into debt which follows them around throughout their lives.

I do agree that teenage motherhood is still viewed badly by society. People assume that if you're a young mother then you must be scrounging off the state and sitting around doing nothing. This is not true, as most young mothers are furthering their education or trying very hard to gain employment.

Conclusion

I feel that there needs to be less talk about policies and more action. The government needs to create a balance between preventing teenage pregnancy and helping and supporting pregnant teens/young mums:

- Educational support for pregnant teens and young mums needs to be increased and there should be a national framework in place for this.
- The government currently sets the amount of income support that young mums 'need' to live on, and this doesn't account for 'luxuries' such as clothes and furniture. This policy needs to be reviewed urgently.

- There needs to be an increased awareness by young mothers of agencies available to support them in their local area.

I think that it is good that support for certain 'groups' of young mums is being looked at with a view to improvement, i.e. care leavers. However, young mums who do not fall into any of these groups need to be supported as well. For example, a 16 year-old mum with no social worker who has lived with her parents in a stable family home until now may not receive the help she needs, as she would not be seen as a 'vulnerable' young mother.

All in all, the chapter covers a lot of policy as well as the opinions of young mums, and hopefully the policy makers will take note and see where they might be going wrong or overlooking areas.

Chapter 13

Growing up caring: Young carers and vulnerability to social exclusion

Chris Dearden and Saul Becker

In this chapter we outline some of the ways in which children and young adults who provide unpaid (informal) care to family members can suffer, or be vulnerable to, social exclusion and how social policies may *exacerbate* this situation. We go on to suggest ways in which young carers may be supported in their caring roles and may be assisted to achieve a better degree of social inclusion.

Young carers are defined as:

> Children and young persons under 18 who provide or intend to provide care, assistance or support to another family member. They carry out, often on a regular basis, significant or substantial caring tasks and assume a level of responsibility which would usually be associated with an adult. The person receiving care is often a parent but can be a sibling, grandparent or other relative who is disabled, has some chronic illness, mental health problem or other condition connected with a need for care, support or supervision.
>
> (Becker 2000a: 378)

In common with most other definitions, this one emphasises the fact that young carers are *children*, i.e. under the age of 18 years old and still, technically, the dependants of adults. However, young people who have provided care throughout part of their childhood rarely cease to be carers once they achieve majority, and caring can have a significant impact on both their childhood and their transition to adulthood.

While young caring has existed for centuries within the private domain of the family, it is only in the past decade or so that it has come to our attention as a social issue and has been identified in legislation, policy and practice. In many ways the notion of children and young adults providing care transgresses social norms: children are supposed to be the *recipients* of care and nurturing from their families, particularly their parents or guardians. While early research into young caring raised awareness of the issue of children having to provide care to other family members, especially to parents, it also led to widespread, often unhelpful media coverage that portrayed young carers as victims and their ill or disabled parents as dependants – the idea that children had become their parents' parents. If young carers are in any sense 'victims', then they are not the victims of dependant or uncaring relatives, but rather of a *system* that relies predominantly on families to provide unpaid care work for other family members, often unsupported and unacknowledged. Ill or disabled parents have also suffered from a community care policy that is underfunded and relies heavily on family, friends and the wider community to provide the care, support and assistance they require to remain within – or to live independently in – their own homes or communities. Furthermore, the emphasis on their social care needs as *individuals* has often ignored their wider needs as *parents* (Social Services Inspectorate 2000). These policies, and how they have exacerbated the position of young carers and their parents, will be discussed in more detail towards the end of this chapter. However, we must not forget the *agency* of young carers and their parents, how they care for each other and shape their lives and experiences, even if these are constrained by factors outside the family (Bibby and Becker 2000).

Young caring in context

It is important to realise that having an ill or disabled parent or other family member will not necessarily result in children within a family becoming carers. It is estimated that 23 per cent of all children in the UK (around three million) live in families where one family member is 'hampered in daily activities' by a chronic physical or mental health problem, illness or disability (Eurostat 1997, cited in Becker *et al* 1998). Secondary analysis of 1985 General Household Survey data suggests that 17 per cent of adult carers aged 16–35 years old (212,000) became carers before the age of 16 years old (Parker 1994), while the NSPCC estimate that four per cent of all 18–24 year olds (173,000) will have regularly cared for an ill or disabled relative during their childhood (Cawson *et al* 2000, Cawson 2002). Recent data from the 2001 Census suggest that there are 174,995 young carers under the age of 18 years old who provide care: 13,029 of these are providing care for 50 hours or more per week (Carers UK 2003). This means that, of the three million children living in families with health problems, just fewer than six per cent (5.83 per cent) are young carers. Prior to these more recent figures the only 'official' estimate was that undertaken by the Office for National Statistics (ONS) on behalf of the Department of Health, which suggested that there were between 19,000 and 51,000 young carers (ages 8–17 years old) nationally (Walker 1996). It is clear from these data, particularly the most recent Census figures, that caring during childhood and young adulthood, while by no means common, is far more prevalent than had previously been thought.

Young carers perform the same tasks as adult carers. These range along a continuum, from basic domestic duties such as shopping, cleaning and cooking to general, nursing-type tasks such as assisting with mobility and giving medication, to emotional support (usually to relatives with mental health problems), through to very intimate personal care such as assisting with toileting, bathing and showering. In addition, some young carers provide child care for younger (well) siblings and some are involved in a range of other tasks such as translating for non-English speaking parents, managing budgets, administrative tasks, etc. Table 13.1 shows the proportions of young carers, aged 18 years old and under, who were providing different types of care in 1995 and 1997. These figures are drawn from two large-scale surveys of young carers supported by dedicated projects around the UK.

The figures in Table 13.1 hide some specific gender- and age-related differences. The 1997 survey showed that girls were more likely to be involved in *all* aspects of care, but particularly domestic and intimate tasks – care work traditionally associated with women. The likelihood of involvement in most tasks, with the exception of child care, increased with age. So, for example, while 21 per cent of 11–15 year olds provided intimate care, 34 per cent of those aged 16 years old and over did so. Fifty-six per cent of 11–15 year olds were involved in general care, compared with 68 per cent of those aged 16 years old and over.

Outcomes for young carers

Qualitative and quantitative research, some of which is briefly outlined below, has highlighted some of the outcomes for children and young people who care. These outcomes include limited opportunities, horizons and aspirations; limited opportunities for social and leisure activities; a lack of understanding from peers and restricted friendships; 'stigma by association', as a result of the often negative connotations attached to disability in general and mental ill health and substance misuse in particular; emotional difficulties; health problems; feelings of exclusion or being outsiders; fear of

Table 13.1 Percentage of young carers providing different caring tasks, 1995 and 1997

Caring tasks	1995 (n = 641)	1997 (n = 2,303)
Domestic	65%	72%
General	61%	57%
Emotional support	25%	43%
Intimate care	23%	21%
Child care	11%	7%
Other	10%	29%

Source: Dearden and Becker 1995, 1998.

what professionals might do; difficulties in their transitions to adulthood; and educational problems and employment difficulties. Taken singularly, but especially in combination, these outcomes or disadvantages can lead to many young carers experiencing social exclusion and detachment from the activities and opportunities that many other children can both enjoy and benefit from. Moreover, they increase young carers' *vulnerability* to social exclusion during their adulthood. In other words, these childhood disadvantages can cast a long shadow forward and exacerbate young carers' vulnerability to social exclusion throughout the life cycle. We will briefly discuss these outcomes in turn.

Limited aspirations

Aldridge and Becker's (1993) early small-scale qualitative research suggested that some young carers had limited aspirations and opportunities. This was partly the result of being needed for care work within the home, but also the result of feeling that the situation was unlikely to change and that they would continue to remain 'available' to their families. More recent research focused on former young carers (Frank *et al* 1999) and 'older' young carers aged 16–25 years old (Dearden and Becker 2000a). These studies found that, as young carers became older, they did indeed continue to limit their horizons, often feeling unable or reluctant to leave home, accepting local employment or training so as to be close, and, in several cases, restricting their employment choices to caring-type roles, often of a low-paid nature. Such research suggests that although young carers are defined by age, i.e. under the age of 18 years old, *children's* experiences as carers go on to affect their transitions to adulthood and their *adult* experiences.

Limited social and leisure activities

All of the research that has been conducted directly with young carers has found evidence of some limitations on their time spent in social and leisure activities. Indeed, one of the most valued aspects of dedicated young carers projects is the provision of such activities (see for example Mahon and Higgins 1995, Social Services Inspectorate 1995, Dearden and Becker 1996, 2000b). The time spent on social and leisure activities may be restricted due to caring commitments, but this is often exacerbated by a lack of money. When such activities are provided by projects, they are usually free of charge or charged at a nominal amount.

Lack of understanding from peers

Linked with the restrictions on the time available for social and leisure activities is a lack of understanding from peers, often associated with restricted friendships. Many young carers express disbelief, and sometimes contempt, at their friends' inability to perform certain tasks that they have been doing for years: e.g. cooking, cleaning and other caring or household responsibilities. Their experiences can make them appear very mature and capable for their ages, which although beneficial in the longer term when they are able to function independently, can also make friendships difficult to sustain as they can find friends of their own age quite immature:

> I think I became an adult overnight when that [stroke] happened to my mam. I think it was just, I was thrown into being responsible then . . . some people my age haven't got a care in the world. I mean, my friend that used to live down the bottom of the street, she's got both parents at home . . . and she still comes home with her laundry and things like that.
>
> (Diana, age 23, quoted in Dearden and Becker 2000a: 41)

> I think I became an adult quite some time ago, when I was sixteen, because of the responsibilities, and I think it just depends on what responsibilities you take on . . . you could be twenty years old and still your mum does everything for you.
>
> (Ravinder, age 19, quoted in Dearden and Becker 2000a: 42)

Health problems

Some young carers may experience emotional difficulties and health problems associated with caring. Emotional problems can be the result of worrying about leaving an ill family member alone, perhaps because they fear an accident, self-harm or an exacerbation of symptoms. This can result in either young people missing school to remain at home or lacking concentration while at school (Dearden and Becker 1995, 2000a, Frank *et al* 1999). Sadly, some young people will experience the early death of a parent or other relative.

In addition to the emotional stress of caring, which can result in depression, physical health problems such as back and joint problems may be experienced as a result of lifting and carrying excessive weights. The strict guidelines relating to moving and handling that apply to adults working in the caring professions are absent in the unregulated sphere of the family home and professionals are reluctant to teach young people how to lift safely as to do so may be seen as condoning such activities.

Stigma

Children and young people can also face 'stigma by association', as a result of the prejudice and discrimination that results from the ignorance surrounding many illnesses and disabilities. This is particularly marked when they have family members suffering from mental ill health. As Aldridge and Becker (2003: 80–81) observe:

> Twelve of the young carers in our sample said they had also experienced stigma by association with their mentally ill parents, in school, among their friends and in local communities. (Other children purposefully kept quiet about their parents' illness, or felt they had no one to talk to who they could trust.)

Professional failings

Furthermore, this stigma is not restricted to peers and the local community, but extends to professionals, who make assumptions about the parenting capacity of mentally ill adults. Many young carers of parents with mental illness have been in and out of the public child care system, while their parents face negative attitudes in relation to their parenting capacity (Aldridge and Becker 2003, Dearden and Becker 2000a).

Perhaps, unsurprisingly given their experiences, some young carers feel isolated and excluded. They have less free time than their peers, they can find friendships difficult, they experience stigma, discrimination and prejudice and are rarely consulted by any professionals with whom they are in contact. The exclusion of young people from discussions with professionals is well documented (Aldridge and Becker 1993, 1994, 2003, Becker *et al* 1998, Dearden and Becker 1998, Frank *et al* 1999) and can lead to frustration and misunderstandings, as well as a sense of being punished for caring. In the absence of explanations relating to medical conditions, young people can draw their own, often erroneous, conclusions about likely outcomes and prognoses. Furthermore, in the absence of a whole-family approach (to assessing children and parents, and in responding to their joint needs), professionals will not know who provides care and to what extent. It is evident that adult services rarely involve themselves with children in a family and that children's services often fail to involve themselves with parents. Moreover, there is little contact between professionals in children's services and those in adult services (SSI 1995, 1996, Aldridge and Becker 2003, Dearden and Becker 2001) and this failure to 'join up' services can lead to many young carers and their parents falling through the gaps. Young people who provide care are often left in the dark about the nature of an illness/disability, about any support services that may be available and about the optimum ways to manage their roles.

The distrust between many young carers and their families and those professionals with whom they come in contact can result in a fear of such professional intervention. Many parents are anxious that should they seek support then they will be judged and found wanting as parents; their biggest fear is that their children will be taken into care. Young people are also fearful of seeking professional help; for some this is based on past experiences:

> Last time she [mother] was ill I don't know whether I did the right thing or not 'cause we could tell, 'cause she gets ill really quickly. And it was about two weeks and on the third week I rang – not the hospital – my mum's psychiatric social worker and told them to check up on my mum and everything. I don't know whether I should have just left it to progress or see to it as soon as possible. Because my mum went into hospital and then me and my sister had to go into foster care, and I feel as though it was all my fault.
> (Laura, age 17, quoted in Dearden and Becker 2000a: 36)

While young people may be admitted to care while their parents are hospitalised, care proceedings are usually a last resort and reserved for children who are considered to be at risk or have been abused in some way. Nevertheless, in 2000, parental ill health was the third most common reason for children entering the public child care system (Department of Health 2001) and for some families this will be a realistic fear. More recently, better recording of reasons for entry into the care system indicate that the proportion of children entering as a result of parental illness has reduced from ten per cent in 2000 to nine per cent in 2002. However, a new category 'family in acute stress' accounts for a further 12 per cent in 2002. It is likely that at least some of these families will be in distress as a result of ill health (Department of Health 2001, 2003). For most, the fear of care proceedings is usually ungrounded, but this anxiety continues to prevent many families from seeking support.

Transitions to adulthood

Transition to adulthood, the process whereby 'young people move away from dependence for primary, emotional and financial support from their childhood family carers' and 'their needs for income, shelter and social life are met from a wider range of sources' (Barnardo's Policy Development Unit 1996: 9), is problematic for many young carers. Their previous experiences of caring, as outlined above, coupled with educational and employment difficulties, can make the transition difficult and precarious. While many recent policies relating to young people, education and employment and benefit receipt have an impact on a range of young people, carers experience particular problems due to the interdependence of their familial relationships and the specific nature of their caring role. For example, leaving the family home can be problematic for those whose relatives have little or no outside support services. Others, particularly those whose parents have mental health problems, may have very painful transitions, often following a history of being in care or having to care for a loved one whose condition and behaviour can be unstable (Dearden and Becker 2000a).

Educational difficulties

The literature on young caring shows evidence of widespread educational difficulties (see for example Marsden 1995, Dearden and Becker 1995, 1998, 2000a, 2003, Frank *et al* 1999). The two large-scale surveys of young carers supported by projects indicate that in 1995, 33 per cent and in 1997, 28 per cent of school-age carers were either missing school as a result of their caring roles, or had other indicators of educational difficulties such as receipt of educational welfare services, educational psychology or were referred to support projects by educationalists (Dearden and Becker 1995, 1998). Educational difficulties can range from mild to severe, encompassing missed school, persistent lateness, lack of concentration, non-submission of course work and homework and, ultimately, a lack of educational qualifications. In some cases, young carers' attendance and course work are so poor that schools do not enter them for formal examinations (Dearden and Becker 2003).

Employment difficulties

The major route out of dependence is an independent income, which comes for most young people when they enter the labour market. However, research indicates that, for some young carers, this route is also problematic. Their previous educational difficulties often result in them leaving school with no, or minimal educational qualifications. They live in families where poverty and reliance on welfare and disability benefits are common (Dearden and Becker 2000a), and the majority of them live in lone parent families (Dearden and Becker 1995, 1998, 2000a) where the parent is ill or disabled and there are no other adults or other family members in paid employment. Although young carers' employment choices may be influenced by their caring experiences – many work or aspire to work in 'caring professions' (Dearden and Becker 2000a, Frank *et al* 1999) – they are also restricted by their lack of qualifications:

> I was enquiring about social work and social services and I know basically you've got to have this, you've got to have that, you've got to have the other. And I was like, 'Oh my God, I haven't got none of those'.
> (Anna, age 19, quoted in Dearden and Becker 2000a: 40)

Although some young carers find the transition to paid employment difficult, many, of course, have been providing *unpaid*, and unrecognised, care work for a considerable time: care work that, if it took place outside the private family sphere, would attract remuneration, albeit often at a low rate (Becker *et al* 2001). The skills that these young people acquire, such as time-management, organisational skills, independence and maturity, are unrecognised and unaccredited although they would be valued by some employers (Dearden and Becker 2000a).

The negative outcomes of caring, coupled with the associated disadvantages in childhood and in early adulthood, and the poverty that young carers and their families endure, result in some carers experiencing social exclusion while many others are at risk of such exclusion.

Government policy and young caring

There are a variety of reasons why some young people become carers, including the nature of family illness/disability; family structure; child–parent relationships; age and ability; gender; family size; and the presence/absence of other carers. However, the major factor is the availability, or lack of availability, of alternative, good-quality services that would support disabled people adequately and reduce young people's caring responsibilities or prevent them from adopting caring roles in the first place. Research indicates that many families lack such support services and lack an adequate income to purchase alternatives (see Dearden and Becker 1995, 1998, 2000a).

Community care policy rests on the assumption that most care will be provided by family, friends and the local community, with the state stepping in to fill the gaps (Becker 1997). The 1990 NHS and Community Care Act allows for ill/disabled adults who meet certain criteria to be assessed for community care support and services. The Act also states that *carers* may request an assessment of their own needs at the time the ill/disabled person is being assessed and that there should be no assumptions made regarding the carer's ability to continue to provide care. However, from the outset, *young* carers under the age of 18 years old were excluded from this Act since it is intended specifically for *adults*. At this time there was little understanding of the needs of younger carers and there was also a generally held assumption that family carers would themselves be adults. The Social Services Inspectorate (SSI) directed social services departments in 1995 to assess young carers as children in need under Section 17 of the Children Act 1989. It was not until the Carers (Recognition and Services) Act 1995 (implemented in 1996) that this anomaly was ended and *all* carers, irrespective of age, could request an assessment of their own needs. In Scotland, carers under the age of 16 years old continued to rely on the Children (Scotland) Act 1995 to have their needs as carers met, since Scottish law does not allow for children under this age to enter a legal transaction. The Carers and Disabled Children Act 2000 allows for carers over the age of 16, who are assessed as needing support, to receive services or direct payments in their own right. This is the first time that carers have been able to access direct payments and is a further acknowledgement of carers' needs and the necessity to meet such needs if community care is to be a reality for those who need it.

Following the collapse of the youth labour market in the 1970s, education and employment policy has increasingly emphasised vocational training and education. Changes to benefit rules in 1988 made it impossible for most young people of 16 and 17 years old to claim any form of social security benefits, and reduced payments were introduced for the under-25s. While education has been emphasised at the expense of paid work, the erosion of maintenance grants and the introduction of student loans and tuition fees further increases young people's financial dependence. Full-time carers aged 16 years old and over who are caring for someone in receipt of disability living allowance may claim carers allowance, but the number of hours they are allowed to spend studying is restricted. This results in many young carers who are in further education being denied the benefit, while it pushes others into benefit reliance and denies them access to the labour market. The extension of education/training increases young people's financial reliance on their families and, in the case of families where there is illness or disability, results in a reliance on welfare and disability benefits, with young carers and their families remaining in or at the margins of poverty (Dearden and Becker 2000a). As young people become increasingly financially dependent on their families for longer periods of time and the period of transition to adulthood extends, so poorer families struggle to maintain their children. Disabled adults are amongst the poorest in society (Becker 2003). Indeed, even previously affluent families will become poor if they rely on benefits for extended periods of time. Dearden and Becker's (2000a) study of 60 young carers' transitions to adulthood found that none of their parents with illness/disability were in paid employment, while in Aldridge and Becker's (2003) study of 40 families where a parent had mental illness, only one parent with severe mental ill health was employed. Thus, young carers are highly likely to live in families with long-term experience of benefit receipt and poverty. Where young people are able to enter the labour market, the minimum wage legislation excludes those under 18 years old and discriminates against those under 21 years old. Again, there is an assumption that young people do not need (or perhaps deserve) a living wage and it is further evidence of their 'partial' citizenship. While they bear adult responsibilities in the home, they are denied adult welfare rights.

Excluding young carers

Social exclusion is a relative concept and can change between societies and over time. A person is socially excluded if they are unable to participate in key activities of the society in which they live. Burchardt *et al* (2002) define such key activities as consumption, production, political engagement and social interaction, while others (Gordon *et al* 2000) suggest different *dimensions* of exclusion, i.e. poverty, exclusion from social relations, service exclusion and labour market exclusion.

Poverty reduces young carers' ability to consume goods and services. This is true not only when they are younger and financially reliant on their parents but also as they grow older, because of their lack of time to engage in part-time paid work while studying (due to caring commitments) and also due to the increasing length of transitions to adulthood and its associated period of dependence. Long-term ill or disabled adults are less able to provide financially for their children because of their own reliance on welfare benefits and the associated costs of disability. Dearden and Becker (2000a: 23) cite the example of Graham who was 16 years old and doing a part-time further education course when he was interviewed. He had no independent income and his disabled mother was in rent arrears:

> My mum gives me two quid for those three days [when in college] . . . it's from her social, from her social security . . . . I mean mum does buy stuff from shopping for us but no, we don't, I mean some weeks, you know, say like one in every four weeks she can afford to give us like two quid. Well that's enough.

We have already discussed the difficulties many young carers face in entering the labour market and becoming 'productive' members of society. Although caring is labour and a productive activity, it is generally unpaid and children's caring labour *always* goes unpaid – at least until they reach the age of 16 years old, when some may claim carers' allowance. Not only is production a means of earning and becoming financially independent, but it is also a way of becoming accepted as a useful part of society as social status often comes from paid employment. Of 24 young carers aged 19–25 years old in Dearden and Becker's (2000a) study, only seven were engaged in the paid labour market alongside their unpaid care work at home. Another four were full-time carers in receipt of carers' benefits, but lacking the income and status that paid employment could confer. A combination of factors serves to exclude many young carers from the labour market.

Little is known about the political engagement of young carers, but if we take a broader definition of 'political' we can see how young carers are marginalised and excluded from services. Their status as children and young people serves to exclude them from discussions with professionals who are involved in service provision to their relatives. Furthermore, a quarter of young carers in the 1997 survey (Dearden and Becker 1998) had no support services (either for themselves or for their relatives with illness/disability) other than their own contact with a designated young carers' project. Indeed, many families only receive social care support services due to the intervention of such projects. While these projects do provide support and services to young carers, they are not available in every local area. In 1992, there were only three projects; by 1995 there were 37 and in 2003 there are more than 250. Although this is a significant increase in a comparatively short period of time, many young carers will not have access to a project in their area. One way in which such projects have increased young carers' political engagement is by involving them in discussions and decisions about family matters, including care, and in enabling them to access the political process by lobbying politicians and others, including local policy makers and professionals who, in the past, had ignored their individual needs and collective presence. Although assessment of young carers, either as children in need under the 1989 Children Act or as carers under the 1995 Carers (Recognition and Services) Act or the 2000 Carers and Disabled Children Act, can lead to service provision, only 11 per cent of the 2,303 carers surveyed in 1997 (Dearden and Becker 1998) had received any form of assessment.

The disadvantages and negative outcomes associated with young caring, which we have outlined above, indicate the extent of young carers' exclusion from social relations. The nature of their social interactions within and outside the home can be restricted because of their caring roles and as a result of their 'difference'. This social isolation is exacerbated by family poverty.

Singularly, any one of these disadvantages can be the crucial determinant of a particular young carer's social exclusion. So, for example, educational disadvantage can be the main factor that excludes some young carers from wider participation and increases the vulnerability to social exclusion of others. In another family, the determining factor may be poverty or low income. In others still, a lack of opportunity to participate in paid work will be the factor that maintains exclusion for younger adult carers. In other cases it will be 'systems failures' that maintain or exacerbate exclusion: for example, where professionals neglect the views and experiences of young carers, or fail to provide suitable alternative care arrangements for families. In any family, one or more of these disadvantages can determine the extent, nature and duration of a young carer's social exclusion. When many factors are present in combination, such as poverty, poor educational attainment, restricted social relations and professional neglect, vulnerability to social exclusion is likely to be severe (see also Becker 2000b).

Including young carers

The research evidence suggests that young carers are likely to experience or be at risk of experiencing some degree of social exclusion. Furthermore, many policies and practices in both health and social care, and in education and employment, exacerbate such exclusion for some families. So, how can we counter the disadvantages and tendencies that work to exclude young carers and their families?

First, community care policy and implementations need to ensure that ill or disabled people receive adequate, affordable, good-quality services and support that reduce their reliance on the 'informal' unpaid care of family (including children), friends and the wider community. This support *must* meet their needs as parents and their social and health care needs. It must also meet carers' needs.

Secondly, children's and young people's ability or willingness to provide care work should *not* be taken into account when assessing disabled adults for support. It is when children's care work is accepted as the norm and goes unchallenged that children and young people end up adopting inappropriate caring roles that can have a negative impact on their childhood and their transitions to adulthood.

Thirdly, when an adult is assessed for community care services the assessment process must be holistic and take into account the needs and wishes of the whole family. Equally, when children are assessed as children in need or as carers, a whole family approach is required. It is impossible to assess the needs of parent or child in isolation and any assessment of one party should automatically trigger an assessment of the other. Such assessments must not breach an individual's confidentiality, but must enable all family members to speak openly and frankly about their wishes and needs. It is not necessary for assessments of parents and children to be conducted together. Indeed, some families may prefer to be assessed individually. Nor is it essential that such assessments be conducted by different agencies/departments; the important factor is that assessments are holistic and family-focused and that the person conducting the assessment is able to understand and appreciate children's needs in addition to those of ill/disabled adults.

Fourthly, there should be some means of acknowledging and accrediting the skills and competencies acquired by young carers, since they add value within the paid arena of work and would be respected by many employers. However, young carers should not be pushed into low-paid, low-status caring jobs simply because of their previous experiences. These skills are transferable to other types of employment and opportunities should not be restricted.

Fifthly, more thought needs to be given to the financial support of young people in the absence of youth employment or the opportunities to engage in paid work because of unpaid care responsibilities in the home. The widespread use of education maintenance payments would help those in further education, but rigid attendance rules may have to be relaxed for young people whose parents have chronic illness or disability. Young people should not be financially penalised for caring for family members. Coupled with this, there needs to be additional flexibility in paying for higher education so as not to exclude young people who experience poverty and social exclusion as a result of long-term illness within the family. Second chances for young people who do not complete courses due to family illness should also be available.

Sixthly, all the above require a re-conceptualisation of the importance and value of unpaid care work within the home. Millions of adults and tens of thousands of children each day provide unpaid care to other family members. That non-family members would be paid to undertake this work poses challenges for policy makers, which, the evidence suggests, they are not yet willing to engage with.

Finally, the emphasis should be on prevention. The adequate support – medical, social and financial – of disabled people would greatly reduce the likelihood of their children becoming young carers. Early interventions that adopt a holistic family approach to disability and care services should mean that young people do not adopt inappropriate caring roles, but provide a level of assistance that would be expected in any other household: on the basis of a gradual adoption of tasks according to age and maturity in preparation for adulthood and independence. Together, these ways forward offer strategies and working practices that will counter the disadvantages that many young carers face, and will help to promote their social inclusion, both during their childhood and into adulthood.

References

Aldridge, J. and Becker, S. (1993) *Children who Care: Inside the world of young carers*, Loughborough: Young Carers Research Group, Loughborough University.

Aldridge, J. and Becker, S. (1994) *My Child, My Carer: The parents' perspective*, Loughborough: Young Carers Research Group, Loughborough University.

Aldridge, J. and Becker, S. (2003) *Children Caring for Parents with Mental Illness: Perspectives of young carers, parents and professionals*, Bristol: The Policy Press.

Barnardo's Policy Development Unit (1996) *Transition to Adulthood*, Ilford: Barnardo's.

Becker, S. (1997) *Responding to Poverty: The Politics of Cash and Care*, London: Longmans.

Becker, S. (2000a) 'Young carers', in M. Davies (ed.), *The Blackwell Encyclopaedia of Social Work*, Oxford: Blackwell.

Becker, S. (2000b) 'Carers and indicators of vulnerability to social exclusion', *Benefits*, 28, (April/May): 1–4.

Becker, S. (2003) '"Security for those who cannot": Labour's neglected welfare principles', in J. Millar (ed.), *Understanding Social Security: Issues for policy and practice*, Bristol: The Policy Press.

Becker, S., Aldridge, J. and Dearden, C. (1998) *Young Carers and their Families*, Oxford: Blackwell Science.

Becker, S., Dearden, C. and Aldridge, J. (2001) 'Children's labour of love? Young carers and care work', in P. Mizen, C. Pole and A. Bolton (eds), *Hidden Hands: International perspectives on children's work and labour*, London: Routledge–Falmer.

Bibby, A. and Becker, S. (2000) *Young Carers in Their Own Words*, London: Calouste Gulbenkian Foundation.

Burchardt, T., Le Grand, J. and Piachaud, D. (2002) 'Degrees of exclusion: developing a dynamic, multidimensional measure', in J. Hills, J. LeGrand and D. Piachaud (eds), *Understanding Social Exclusion*, New York: Oxford University Press.

Carers and Disabled Children Act 2000, London: The Stationery Office.

Carers (Recognition and Services) Act 1995, London: HMSO.

Carers UK (2003) *Census 2001 and Carers – Results from around the UK*, Policy Briefing, London: Carers UK.

Cawson, P. (2002) *Child Maltreatment in the Family: The experience of a national sample of young people*, London: NSPCC.

Cawson, P., Wattam, C., Brooker, S. *et al.* (2000) *Child Maltreatment in the United Kingdom: A study of the prevalence of child abuse and neglect*, London: NSPCC.

Children Act 1989, London: HMSO.

Children (Scotland) Act 1995, London: HMSO.

Dearden, C. and Becker, S. (1995) *Young Carers – The facts*, Sutton: Reed Business Publishing.

Dearden, C. and Becker, S. (1996) *Young Carers at the Crossroads: An evaluation of the Nottingham Young Carers Project*, Loughborough. Young Carers Research Group, Loughborough University.

Dearden, C. and Becker, S. (1998) *Young Carers in the United Kingdom: A profile*, London: Carers National Association.

Dearden, C. and Becker, S. (2000a) *Growing up Caring: Vulnerability and transition to adulthood – young carers' experiences*, Leicester: Youth Work Press.

Dearden, C. and Becker, S. (2000b) *Meeting Young Carers' Needs: An evaluation of the Sheffield Young Carers Project*, Loughborough: Young Carers Research Group, Loughborough University.

Dearden, C. and Becker, S. (2001) 'Young carers: needs, rights and assessments', in J. Horwath (ed.), *The Child's World: Assessing children in need*, London: Jessica Kingsley.

Dearden, C. and Becker, S. (2003) *Young Carers and Education*, available at: *www.carersonline.org.uk*

Department of Health (2001) *Children Looked After by Local Authorities, Year Ending 31 March 2000*, England, London: Department of Health.

Department of Health (2003) *Children Looked After by Local Authorities, Year Ending 31 March 2002, England, Volume 1*, London: Department of Health.

Frank, J., Tatum, C. and Tucker, S. (1999) *On Small Shoulders: Learning from the experiences of former young carers*, London: The Children's Society.

Gordon, D., Adelman, L., Ashworth, K., *et al* (2000) *Poverty and Social Exclusion in Britain*, York: Joseph Rowntree Foundation.

Mahon, A. and Higgins, J. (1995) '. . .*A Life of our Own' Young Carers: An evaluation of three RHA funded projects in Merseyside*, Manchester: Health Services Research Unit, University of Manchester.

Marsden, R. (1995) *Young Carers and Education*, London: Borough of Enfield Education Department.

National Health Service and Community Care Act 1990, London: HMSO.

Parker, G. (1994) *Where Next for Research on Carers?*, Leicester: Nuffield Community Care Studies Centre.

Social Services Inspectorate (1995) *Young Carers: Something to think about*, London: Department of Health.

Social Services Inspectorate (2000) *A Jigsaw of services: Inspection of services to support disabled adults in their parenting role*, London: Department of Health.

Walker, A. (1996) *Young Carers and Their Families*, London: The Stationery Office.

Postscript on young carers

Jennifer Henry and Brad Morton

My name is Jennifer. I'm 15 years old and a carer for my mother who is a mentally ill alcoholic. The majority of caring that I do is emotional support, involving me with my mother's emotions and abuse of alcohol. I'm determined to succeed in life, as I am so fed up of living in poverty.

I am called Brad and I am 17. I have cared for my mentally ill father since I was about 11 but have only been at the Young Carers Project in Sheffield for the last three years. It has boosted up my self-esteem and guided me so far through life, for which I am grateful, and has given me a better understanding of what other people go through similar to me. I am an ambitious rapper who has always used music as a gateway to escape and always wanted to work somewhere in the music industry. I feel the Young Carers Project has helped me express my mind and thoughts and see more clearly through the mist ahead.

We wanted to write about our caring experiences so that professionals can have a better understanding of what our lives are really like. We care for a mother who is a mentally ill alcoholic and a father who is mentally ill. Because of this we feel our lives have never been average or normal. We do jobs such as shopping and make decisions, like about what we eat and when we eat. We cook, clean, face the people in housing and council departments when our parents can't or won't do it. We face teachers and our friends and deal with keeping our home lives secret because there is no protection for us at school or in society. Our experience of being young carers is that we feel neglected: our parents have difficulty caring for us, and they themselves do not get much outside support:

Jen: But also nobody officially ever asked me or my brother and sisters how we were or what we wanted to do about the situation at home. My mother's social worker never bothered trying to even speak to us. I feel that caring is a negative thing, as I would have preferred to live in a normal '2.4 person' household, or something similar, and would possibly have wanted to seem ignorant and selfish, rather than learning how to cook, understand mental illness and survive my life on my own. School is particularly difficult for us although we are determined to do well and definitely do not want to be carers for the rest of our lives. Teachers shout if you are late, but you cannot stand in the middle of class saying you have helped your mentally ill dad or mum because you'll be mocked and bullied. I felt isolated from my friends as I hardly ever saw them at school, and never saw them out of school, as I was far too tired, busy or had no money, due to my parents being on benefits or money being spent on alcohol.

Brad: Some of us as young carers do not have a choice whether we want to care or not. I do not think it's fair because it can spoil your path in life, having to stay in every night to care for the person who needs help and not having the choice or option to become a doctor or singer or whatever people's dreams are.

Jen: The caring that we do has sometimes very negative effects on us. We experience the depression, the emotions and the abuse of our parents' situations. Because of this we have to depend on other people for our needs. I turn to my sister who deserves a medal and a better life.

We both related to the sections in the chapter on financial matters. Lack of money and lack of opportunities are often common problems for young carers. We have experienced little support and have often had to get by on very little money. We can't really go travelling like other young people or just be silly like others. The worst thing is that young carers are not recognised enough, it is not acknowledged that we care, we are not recognised for the support we give and are rarely asked about the issues that affect our social lives.

Ways forward

Young carers and anyone else who deals with an issue should be shown consideration and a better understanding by policy makers, agencies and society generally. The worst thing is that young carers are not recognised enough, in terms of what affects our social lives and the issues we go through.

Young carers should receive more moral support in life because there are some children and young people who do not get recognised as Young Carers and are not as lucky as some of us to get opportunities to go out and do activities that other young people do because they are at home caring.

The government should provide a carer for the parents because young carers have to stay in and they can't live their lives imprisoned in their houses.

Awareness needs to be raised on the issues affecting young people; we get classed as thugs because we wear baseball caps and hang about with our mates on the street, which can make older people feel intimidated. We are each very unique and people should not assume, because we are young people or young carers, that we have no future. We can and do accomplish achievements, like appearing in a book like this:

Jen: I think this book is an excellent way of opening all people's minds, possibly helping non-carers to understand what's going on. The chapter made me realise that caring is a problem that is only just starting to be resolved. Also I didn't know that there were anywhere near that amount of carers. The chapter to me was shocking but truthful. I would like to thank Chris Dearden and Saul Becker for producing this chapter, as reading it made me feel even more determined to do well, and writing this postscript made me feel relieved and at last able to give my side of the story.

Brad: The Young Carers Project in Sheffield provides us with opportunities to do activities, to talk about issues that worry us and to give our side of the story, so that our tiny voices can be heard in this massive world.

Chapter 14

Rebel yell: Young people and substance misuse

Rowdy Yates

Introduction

Young people's use of drugs terrifies most of adult society. Inglis (1975) has noted that our response to drug problems[1] as a society is founded largely upon a fear of the unknown, with little room for objective scientific analysis. Others (Peele 1985, Yates 1984) have suggested that the near hysterical response in Western society to drug problems amongst young people appears to owe much to an atavistic belief in possession by devils. Drugs (particularly those from outside our culture – those embedded within our culture such as alcohol, are largely tolerated or ignored) conjure up '. . .the spectre of addiction, psychosis, alienation and rebellion' (Glassner and Loughlin 1990). Drugs will, we are told, rob us of our children and rob them of their dignity, their reason, even their minds.

But little is known about young people's drug use. Most studies have focused on the misuse of drugs by adults, generally reviewing the lives of those already known to treatment services and thus, by definition, already experiencing problems. A brief review of the literature suggests that most studies and, importantly, the way in which they have been undertaken, have largely been reflective of contemporary social policy.

Thus, early American research from the 1940s to the 1960s[2] is largely reflective of the political and social view of drug misuse at that time. Drug misuse was seen as a disease, a generally incurable disease, which needed to be contained. Moreover, it was a disease that particularly afflicted poor, minority ethnic groups. As a consequence, most of these early studies were epidemiological in structure and focused almost exclusively on blacks, Mexicans and Puerto Ricans within the criminal justice system (Ball and Chambers 1970). Drug misuse was a small but persistent problem which, like tuberculosis, thrived on poverty, spread through physical or social contact and, once contracted, would proceed inexorably to the debilitating latter stages of the disease. Ball and Chambers (1970) note the similarities in construction between these studies and those examining the prevalence of syphilis, tuberculosis and smallpox.

Later American studies explored the drug use phenomenon through a more political model. These studies viewed the terminologies of drug policy as largely social constructions and examined the ways in which these definitions were developed and how they affected the protagonists. Such studies (Barber 1967, Lindesmith, 1965) recognised both that some drug use might be 'recreational' and comparable to 'social drinking'; and that the illegality of certain drugs – and thus societal disapproval of their use – itself had a significant impact upon the individual's experience of them. Whilst these studies continued to focus upon the use of illegal drugs by (mainly) adults, they were significant in recognising the importance of the social context within which drug use takes place. Thus, the work of Robins *et al* (1977), in particular, in uncovering substantially higher than expected recovery rates amongst returned Vietnam veterans, was an important milestone in extending the research debate beyond a simple mapping of the spread of an epidemic.

Finally, more recent studies, building upon the work of those such as Peele and Brodsky (1975) and Zinberg (1984) who highlighted the importance of the individual – his culture, background, feelings about himself, etc. – as an equally significant factor in the drug problem equation, have attempted to enter the world of the young drug user and describe it 'from the inside'. This represents a rich seam of information originating in earlier, classic studies such as Becker's (1953) study of marijuana smokers, Carey's (1968) portrait of American college kids, Auld's (1981) review of drug use amongst English university students and Cohen's (1972) examination of the lives of disaffected English youth. Studies of this type have generally sought to report the world of young drug users from their own perspective. However, with a few exceptions (Cohen 1972, Glassner and Loughlin 1990), the majority of these studies have concentrated entirely upon the use of drugs within these groups and rarely report this phenomenon with a view to its relative place in the totality of young people's lives. Moreover, most (although Glassner and Loughlin 1990 are a significant exception in this respect) have considered the worlds of young adults of 18 years old and above.

Studies which consider the use of drugs and alcohol by young people, the role they play in young people's lives and their views about the use and misuse of drugs and alcohol are surprisingly rare. Whilst we know a great deal about the drugs which they use, the ages at which they begin to use them and their attitudes to these and other drugs, much of this information is gleaned from prevalence studies designed to calculate the extent of 'the problem' and from initiatives established to estimate the relative success (or otherwise) of various drug 'education' programmes in reducing the apparently steadily increasing rate of recruitment of young people into drug use. Few have gone beyond these primary aims to examine *why* some young people say yes whilst others do not; why some limit their use of drugs in such a way that it rarely constitutes a problem (for them); the function or functions these substances have in their everyday lives; and what factors are involved in cessation of use by young people.

Current trends in young people's drug and alcohol use

In the UK between the late 1960s and the mid 1980s, public and political concern at the escalation in drug use amongst the young led to the development of a network of specialist treatment services (Strang 1989, Turner 1994) and a wholesale revision of the legislative framework (Glatt et al 1967, Yates 2002). However, the major concern during this period was a small but rapidly increasing group of young drug injectors, mainly within the London area, and this reinforced the development of treatment and policy in the UK around a severely restricted list of illicit substances, most consistently heroin and cocaine (Yates 1999). This in turn has led to young people's use of some substances such as volatile solvents (Ives and Tasker 1999), amphetamines (Klee 1997) and alcohol (Plant et al 1985) being largely ignored by drug treatment services and policy makers. The narrow focus of drug treatment services has proved to be a self-perpetuating limitation in the evidence base, since the bulk of research has tended to be conducted with drug users already in treatment (Yates 1999, Klee 1997).

Balding (1997) has estimated that one in every two or three children in the UK will have used an illegal drug by the age of 15 years old. Ramsay and Spiller (1997) found that 42 per cent of young people between the ages of 16 and 19 years old had experimented with illicit substances. Barnard et al (1996), in a survey of Scottish schoolchildren, found similar levels and little indication that these levels were confined to urban 'hot-spots'. A survey of detached youth workers in Scotland (in both rural and urban settings) found that 20 per cent of respondents were spending at least half their time dealing with drug-related issues. Moreover, 35 per cent of respondents reported dealing with usage which they categorised as 'problematic' (Fast Forward 1997). Recent figures from St. George's Hospital Medical School show that a total of 73 deaths in the UK in 1999 were associated with the inhalation of volatile solvents. One-third were of young people under 18 years old, and Scotland appears to account for a disproportionate number of these deaths (Esmail et al 1997). The majority of deaths continue to be amongst teenagers and go largely unreported (Ives and Tasker 1999) and there is little evidence of those with volatile solvent problems presenting to substance misuse services.

The last two decades has been marked by a seemingly inexorable rise in the numbers of young people using drugs of all kinds. Further, there has been an apparent overall lowering of the age of recruitment into drug use

(Drugscope 2000), often preceded by early introduction to tobacco and alcohol. This has resulted in a growing awareness of the need to broaden our focus and develop new, more eclectic responses to a complex and constantly shifting problem (HM Government 1998). As a result, attention has now turned to the nature of young people's drug use and the services they require. In recent years, a number of UK reports have examined this question in some detail. The Standing Conference on Drug Abuse (SCODA – now Drugscope) and The Children's Legal Centre have published detailed guidance on intervening in young people's drug use in England and Wales (1999) and the Scottish Executive has commissioned similar research publications for Scotland (Burniston *et al* 2002, Effective Interventions Unit and Partnership Drugs Initiative 2002b). In addition, a great deal of work has been undertaken in recent years, examining young people's routes into drug use (Pudney 2002) and the impact of drug use by other family members (ACMD 2003).

The influences on young people

Whilst the literature on young people's drug use remains sparse, a great deal is now known about those young people whose drug use becomes problematic, particularly those whose drugs of choice ensure that they naturally gravitate towards specialist services. The existence of recreational or non-dependent forms of drug use – broadly parallel to the concept of social drinking in the alcohol misuse field – has been recorded since at least the late 1970s (Yates 1979, Zinberg 1984), as has the range of influences which have significance both in respect of recruitment into drugs and the escalation of recreational use into dependence. Some of these influences, such as early childhood trauma (Briere 1988, Najavits *et al* 1997, Yates and Wilson 2001), psychiatric co-morbidity (Anthony and Helzer 1991, Farrell *et al* 1998) and homelessness (Flemen 1997, Klee and Reid 1998), have been extensively researched. Others such as ethnicity have been widely studied in the USA (Barrera *et al* 1999, Hoffman *et al* 2000) but have received considerably less attention in Europe.

Much of the literature examining the use of drugs by young people assumes either that they have not yet been exposed to drug use and therefore require interventions aimed at prevention through the development of resilience (Bradshaw 2000, Fountain *et al* 1999), or that their use of drugs is experimental/recreational and that what is required is health information (Boys *et al* 1998). However, there is strong evidence to indicate that this view is increasingly out of touch with reality: that young people's experimentation with drugs of all kinds frequently dips in and out of dependence, that the mechanisms for these changes are extraordinarily complex and that the UK has some of the highest rates of both experimentation and problem use amongst young people in Europe (Drugscope 2001, EORG 2002, Measham *et al* 1998).

Most studies agree that it is generally the most vulnerable children whose early experimentation with drugs spirals out of control and becomes a major problem for the individual and those around them. Amongst the most vulnerable groups are those children or young people who were recruited into regular use of alcohol and tobacco at an early age; who have been or are currently excluded from school; those with a record of petty offences; homeless, runaway and looked-after children; children of drug – or alcohol-misusing parents; or children who have been subjected to physical or sexual abuse (Barnard 1999, Cadoret 1992, McKeganey and Beaton 2001, McKeganey *et al* 2003, Melrose and Brodie 2000, Yates *et al* 2002a).

This echoes findings in studies of young people's lives in general, where, although boredom was most often cited as the primary reason for initially experimenting with drugs, it was usually feelings of depression, loneliness and helplessness which triggered the escalation into more extensive or chaotic use (Glassner and Loughlin 1990). Moreover, what evidence there is of dependent drug use by young people appears to point to a more opportunistic and fluid approach to drug use than that presented by their adult counterparts (Measham *et al* 1998) and young people will frequently dip in and out of drug use; reducing their intake of one drug whilst significantly increasing their use of another and sometimes ceasing to use some drugs altogether (Ward *et al* 2003).

Young people are also extraordinarily resilient and, even amongst the most vulnerable groups, some studies have shown that there remains a core of young people who are resolutely determined to ensure either that they do not use drugs at all or that their use of drugs remains firmly under their control. A study by Ward *et al* (2003) of the experiences of 200 young people leaving care found that, in terms of ASMA categorisation[3], 29 per cent had either never used an illegal drug or were current abstainers. This resilience amongst a small but significant subgroup was also reflected in their refusal to use, or their modification of prior use of, tobacco and alcohol. Here, eight per cent had never smoked and a further 19 per cent had smoked in the past but had since given up. A total of 14 per cent had either never drunk alcohol or had stopped drinking, whilst a further 29 per cent described themselves as drinking less than before. Although these figures are lower than those found in studies concerning the drug and alcohol usage of young people generally, the findings do illustrate that vulnerability does not make drug use inevitable; nor does it preclude recovery.

Much of UK drug policy for the past 100 years has concentrated upon the relatively simple notion of restricting access (particularly amongst the young) to both illicit and licit drugs and 'peer pressure' appears to be the most popularly accepted explanation for the recruitment of young people into drugs. However, studies of non-users have found that they are just as peer-oriented as their drug-using contemporaries. Glassner and Loughlin's study (1990) of a group of adolescents in mid-West America found that the non-users they interviewed spend substantial portions of their leisure time playing computer games and/or discussing these games with their peers. The authors point out that although there is much media discussion around the preoccupation of young people with such activities and even suggestions that they can be addictive, peer pressure is almost never cited as a reason for recruitment and maintenance. The concept of peer pressure appears to be one of which adults are selective in their use of and, ultimately, a concept that is little more than a sophisticated version of the simplistic notion of accessibility.

For most non-using children and young people, pressure – either to use or to consciously avoid the use of drugs or alcohol – may come not from peers, but from members of their own family. Orford (1985) has noted that children of heavy drinkers often experience violence, fear, anxiety and embarrassment. As a result, they are often socially isolated and report feelings of depression and unhappiness (Johnson and Rolf 1990, Laybourn *et al* 1996). The National Association for the Children of Alcoholics estimates that some 920,000 dependent children are living with a parent who drinks heavily and that over six per cent of the adult population grew up in families where heavy drinking was the norm (NACOA 2000). The National Society for the Prevention of Cruelty to Children has reported that calls to its helpline indicate that misuse of alcohol is a significant factor in 23 per cent of calls relating to emotional abuse (NSPCC 1997). Studies have shown that children of problem drinkers have a significantly higher risk of early onset of psychiatric disorders (Lynskey *et al* 1994) and are twice as likely to become alcoholics themselves at an early age (NACOA 2000).

The Advisory Council on the Misuse of Drugs (2003) estimates that there are some 200,000–300,000 children of dependent drug users in England and Wales (two to three per cent of all children under 16 years old) although around half of these will be living elsewhere; generally with other relatives or in the care of a local authority. In Scotland, there are an estimated 41,000–59,000 children of problem drug users (four to six per cent of all children under 16 years old) with an estimated 10,000–19,000 living with their parents. Little is known at this stage of the long-term impacts of growing up in a family where one or both parents is drug dependent, but some studies have indicated that young people from such backgrounds are significantly more likely than their peers to initiate illicit drug taking (Cadoret 1992, McKeganey *et al* 2003).

Whilst there have been a number of European studies, dating back to the early 1960s, which have examined the use of drugs by siblings, most have been biologically based studies of predisposition to alcoholism amongst twins and adopted children. These studies represent a school of study – most prevalent in the 1970s – which sought to establish a genetic component or 'footprint' to the apparent existence of a familial inheritance of drug/alcohol problems (Goodwin 1990, Murray and Gurlin 1983).

Other studies, mostly undertaken in the USA, indicate a high correlation between drug use by an older sibling and psychiatric co-morbidity (Luthar and Rounsaville 1993, Najavits *et al* 1997) and some (Boyd and Guthrie 1996; Catalano *et al* 1992) have found significant ethnic and gender differences. Rowe and Gulley (1992) found that the nature of the relationship (with the drug-using sibling) was significant, with factors such as the warmth between the siblings and the existence of mutual friends positively correlated with recruitment into drug use. However, the authors also noted that conflict within the relationship could reinforce non-use. Indeed, a number of other studies have also noted the influence of elder siblings (usually brothers) in the development of resilience and the progress of therapeutic intervention (Brook *et al* 1991, Cleveland 1981, Glaser *et al* 1971). As with more general surveys of youth involvement with substance misuse though, much of the research in this area appears to have concentrated upon the influence of older (usually male) siblings in the recruitment of young people into drug use, with a general agreement that this is a powerful factor, second only to the influence of the peer group (McKillip *et al* 1973, Stillwell *et al* 1999).

One large European-wide study found significant correlation between drug dependents entering residential treatment and extensive familial and sibling use coupled with high levels of early neglect or abuse (Kaplan *et al* 1999). In a recent small study in the West of Scotland, a sample of homeless drug and alcohol misusers were interviewed using the European Addiction Severity Index (ASI-X) (Blanken *et al* 1995, Fureman *et al* 1990). Although this was a small sample, virtually all respondents cited drug and alcohol misuse amongst siblings and other family members (Yates *et al* 2002a).

Young people's access to drug and alcohol services

Specialist services for young people – both users and non-users – are relatively rare. In most of the UK, young people will be faced with the choice of either presenting to generic youth services where staff have severely limited training and experience of drug and alcohol issues, or to specialist addiction services where staff are skilled in dealing with an adult clientele but may have little experience of working with young users and little in the way of separate facilities and resources (Burniston *et al* 2002, Yates 1999).

Moreover, given the current focus in many specialist treatment agencies on substitute prescribing approaches and the fluidity of many young people's drug taking, specialist services may have a limited value for this group. Ideally, young people experiencing problems with drugs and alcohol should be able to turn to those non-specialist services with which they are already in contact: usually youth services and social work. However, staff in such services have often received very little instruction in addictions issues within their professional training. Drug and alcohol issues continue to be given scant attention in most professional qualifying courses, with the emphasis remaining on short course in-service interventions. Thus, for example, most social work qualifying courses include addiction issues as a marginal subject area, generally delivered by an external lecturer who is usually a staff member in a drug or alcohol treatment service.

Specialist services in particular are often wary of providing treatment and other interventions for young people, given the current complexity of the legal position. Much of the uncertainty is centred upon the issue of what service or services may be provided by an agency to young people without parental consent or knowledge. Advice and information on drugs and alcohol can be provided without parental consent and agencies are under no obligation to inform any third party that such services have been offered. However, any professional considering the provision of physically invasive treatment (including medication) will need to ensure that this is given with the consent of the patient. Absence of informed consent in such circumstances would constitute a physical assault in law (Standing Conference on Drug Abuse and The Children's Legal Centre 1999). Under the Family Law Reform Act 1987 (Section 8) in England and Wales, young people from 16–18 years of age are normally regarded as competent to provide consent to treatment (Standing Conference on Drug Abuse and The Children's Legal Centre 1999). In Scotland, similar provisions exist under the Age of Legal Capacity Act (Scotland) 1991 (Effective Interventions Unit and Partnership Drugs Initiative 2002b). In addition, across the UK, services would be expected to ensure that their dealings with children and young people are in line with the United Nations Convention on the Rights of the Child 1989, to which the UK is a signatory.

Below the age of 16 years old, however, the legal position becomes much less clear. The Children Act 1989, and in Scotland, the Children (Scotland) Act 1995, clearly state that responsibility for the welfare of the child will normally rest with the parent or parents and that consent to treatment should normally be a matter for them. However, the judgement in the House of Lords in Gillick[4] has indicated that in certain circumstances, medical practitioners may provide treatment to a person below 16 years old without parental consent and this provision has been extended by analogy to other professionals, including psychologists and counsellors. In order to proceed with any proposed treatment intervention, the treatment provider must ensure that the young person in question is 'Gillick competent' to give informed consent to that treatment. 'Gillick competence' must be assessed in each individual case and the ruling does not provide any firm criteria for such an assessment. The general guidance for such assessments are that they should take into account the perceived maturity of the patient (or proposed patient); the child's level of understanding of his/her actions; his/her understanding of the consequences or potential consequences of the treatment proposed; the extent to which other factors (such as intoxication) might affect the child's judgement at the time of consent; and the nature of the proposed treatment and its level of invasiveness. Assessment procedures are also required to recognise that the child's competence to consent may not remain constant, and provision should be available for such decisions to be routinely reviewed (Standing Conference on Drug Abuse and The Children's Legal Centre 1999, Effective Interventions Unit 2002a).

UK guidance in respect of treatment services for young people with drug or alcohol problems (whether in respect of their own misuse or misuse by a family member) suggests that services be provided in four tiers according to need (Health Advisory Service 1996, Standing Conference on Drug Abuse and The Children's Legal Centre 1999). The first tier includes the provision of drugs education, advice and further referral. The second tier includes all of Tier One in addition to the provision of prevention interventions and counselling. Tier Three covers services providing specialist drug or alcohol interventions, generally in multi-disciplinary settings, whilst Tier Four involves the provision of intensive forms of treatment in complex cases, including residential treatment and rehabilitation. Drug Action Teams (see HM Government 1998) are expected to ensure that these levels of treatment are available in their areas and that all staff are competent to assess which tier is appropriate in each individual case (Health Advisory Service 1996, Standing Conference on Drug Abuse and The Children's Legal Centre 1999). Further advice suggests that treatment services should ensure that treatment provision is available at appropriate times (generally outwith school or college times), that supplementary reading materials (both those provided alongside treatment interventions and general materials available in waiting areas) are suitable for young people and that, where necessary, steps are taken to limit contact with adults also receiving treatment (Health Advisory Service 1996, Standing Conference on Drug Abuse and The Children's Legal Centre 1999).

Problems of exclusion: Drug-taking as the new normality?

The extent to which substance use and misuse by young people is likely to lead to social exclusion or, conversely, is itself a result of such exclusion, is extraordinarily complex. Gilman (1998) has argued that the term *social exclusion* is merely a polite way of describing the *underclass* defined by authors such as Murray (1984, 1990) and Gordon (1994). Several authors have noted that drug misuse tends to flourish in areas of high social and economic deprivation (Currie 1993, Pearson 1995) with some (e.g. Wilson 1996) arguing that in areas of high unemployment, the illicit drug economy has replaced employment as a provider of occupation and status.

However, much of this work has concentrated upon particular forms of drug misuse – extensive daily consumption, generally of opioids or cocaine, which are routinely accompanied by acquisitive criminal activity in order to raise the required finances and occasionally by violent crime whilst intoxicated. But, numerous surveys have found that this form of drug taking amongst young people is very rare. According to the 1994 British Crime Survey (Ramsay and Percy 1996) less than one per cent of young people between the ages of 16 and 24 years old have ever used heroin. The figure for cocaine was three per cent Surveys of drug use amongst young people invariably list cannabis as the most commonly used illicit drug, with amphetamine, the second-most popular, lagging some way behind, and the so-called *hard* drugs such as heroin and cocaine, almost non-existent (Barnard *et al* 1996, Drugscope 2000, 2001, Graham and Bowling 1995, Ramsay and Percy 1996, 1997).

However, drug use among young people is not just restricted to areas of multiple deprivation. The 1998 British Crime Survey found that those living in 'rising' areas (standard ACORN classification[5]), were approximately twice as likely to have used a drug in the last year. In fact, this statistic remained even when the more conservative measure of 'drugs used in the past month' was employed. In many respects, illicit drugs have become almost commonplace. They appear to be readily available in many areas of the UK and available with the minimum of effort in others. This easy accessibility, coupled with a range of surveys showing increasing experimentation by young people, has led some authors (Parker and Measham 1994, Parker *et al* 1995, Redhead 1991) to conclude that what is being witnessed is the *normalisation* of drugs in a postmodern culture where epochal changes in the attitudes of young people to drugs have rendered the divisions between the licit and illicit markets almost meaningless. Parker *et al* (1995) argue that the use of some drugs is now so commonplace that we have almost reached a point where abstention becomes the deviant position.

This, however, fundamentally misreads the meaning of *normal* and exaggerates the extent of drug consumption. An analysis of the surveys over the second half of the 20th century shows a steady increase in those professing to have 'ever used' and a slightly less marked increase in those who have 'recently used' (surveys vary in their interpretation of this with the majority asking about either drug use over the previous year or, occasionally, over the previous month) (Shiner and Newburn 1999). Even so, this trend tends to disguise a number of interesting findings which undermine the normalisation hypothesis. At no point does the number of those who have ever used drugs exceed those who have not; even within the peak age range of 16 to 19 years old. Indeed, those who are *currently* abstaining far outnumber the others. Moreover, since other studies would indicate a dramatic increase in availability over this period (Drugscope 2000, 2001), it would seem probable that amongst those who have never used drugs, there may be a significant and increasing group whose abstention is the result of actually saying no rather than a default position due to lack of access (Shiner and Newburn 1999). Finally, the increase over the past 50 years has been relatively even, with no evidence of the watershed change proposed by many postmodernists.

Normalisation is not simply about critical mass. The process whereby certain activities become redefined as *normal* requires also that attitudes towards that activity also change in a fundamental way within the relevant audience. Here, there is clear evidence that young people in the UK continue to regard drug use as deviant. In one study of 1000 young people aged 12–15 years old (Dowds and Redfern 1994), approximately 65 per cent considered cannabis use to be a serious offence. Shiner and Newburn (1996) in their study of attitudes amongst young Londoners found that many respondents expressed concerns about drugs, including costs, health risks and the prospect of being drawn into criminal activity. Although these concerns were strongest amongst those who did not use drugs, they were by no means absent from the thoughts of those who did. Even those respondents who used drugs regularly told of strategies to avoid interaction with heavier users or users of other drugs which they perceived to be more problematic. This finding echoes that of the American study undertaken by Glassner and Loughlin (1990), who found that both users and non-users would often avoid contact with other young people whose use of drugs or alcohol was felt to go beyond accepted standards.

Thus, the argument that drug use amongst young people has become a normalised activity probably overestimates current levels of use and underestimates the number and meaning of refusals. Also, whilst there is a substantial body of evidence to suggest that the use of certain drugs has become synonymous with areas of social deprivation, this is by no means true of all drugs or of all young drug users.

There remains the question of those young people whose parents or other family members are misusers of alcohol and drugs. Here, the evidence is somewhat sparse, but McKeganey *et al* (2003), in respect of drugs, and Orford (1985), in respect of alcohol, have found that some young people in this situation will often become excluded, or will exclude themselves to avoid embarrassment and humiliation. These are the young people who avoid inviting their peers to the family home or who 'lose' the school letter inviting parents to various school events.

Conclusion

Teenage years and early adulthood represent an extraordinarily difficult time for young people and they will often 'test the limits' by engaging in activities, including drug and alcohol use, in ways which are problematic both for them and for others around them (Balding 1997, Barnard *et al* 1996, Glassner and Loughlin 1990, Ramsey and Spiller 1997). Whilst much of this activity represents a real and meaningful immediate danger, the consequences of most youthful experimentation will have only limited long-term significance. Some young people, however, are particularly vulnerable to exploitation, physical and social negative consequences and, for a few, long-term problems of dependence and associated problematic behaviour.

Services for young people with drug or alcohol problems are sparse in most areas, although the position is improving. One study in Scotland (Burniston *et al* 2002) found 42 relevant services although services were located in only 12 of the 22 Scottish Drug Action Team areas. The legal position regarding the treatment of young people is often unclear and many professionals are reluctant to provide services without parental consent. Generally, the more invasive the proposed treatment, the less likely it is that a young person under the age of 16 years old would be adjudged as competent to give informed consent.

Within the past decade, the issue of drug and alcohol misuse by young people has become one of real concern and there has been much good work undertaken in the UK to develop appropriate services, provide relevant educational inputs, identify vulnerable groups and ensure that the relevant professionals are given appropriate training and support to offer services to this group. However, support and advice for young (non-using) people affected by the use of drugs and alcohol by others around them is less readily available. Little is understood regarding the resilience of young people to drug or alcohol misuse and few services are in a position to provide services which might strengthen this resolve.

Youth is a time when many individuals struggle to understand their position in the family and within the wider community: they are too old to be included as children and yet, for many, they are denied the resources and independence normally assigned to adults. For many, experimentation with drugs and alcohol represents a way of impressing their peers, of rebelling against parental control and restraint or of simply occupying time with a pleasurable – usually communal – activity. Most will suffer little long-term damage and will probably reduce their involvement naturally in later years. However, it is clear too that in some cases, for some individuals, such activities can result in dislocation from the mainstream or deepen an already existing gulf.

Endnotes

1 The definition of problem drug use used throughout this chapter is that set down by the Advisory Council on the Misuse of Drugs (ACMD) in its 1982 report, *Treatment and Rehabilitation*. This definition states: 'Thus a problem drug taker would be any person who experiences social, psychological, physical or legal problems related to intoxication and/or regular excessive consumption and/or dependence as a consequence of his own use of drugs or other chemical substances' (ACMD 1982).

2 There are few, if any, examples of European or UK studies during this period and given the later recognition of drug use as problematic, such studies, when they do appear, in the 1960s, generally follow a logically later timescale than their American counterparts.
3 Assessment of Substance Misuse in Adolescence (ASMA) is a brief screening instrument developed by Swadi (1997) and modified by Willner (2000) in order to test frequency and severity of licit and illicit drugs in young people.
4 Gillick [1985] 3 All ER 402 – This ruling arises out of a legal action raised by the campaigner Victoria Gillick in respect of the provision (without her consent) of contraceptive medication to her daughter. Whilst the Lords decision was specific to the particular case, the guidance provided is universally accepted to pertain to all types of medical intervention.
5 ACORN – standardised classification of residential areas developed by CACI Limited (www.caci.co.uk/acorn/acornmap.asp) and categorising areas according to various Census characteristics such as unemployment, poverty, number of single-parent households, etc.

References

Advisory Council on the Misuse of Drugs (ACMD) (1982) *Treatment and Rehabilitation*, London: HMSO.
Advisory Council on the Misuse of Drugs (ACMD) (2003) *Hidden Harm: Responding to the needs of children of problem drug users*, London: HMSO.
Anthony, J.C. and Helzer, J.E. (1991) 'Syndromes of drug abuse and dependence', in L. Robins and D. Regier (eds), *Psychiatric Disorders in America: The Epidemological Catchment Area Study*, New York: Free Press.
Auld, J. (1981) *Marijuana Use and Social Control*, New York: Academic Press.
Balding, J. (1997) *Young People and Illegal Drugs in 1996*, Exeter: Schools Health Education Unit.
Ball, J. and Chambers, C. (eds) (1970) *The Epidemiology of Opiate Addiction in the United States*, Illinois: Charles Thomas.
Barber, B. (1967) *Drugs and Society*, New York: Russell Sage.
Barnard, M. (1999) 'Forbidden questions: drug dependent parents and the welfare of their children', *Addiction*, 94: 1109–1111.
Barnard, M., Forsyth, A. and McKeganey, N. (1996) 'Levels of drug use among a sample of Scottish schoolchildren', *Drugs Education, Prevention and Policy*, 3: 81–89.
Barrera, M., Castro, F. and Biglan, A. (1999) 'Ethnicity, substance use and development: Exemplars for exploring group differences and similarities', *Development and Psychopathology*, 11: 805–822.
Becker, H. (1953) 'Becoming a marijuana user', *American Journal of Sociology*, 59: 235–243.
Blanken, P., Hendricks, V., Pozzi, G., et al. (1995) *European Addiction Severity Index: A guide to training and administering EuropASI Interviews*, Lisbon: COST A6 Working Group.
Boyd, C. and Guthrie, B. (1996) 'Women, their significant others and crack cocaine', *American Journal of Addiction*, 5: 156–166.
Boys, A., Fountain, J., Griffiths, P., et al. (1998) *Making Decisions: A qualitative study of young people, drugs and alcohol*, London: Health Education Authority.

Bradshaw, J. (2000) 'Regaining lost youth: Youth workers success with drug users', *Druglink* 15: 9–11.

Briere, J. (1988) 'The long term clinical correlates of childhood sexual victimisation', *Annals of the New York Academy of Sciences*, 528.

Brook, J., Whiteman, M. Brook, D. *et al.* (1991) 'Sibling influences on adolescent drug use: Older brothers on younger brothers', *Journal of the American Academy of Child and Adolescent Psychiatry*, 30: 958–966.

Burniston, S., Dodd, M., Elliott, L. *et al.* (2002) *Drug Treatment Services for Young People: A research review,* Edinburgh: Effective Interventions Unit, Scottish Executive.

Cadoret, R. (1992) 'Genetic and environmental factors in the initiation of drug use and the transition to abuse', in M. Glantz and R. Pickens (eds), *Vulnerability in Drug Use*, New York: American Psychological Association.

Carey, J.T., *The College Drugs Scene*, Englewood Cliffs, N.J.: Prentice-Hall.

Catalano, R.F., Morrison D.M., Wells E.A., *et al.* (1992) 'Ethnic differences in family factors related to early drug initiation', *Journal of Studies in Alcoholism*, 53: 208–217.

Cleveland, M. (1981) 'Families and adolescent drug abuse: Structural analysis of children's roles', *Family Process*, 20: 295–304.

Cohen, S. (1972) *Folk Devils and Moral Panics*, London: MacGibbon and Kee.

Currie, E. (1993) *Reckoning: Drugs, the cities and the American future*, New York: Free Press.

Dowds, L., Redfern, J., (1994) *Drug Education Amongst Teenagers: a 1992 British Crime Survey Analysis*, London: Home Office, Research and Planning Unit.

Drugscope (2000) *UK Drug Situation 2000: The UK Report to the European Monitoring Centre for Drugs and Drug Addiction (EMCDDA)*, London: Drugscope.
www.stir.ac.uk/Departments/HumanSciences/AppSocSci/DRUGS/drugreport.pdf

Drugscope (2001) *UK Drug Situation 2001: The UK Report to the European Monitoring Centre for Drugs and Drug Addiction (EMCDDA)*, London: Drugscope.
www.stir.ac.uk/Departments/HumanSciences/AppSocSci/DRUGS/uk2001.pdf

Effective Interventions Unit (2002a) *Drug Treatment Services for Young People: A systematic review of effectiveness and the legal framework*, Edinburgh: Effective Interventions Unit, Scottish Executive.

Effective Interventions Unit and Partnership Drugs Initiative (2002b) *Services for Young People with Problematic Drug Misuse: A guide to principles and practice*, Edinburgh: Effective Interventions Unit, Scottish Executive.

Esmail, A., Warburton, B., Bland, J., *et al.* (1997) 'Regional variations in deaths from volatile solvent abuse in Great Britain', *Addiction* 92: 1765–1771.

European Opinion Research Group (EORG) (2002) *Attitudes and Opinions of Young People in the European Union on Drugs: Eurobarometer 57.2, Special Eurobarometer 172*, Brussels: Directorate-General for Justice and Home Affairs.

Farrell, M., Howes, S., Taylor, C., *et al.* (1998) 'Substance misuse and psychiatric comorbidity: An overview of the OPCS National Psychiatric Morbidity Survey', *Journal of Addictive Behaviour*, 23: 909–918.

Fast Forward (1997) *Out There with Us: Young people, drugs and the role of the detached youth worker*, Edinburgh: Health Education Board for Scotland.

Flemen, K. (1997) *Smoke and Whispers: Drugs and youth homelessness in central London*, London: The Hungerford Drug Project.

Fountain, J., Bartlett, H., Griffiths, P., *et al* (1999) 'Why say no? Reasons given by young people for not using drugs', *Addiction Research* 7: 339–353.

Fureman, B., Parikh, H., Bragg, A. *et al.* (1990) *Addiction Severity Index: A guide to training and supervising ASI interviews based on the past ten years*, Pennsylvania: The University of Pennsylvania/Veterans Administration, Center for Studies of Addiction.

Gilman, M. (1998) 'Onion rings to go: Drugs and social exclusion, *Druglink* 13(3): 15–17.

Glaser, D., Lander, B. and Abbott, W. (1971) 'Opiate addicted and non addicted siblings in a slum area', *Social Problems*, 18: 510–521.

Glassner, B. and Loughlin J. (1990) *Drugs in Adolescent Worlds: Burnouts to straights*, London: Macmillan.

Glatt, M., Pittman, D., Gillespie, D. *et al.* (1967) *The Drug Scene in Great Britain: Journey into loneliness*, London: Edward Arnold.

Goodwin, D. (1990) 'Evidence for a genetic factor in alcoholism', in R. Engs (ed.), *Controversies in the Addiction Field*, Dubuque: Kendall Hunt.
http://www.indiana.edu/~engs/cbook/index.html

Gordon, D. (1994) *The Return of the Dangerous Classes: Drug prohibition and policy politics*, New York: W. W. Norton.

Graham, J. and Bowling, B. (1995) *Young People and Crime*, London: Home Office.

Health Advisory Service (1996) Children and Young People: Substance misuse services – the substance of young need, London: HMSO.

HM Government (1998) *Tackling Drugs To Build A Better Britain: The Governments ten year strategy for tackling drug misuse*, London: HMSO.
http://www.official-documents.co.uk/document/cm39/3945/3945.htm

Hoffman, J., Barnes, G., Welte, J. *et al.* (2000) 'Trends in combinational use of alcohol and illicit drugs among minority adolescents, 1983–1994', *American Journal of Drug and Alcohol Abuse*, 26: 311–324.

Inglis, B. (1975) *The Forbidden Game: A social history of drugs*, London: Hodder and Stoughton.

Ives, R. and Tasker, T. (1999) *Volatile Substance Abuse: A report on survey evidence*, London: Health Education Authority.

Johnson, J. and Rolf, J. (1990) 'When children change: Research perspectives on children of alcoholics', in R. Collins, K. Leonard and J. Searles (eds), *Alcohol and the Family*, London: Guilford Press.

Kaplan, C., Broekaert, E. and Frank, O. (1999) *Biomed 2 IPTRP Project on Improving Psychiatric Treatment in Residential Programmes for Emerging Dependency Groups: Final Report 1996–1999*, Maastricht: University of Maastricht.

Klee, H. (1997) *Amphetamine Misuse: International perspectives on current trends*, London: Harwood Academic.

Klee, H. and Reid, P. (1998) 'Drugs and youth homelessness: Reducing the risk', *Drugs Education Prevention and Policy*, 5: 269–280.

Laybourn, A., Brown, J. and Hill, M. (1996) *Hurting on the Inside; Children's experiences of parental alcohol misuse*, Aldershot: Avebury.

Lindesmith, A. (1965) *The Addict and the Law*, New York: Random House.

Luthar, S. and Rounsaville, B. (1993) 'Substance misuse and comorbid psychopathology in a high risk group: A study of siblings of cocaine misusers', *International Journal of Addiction*, 28:415–434.

Lynskey, M., Fergusson, D. and Horwood, J. (1994) 'The effects of parental alcohol problems on rates of adolescent psychiatric disorders', *Addiction*, 89: 1277–1286.

McKeganey, N. and Beaton, K. (2001) *Drug and alcohol use amongst a sample of looked after children in Scotland*, Unpublished Report.

McKeganey, N., McIntosh, I. and MacDonald, F. (2003) 'Young people's experience of illegal drug use in the family', *Drugs Education, Prevention and Policy*, 10: 169–184.

McKillip, J., Johnson, J. and Petzel, T. (1973) 'Patterns and correlates of drug use among urban high school students', *Journal of Drug Education*, 3: 1–12.

Measham, F., Parker, H. and Aldridge, J. (1998) *Staring, Switching, Slowing and Stopping: Report for the Drugs Prevention Initiative Integrated Programme*, London: HMSO.

Melrose, M. and Brodie, I. (2000) 'Vulnerable young people and their vulnerability to drug misuse', in Drugscope and Department of Health (eds), *Vulnerability Young People and Drugs: Opportunities to tackle inequalities*, London: Drugscope.

Murray, C. (1984) *Losing Ground: American social policy*, New York: Basic Books.

Murray, C. (1990) *The Emerging British Underclass (Choice in Welfare Series, No. 2)*, London: Institute of Economic Affairs.

Murray, R. and Gurlin, C. (1983) 'Twin and alcoholism studies', in M. Galanter (ed.), *Recent Developments in Alcoholism*, New York: Gardner Press.

NACOA (2000) *Preliminary Survey Findings*, Bristol: NACOA.

NSPCC (2000) *NSPCC Calls for New Year's Resolution on Drinking*, London, Press release dated 30th December 1997.

Najavits, L. M., Weiss, R. D. and Shaw, S. R. (1997) 'The link between substance abuse and post traumatic stress disorder in women: a research review', *American Journal on Addictions*, 6: 273–283.

Orford, J. (1985) 'Alcohol problems and the family', in J. Lishman and G. Horobin (eds), *Approaches to Addiction*, London: Kogan Page.

Parker, H. and Measham, F. (1994) 'Pick 'n' mix: Changing patterns of illicit drug use among 1990s adolescents', *Drugs Education, Prevention and Policy*, 1: 5–13.

Parker, H., Measham, F. and Aldridge, J. (1995) *Drugs Futures: Changing Patterns of drug use amongst English youth*, London: Institute for the Study of Drug Dependence.

Pearson, G. (1995) 'City of darkness, city of light: Crime, drugs and disorder in London and New York', in S. MacGregor and A. Lipow (eds), *The Other City: People and politics in New York and London*, Atlantic Highlands: Humanities Press.

Peele, S. (1985) *The Meaning of Addiction: Compulsive experience and its interpretation*, Lexington: Lexington Books.

Peele, S. and Brodsky, A. (1975) *Love and Addiction*, New York: Taplinger Publishing.

Plant, M., Peck, D. and Samuel, E. (1985) *Alcohol, Drugs and School Leavers*, London: Tavistock.

Pudney, S. (2002) *The Road to Ruin? Sequences of Initiation into Drug Use and Offending by Young People in Britain*, London: Home Office Research, Development and Statistics Directorate.

Ramsay, M. and Percy, A., (1996) *Drug Misuse Declared: Results from the 1994 British Crime Survey*, London: Home Office Research and Statistics Department.

Ramsay, M. and Spiller, J. (1997) *Drug Misuse Declared in 1996: Latest results from the British Crime Survey*, London: Home Office Research and Statistics Department.

Redhead, S. (1991) 'Rave off: Youth subculture and the law', *Social Studies Review*, 6: 92–94.

Robins, L., Helzer, J., Hesselbrock, M., *et al.* (1977) Vietnam veterans three years after Vietnam, in L. Harris (ed), *Problems of Drug Dependence*, Washington: National Academy of Sciences.

Rowe, D. and Gulley, B. (1992) 'Sibling effects on substance use and delinquency', *Criminology*, 30: 217–233.

Shiner, M. and Newburn, T. (1999) 'Taking tea with Noel: The place and meaning of drug use in everyday life', in N. South (ed.), *Drugs: Cultures, controls and everyday life*, London: Sage Publications Ltd.

Standing Conference on Drug Abuse and The Children's Legal Centre (1999) *Young People and Drugs: Policy guidance for drug interventions*, London: SCODA.

Stillwell, G., Hunt, N., Taylor, C. and Griffiths, P. (1999) 'The modelling of injecting behaviour and initiation into injecting', *Addiction Research*, 7: 447–459.

Strang, J. (1989) 'The British System: Past, present and future', *International Review of Psychiatry*, 1: 109–120.

Swadi, H. (1997) 'Substance misuse in adolescence questionnaire (SMAQ): A pilot study of a screening instrument for problematic use of drugs and volatile solvents in adolescents', *Child Psychology and Psychiatry Review* 2: 63–69.

Turner, D., (1994) 'The development of the voluntary sector, no further need for pioneers', in J. Strang and M. Gossop (eds), *Heroin Addiction and Drug Policy: The British System*, Oxford: Oxford University Press.

Ward, J., Henderson, Z., Pearson, G., (2003) One Problem Among Many: Drug use among care leavers in transition to independent living, London: Home Office Public Policy Research Unit, Goldsmiths College.

Willner, P. (2000) 'Further validation and development of a screening instrument for the assessment of substance misuse in adolescents', *Addiction*, 95: 1691–1698.

Wilson, W. J. (1996) *When Work Disappears: The world of the new urban poor*, New York: Alfred A. Knopf.

Yates, R. (1979) *Recreation or Desperation*, Manchester: Lifeline Project.

Yates, R. (1984) 'Addiction: An everyday disease', in J. Lishman and G. Horobin (eds), *Approaches to Addiction*, London: Kogan Page.

Yates, R. (1999) 'Only Available in Black: The limiting of addiction services in the twentieth century', *Uteseksjonen 30 Ar Pa Gata*, November 1999, Oslo: Uteseksjonen.

Yates, R. (2002) 'A brief history of British drug policy', 1950–2001, *Drugs Education, Prevention and Policy*, 9: 113–124.

Yates, R. and Wilson, J. (2001) 'The modern therapeutic community: Dual diagnosis and the process of change', in B. Rawlings and R. Yates (eds), *Therapeutic Communities for the Treatment of Drug Users*, London: Jessica Kingsley.

Yates, R., Anderson, I., Wilson, J., *et al.* (2002) *Trouble Every Way I Turn: Homelessness and substance misuse in East Renfrewshire*, Study commissioned by East Renfrewshire Council.

Zinberg, N. (1984) *Drug, Set and Setting: The basis for controlled intoxicant use*, New Haven: Yale University Press'.

Postscript on substance misuse

Jean-Paul Duffy and Daniel Raffell

Jean-Paul Duffy

My name is Jean-Paul Duffy, known to my friends as J-P. I am 26 and work with the homeless as a Project Worker. I live in Edinburgh and have done for the past three years. It has been over these three 'drug-free' years that I have investigated and reflected upon, in depth, my own drug use, which finally led to a heroin addiction.

I work with the homeless and I have recognised that a very large majority of them have addiction issues. Now, of the ones who have addictions, there are many similarities/common denominators. Many have grown up in impoverished areas. Many have grown up in single-parent families or broken homes. Many have been witness to the use of substances from an early age and many have themselves used from an early age. These facts have indicated to me that it is the lower classes within society that are more commonly affected in the long term by substance use/misuse. But drugs are everywhere and don't distinguish by class, so why do the relatively poor appear to suffer the most?

Often, for a youth living in a not so deprived area, this is not experienced to the same degree. They may be witness to better role models and have a more settled home life. But the main reason, I think, may be that the level of expectation on these youths to succeed to a level that society considers acceptable is far greater. Their parents might be that little bit more involved as they encourage and expect their child to succeed. Those youths also learned a pattern to live by and drug misuse may be recognised as a threat to the realisation of their ambitions.

Through a previous job doing street work (working with youths on the street in 'poor areas'), I was able to identify what could be some of the contributing factors as to why poorer young people are more likely to get into drugs. Most of these kids didn't have any ambition to make a better future for themselves. They didn't apply themselves at school and their parents didn't seem to be very encouraging. I think that they were missing a positive role model. Sadly, the only role models they had were their parents or the older youths who had been raised similarly and were demonstrating destructive lifestyles. This is not a generalisation and of course I am not suggesting that everyone who lives in these communities is the same but there is a considerable percentage that is caught in this cycle and learned behaviour is demonstrated.

To address my own drug addiction, I was forced to leave my home in Fife and move to Edinburgh. This was due to the limited services available in Fife. It was very difficult for me to access a relevant service, as they are few in number and have very long waiting lists. Also, it appeared that, unless the application was prompted by the criminal justice system, then the chances of addressing my problem were effectively halved at best. Unless your addiction caused you to repeatedly offend, i.e. shoplift, house break, rob, etc., then the provision to address the core problem (addiction) was minimal. This isn't to say that I was not involved in criminal activity. I was, and I do have a criminal record. I was just never caught as often as I should have been, or was not yet seen by the criminal justice system as a serious problem to society.

Why is there more help available to someone who has reached the point where their drug use has spiralled out of their control? Should there not be more services available (in the community) to help those who have recognised that they may be developing a problem? I think there should. Consider the young person, the teenager: for some it may be considered cool to use drugs/alcohol and done to impress friends or the opposite sex. Or maybe it is a coping mechanism to help them deal with their home life, which may be troubled, or to help them with the pressures of exams. Where can these kids go to get help, especially if they are under 16? Approaching a teacher could result in parents being called in. Speaking to friends may cause them to look uncool or weak. Services have to be easily accessible to both adults and young people. They have to be found in the community and they must not be unwelcoming. When trying to target youths, maybe peer educators could be employed: young adults with relevant experience who can connect with the youths on their level.

I am aware that these strategies are already used by many different organisations but in my opinion not nearly enough. The government needs to invest a lot more of its time and money to address the rising drug problem among the youth population of today.

Daniel Raffell

My name is Danny Raffell. I am 25 and have lived in Edinburgh for the last two years. I have worked most of my working life (mainly as a qualified landscape gardener and golf caddying), and am now working in two voluntary organisations. One is a drop-in centre for homeless people and the other is educating people on drugs and alcohol awareness, sexual health and facilitating workshops. I am passionate about the drugs problem and want to continue using my experiences of drugs to try and help others.

The issues that surround drugs are deep and complex. Society as a whole tends to stereotype drug users and addicts, which I find not only unhelpful but sometimes hindering, naive and dangerous. I believe drug use and addiction is more about individuality than a collective issue and this needs to be looked at. Adults in society tend to want to bury their heads in the sand and try and wish away the problem. Wake up! it's happening and it will continue to go on. It seems to be only a handful of people that actually have an open mind and have practical views on these issues.

My experience of having been a regular drug user, up to the point of having a dependency for drugs spanning over the last 11 years, leaves me with varied knowledge and first-hand views on such a subject, although as I mentioned it is an individual thing and it is only one person's experience. Having come from a loving family and with no experience of abuse of any kind, it is hard to pinpoint any specific reason for my drug taking. There are many factors that may have contributed, from peer pressure (which can be a very powerful factor) to having older brothers (who have been in similar situations before me). But let's be honest: a simple thing such as boredom was probably a main reason, and if I were to be completely honest it was fun and I enjoyed it immensely. I took drugs for five to six years before I even came close to realising I had a problem, and when I reached this point my attitude and my characteristics had changed probably without me consciously knowing. My self-esteem was low, I had little confidence in society and felt I had nowhere to turn for help or support. I felt alone and a little scared to talk to anyone in the beginning due to the view people have on drugs, and this led me to become more private and reclusive, and then carrying on thinking it was just my lot in life.

I progressed from buzzing solvents to smoking cannabis, taking LSD, cocaine, amphetamines and ecstasy, leading to depressants like valium, temazipam and heroin. I felt I didn't have a problem with drugs, even up to the point of taking heroin on a daily basis. I certainly did not have as bad an addiction as I did after I got introduced to the methadone programme – the idea of having free drugs sounded good but I felt that it kept me in addiction longer. For four to five years I struggled to come off the heroin substitute, and in some ways I wish I had never been introduced to it. At this time I felt I received little help from drug counsellors and, even the few times I did come into contact with them, automatically there were barriers up as I knew they did not really understand the situation people go through. I do realise this is not the case with all services but true empathy is hard to find when you have not experienced such things yourself, but it is a very important factor, I feel, in helping to improve the situation. Having more ex-addicts can be an effective way of helping ease some situations, not only in supporting or giving counsel to other drug users but also by allowing them to educate and train parents, teachers and youth workers in prevention, harm reduction and other information on what a drug-using lifestyle has to offer. We cannot carry on with this ignorant way we try to deal with the issues young people face today.

It is important that young people growing up are allowed their own freedom to make choices and inevitably make their own mistakes. Having parental restrictions and rules are vital but children tend to be rebellious in some ways and being too over protective can work in the opposite way. Restricted access and availability to some drugs and the surrounding lifestyle is important, but we are living in the real world and have to wake up to the real problems. Because drugs can be a big part of growing up for some people, we need to have in place services to educate and train youngsters and adults in making the correct decisions. We need to offer support to youngsters involved in drug experimentation, without the need for parental consent, as sometimes this can scare young people to keep it to themselves and become more private and then parents loose contact with the severity of the issue.

Fortunately for me, I have come through a tough process of recovery and know how hard it is to escape such a lifestyle. However, I feel that if there were services as mentioned earlier, even someone to share things with a little more in depth than was offered to me or even just to show me a little of the life I was getting myself into, things may have been a little different and a lot less painful. I now seek to use my experiences in a way to help other people not only in addiction but in trying to prevent people making these mistakes in the first place. As I also mentioned earlier, I feel someone who has experienced these things can sometimes have more to offer their peers than some professional services. I just hope the government can wake up to this escalating problem and put practical things in place to try and combat this difficult issue of drugs.

Chapter 15

Conclusions

Monica Barry

The aim of this book has been to explore varying perceptions on youth policy and social inclusion in the UK, including the perceptions of young people themselves. What this book has highlighted is the possible discriminatory attitudes and practices of 'adults' which may serve to exacerbate rather than alleviate young people's social exclusion from the wider society. The postscripts to each chapter challenge orthodox views about youth policy, whilst confirming the fact that such policies are often misplaced in attempting to engage and integrate young people in our society.

Involving young people in the postscripts has emphasised their role as 'expert witnesses', based on their direct experience of issues such as homelessness, crime, poverty and unemployment. The book offers young people the opportunity to voice their opinions and concerns on current thinking about particular issues. Together with the academic contributions in this volume, which also draw extensively on qualitative research with particular groups of disadvantaged young people, these postscripts give significantly greater weight to the concerns of many academics and young people about youth policy and social inclusion.

This concluding chapter concentrates on the unique contribution of the young people. It will not endeavour to summarise the academic contributions, partly because the authors have drawn conclusions themselves within each chapter, but also because there are striking similarities between the chapter authors' views and those of the young people in addressing the various issues. Throughout this chapter, the names of the young people will be given in full; chapter authors will only be referred to as 'the author of chapter . . .'.

Tajfel (1982: 502) has commented that:

> One of the few privileges associated with the task of an editor consists perhaps of being able to look back from some small distance at the various arguments developed in a book in order to see if some kind of a common perspective can sometimes emerge from viewpoints which appear to be diametrically opposed.

Fortunately in one sense, the ideas contained in these chapters and post-scripts do not appear to be diametrically opposed, thus making my task as editor much easier. However, the consistently repeated suggestions within this book of discrimination and disrespect of young people are nothing to be proud of. Musgrove (1964) suggested some 40 years ago that youth was an oppressed group that had been rejected by adults at a time when young people should have been protected and integrated within society. He con-cluded that the situation for young people was unlikely to improve. It seems that his pessimism has, regrettably, stood the test of time. Certain themes have emerged from the chapters and postscripts in this book which reflect the current pessimism of many academics and young people: namely, issues of practical support (services, advice and publicity) and what I term 'rela-tional' support (the status of young people in society vis-à-vis their older counterparts). Within both of these themes runs a strong element of discrimination, not only by class but also by age.

Elsewhere, I have suggested (Barry 2004) that the politicisation of youth and the criminalisation of young people has masked structural and age-related inequalities in society and led many young people to view their own transition to adulthood as a personal problem. Wyn and White (1997), for example, note the state's marginalisation and criminalisation of young peo-ple, because of their young age, low status and lack of citizenship, as a deliberate means of deflecting attention away from issues of poverty and unemployment as well as wider structural inequalities. This chapter now describes the current context within which such discrimination of young people occurs, using the two themes of practical support and relational support as terms of reference.

Practical support

Three issues emerged from the postscripts which related to practical sup-port – the fact that many services for young people are reactive rather than proactive in nature; that they are often inappropriate to the needs and wishes of young people most in need of them; and that they are inade-quately publicised to make them accessible to those young people who most want them. These are explored in further detail below.

Reactive services

Many of the contributions in this book note that it is the most socially excluded young people who receive the least support and are least likely to meet the stringent criteria prescribed by policy initiatives. Ellen Leaver and Regan Tammi (Chapter 4) note that those who are in most need of educa-tion, for example, are those most likely to be excluded, and the author of Chapter 12 suggests that, in relation to young mothers, those 'who have the least resources are frequently those to whom the least is offered'. And yet, several of the postscripts draw attention to the anomaly that unless a young person has existing problems that are known to professional agencies, they are unlikely to receive appropriate support or services. Annmarie Fraser and Stephanie George (Chapter 12) highlight the fact that support is less likely to be forthcoming for teenage mothers *unless* they have existing social work involvement. This was reiterated by Jean-Paul Duffy (Chapter 14) when he notes that young people can only readily access treatment for drug problems if they first come to the attention of the criminal justice system because of persistent offending. Jon Paterson and Julie Johnson (Chapter 9) also state, in relation to homelessness: 'we were in 'crisis' before any support was offered'. Thus, as many of the postscript contributors imply, services offer 'too little too late' to prevent crises and to minimise the impact of such difficulties on young people's lives.

More preventative services and proactive support at an earlier age or stage in their lives are therefore needed before young people's situations become critical. There is also a need for support which takes into account both structural inequalities and individual need.

Inappropriate services

Several postscript contributors agree with the chapter authors that many services for young people are inappropriate and inaccessible. Their reasons for this are because such services:

- do not target the needs and wishes of young people;
- do not utilise the expertise and empathy of other young people with similar past experiences of the difficulties being faced;
- apply criteria for eligibility which are convoluted or overly narrow in focus; or
- are seen by many young people as tokenistic and short-lived.

In relation to the appropriateness of the target group for many services, education is singled out by young people as failing them in terms of current and future needs. Heather Barnshaw and Mary Ho (Chapter 5) and Charlotte Ali (Chapter 8) stress the importance of offering a wider set of curricular activities in consultation with pupils rather than channelling them down either academic or vocational routes dependent on qualifications and ability.

Many of the postscript contributors have been, or are currently, working with other young people, thus capitalising on their own experiences. For example, Jean-Paul Duffy and Daniel Raffell (Chapter 14) advocate the employment of young people with past experience of substance misuse as peer educators, trainers or mentors to ensure some sense of understanding and empathy for young people's lived experiences.

Many policies emanating from governments of all political persuasions by definition are short-term and expedient. However, the inflexible, over-coercive and myopic nature of many policies relating to young people in particular tends to dilute their effectiveness with those most susceptible to multiple disadvantage. Several chapter authors have noted the short-term nature of much youth policy, notably the New Deal, which defines sustainable employment as that continuing beyond 13 weeks in duration (see Chapter 8). In the postscripts on asylum seekers, youth justice and young mothers, it is also suggested that once a young person reaches a certain age, their entitlement to certain services is restricted – or in the case of youth justice, that the emphasis changes from welfare to punishment. This can often have a debilitating effect on young people who rely on the continuity of a service to support them throughout difficult times, irrespective of their age.

There is also an expectation by policy makers that young people will 'fit' their criteria, highlighting what the author of Chapter 2 describes as 'an absurd sense of urgency' by government to demonstrate success. Thus, as Kieran Marshall (Chapter 2) suggests, there is an increasing preoccupation with a 'tick box mentality' by both policy makers and practitioners at the expense of effective interventions once the young person is 'through the door'. However, many young people have neither the wherewithal nor the self-determination to slot readily into rigid categories, but require a more holistic, longer-term and 'joined up' response which they perceive as appropriate and effective in addressing *their* issues. As Steven Kidd (Chapter 2) remarks: 'a young person is not a statistic, but a complex collection of skills, abilities, needs and desires, and services directed towards young people would do well to take this on board'.

Publicity

Publicity was seen as an issue for many young people, for two reasons. First, much media coverage of youth issues, as Steven Kidd suggests in Chapter 2, has portrayed young people in a negative light and tended to sensationalise problems and stigmatise young people as a result. Jennifer Henry and Brad Morton (Chapter 13) argue that public awareness needs to be raised of the issues affecting young people and Mustajab Malikzada and Ahmad Qadri (Chapter 10) suggest that there is 'widespread prejudice' about asylum seekers which is fuelled by racist media coverage. If the media was to give as much attention to the positive contributions that young people make within their communities (from an education, employment, leisure or voluntary perspective, for example), this would raise public awareness of young people's responsibilities and enhance their social inclusion.

Secondly, general publicity, notably in the form of sharing information and giving advice about certain services, is often inappropriate or inaccessible to young people. This also relates to the lack of participation generally of young people in youth policy matters (see below), but is exacerbated by policies and services being inappropriately or poorly publicised. Young people want constructive advice that is relevant to them and expressed in their terms, in order to negotiate their way through the labyrinth of legislation, documentation and services purportedly designed to meet their current and future needs.

Relational support

Given that the period in one's life from the age of 15–25 years old is one when many fundamental changes and decisions have to be made that influence the rest of one's life, it is crucial for young people to have practical support at this time. However, without a wider social environment that is conducive to this process of change, then some young people are more likely to feel constrained and isolated. Several issues are explored within this relational context: namely, a consideration of the 'deficit model' of youth; discrimination by age; the criminalisation of young people; their opportunities for participation; and their need for recognition.

A deficit model of youth

Young (1999: 52) suggests that any 'deficit' model pertains to the lack of morals or normative values of individuals, rather than to structural inequalities within society. He cites criminality, in particular, as involving 'a loss and an individualistic response'. It is this individualistic response that puts into question the pertinence of much contemporary youth policy. Many of the authors and postscript contributors in this volume have suggested that policy and practice view young people as being 'in deficit'. Because policy tends to blame young people for their own circumstances, it can thus focus on reducing 'push' factors rather than offering 'pull' factors (see Chapter 2).

Chapter 3 raises the notion of the 'deficient citizen' and Tom Burke, in his postscript to this chapter, questions the validity of such a model: what 'deficiency' actually means and who defines it. The discussion of education policy in Chapter 5 implies a deficit model by seeing education as a means of furnishing young people with skills for the future rather than acknowledging or focusing on their current skills. Chapter 6 also suggests that young people's current skills and responsibilities tend to be ignored by parents, practitioners and employers alike, making it more likely that such young people will internalise and blame themselves for their perceived deficiencies. Youth education and employment schemes (the New Deal being a case in point) are publicised as 'training' young people to be employable in the future, conveniently masking the thorny issue of changed labour market priorities which see young people as surplus to requirements. In Chapter 8, it is argued that youth unemployment is explained by policy makers in

terms of a deficit in labour supply rather than labour demand, and likewise
Cohen (1982: 45, quoted in Muncie 1999: 220), sees many youth training
schemes as tending to 'blame the victim' by representing youth employment
as:

> . . . a problem of faulty supply rather than demand; a failure of the edu-
> cational system rather than capitalism; a personal problem of jobless-
> ness due to lack of motivation, experience or skill, rather than the
> position youth occupies in the market economy.

It is argued by policy makers that increasing young people's skills will solve
the problem; however, there are still no opportunities for them to use those
additional skills. There is a dogmatic culture of blame in relation to young
people that focuses on the individual's deficiencies: for example, in being
unemployed, resorting to drug taking or offending more generally, seeking
asylum or being homeless.

In terms of teenage pregnancy and young motherhood, it is suggested
that policy makers blame young people for inappropriate sexual behaviour
(for their age) rather than supporting young mothers as parents whilst
enabling them to further their careers. Professionals see young people as
unlikely to succeed if they become mothers at a young age, as 17-year-old
Ebele (quoted in Chapter 12) explains: 'That's the automatic stereotype,
like a game of dominoes, you do this, this will happen, this will happen, this
will happen' – and the inference is that 'this' is always negative.

Several chapters in this volume have suggested that young people blame
themselves for 'deficiencies', either seeing themselves as second-class citizens or viewing their current predicament as a result of their own failings
in the past. Indeed, Bates and Riseborough (1993) argue that the social construction of age itself, coupled with the individualisation focus of much
postmodern thinking, has lessened the political relevance of class inequalities and resulted in young people viewing their marginalisation as a
personal problem rather than a public issue.

This self-blame can often become internalised: Annmarie Fraser (Chapter
12) suggests that, in relation to young mothers, 'It has always been drummed
into their heads that they can't do any better' and Tom Burke (Chapter 3)
argues that the criminalisation of young people has meant that many young
people 'have started to believe . . . the hype and propaganda that they are second class'. Young people who do not have encouragement or resources to
succeed may lack aspirations and motivation and it becomes a self-fulfilling
prophecy that they will not succeed. The author of Chapter 9 also suggests
that such self-blame can result in an increased loss of self-esteem and self-
confidence amongst young people. Steven Kidd (Chapter 2) suggests that the
government is now moving away from a 'problem-oriented' deficit model of
youth, although the extent to which there is merely a shift of focus from

young people – to their parents, for example – is a moot point, since the following discussion of discrimination and the criminalisation of youth suggests that the deficit model is still alive and well.

Discrimination

There have been numerous examples in this book of active discrimination of young people by adults, resulting in such discrimination being a major obstacle to young people's quest for social inclusion. In Chapter 3, for example, the different views of adults and young people are highlighted in relation to citizenship, suggesting that adults see young people as wanting rights rather than responsibilities, whereas young people see responsibilities as a greater priority. Adults see young people as apathetic and disengaged and yet many young people are concerned about and constructively engaged in their communities through, for example, voluntary or campaigning activities.

Whilst it is acknowledged that many adults experience discrimination in society, young people tend to be treated as a homogeneous group within much social policy. Chapter 8 highlights discriminatory attitudes to young people in the workplace, through earnings inequalities, whilst Chapter 9 notes that homeless young people are denied access to affordable housing and adequate state benefits. Chapter 11 suggests that increased surveillance and punishment of young offenders is not commensurate with the decrease in the frequency and seriousness of youth offending overall: the prison population rose by 20 per cent since New Labour came to power in 1997, and yet the crime rate fell by some 25 per cent in the same period. Chapter 13 notes that young carers often perform the same tasks as adult carers but are rarely recognised or rewarded for such work.

According to Bromley (1993), an approved role within the wider community can enable one to develop a sense of self-worth and security, whereas a lack of such responsibility can result in increased alienation:

> Failure to establish an approved role in society, through educational failure and unemployment for example, leads some people to suppose that they have little to lose from antisocial behaviour . . . Conversely, people with an established approved role in society have a lot to lose.
> (Bromley, 1993: 62).

Our self-identity, self-esteem and self-confidence are formulated and modelled on others' views of us and, in turn, such views are based on one's ability or otherwise to contribute towards the 'common good'. Passive discrimination could therefore be experienced by young people as a result of feeling ignored or not being acknowledged by professionals for the contributions that they make. The author of Chapter 2 talks of 'status zer0' youth as 'young people who apparently counted for nothing' and Chapter 6 depicts a 'liminal phase' in youth where young people are in a state of limbo between having the protection of childhood and the autonomy of adulthood. Chapter 10 also suggests that young asylum seekers are in limbo whilst awaiting often lengthy decisions on their futures. It is hardly surprising, as the author of Chapter 14 points out, that many young people, as a result of such uncertainties in transition, 'struggle to understand their position in the family and within the wider community'.

The criminalisation of young people

In Chapter 11, it is suggested that youth justice policy could soon offer 'nothing but coercion, surveillance and punishment'; such a description could equally apply to certain youth policy initiatives in other topic areas. Policies can both punish and control young people, but rarely offer encouragement and appropriate support. As Michael Fadipe (Chapter 11) suggests, agencies are often 'nosey' and penalise young people through such intrusive surveillance. Social policy has criminalised young people and set them apart from adult society, thus further exacerbating their social exclusion. As Tom Burke (Chapter 3) suggests, young people's rights to citizenship are being violated through the criminalisation of their attitudes and behaviour.

Several of the postscript contributors – for example, Lindsay Kelly and Jackie Mooney (Chapter 6), Mustajab Malikzada and Ahmad Qadri (Chapter 10), Michael Fadipe and Lance Gittens-Bernard (Chapter 11) and Daniel Raffell (Chapter 14) – also imply that an overemphasis on controlling or penalising young people can be counterproductive, resulting in rebellion or, in asylum terms, 'going underground'. In relation to asylum seekers, for example, it is suggested that there is an overt strategy to criminalise young people by giving them fewer rights and entitlements as a means of deterring others from seeking asylum in the UK. Equally, in the postscript to this chapter, it is further suggested that young asylum seekers are purposefully 'locked up in the legal system' to reduce and delay their opportunities for integration and social inclusion.

Participation

The strong desire of young people for more genuine involvement in decisions that affect their lives and greater respect through having their voices heard has also been highlighted by the postscript contributors. These young people suggest that they should be consulted more systematically and more effectively in order that youth policy is relevant and appropriate to their needs. For example, in relation to opportunities for leisure (Carys Lovering, Chapter 7) and employment (Charlotte Ali, Chapter 8), it is suggested that young people are rarely consulted about what they require: what they want from services and what they receive often seem to them to be incompatible. Without direct involvement in the planning and implementation of services, young people's self-esteem and self-confidence can also suffer and their social exclusion become further exacerbated. Youth policy needs to adopt a more holistic approach in order – as Michael Fadipe (Chapter 11) suggests – to see 'the bigger picture' of young people's circumstances.

The need for recognition

It has been argued here that young people are often denied access to social capital, financial resources, services and opportunities because of their limited status in an age- and power-oriented hierarchy, and therefore have few legitimate means to achieving recognition within society. Many of the postscript contributors mention this lack of recognition for achievements they have made or work they have undertaken in the past. The valuable work of young carers is an obvious example of this. Many of the young people in this book have been involved in voluntary activities which have furnished them with skills and knowledge, but they often feel that this experience holds little sway with, for example, potential employers. Equally, when they do find paid work, their remuneration is often less than that given to adults who do the same tasks.

Thus, young people may take on varying levels of responsibility, not always commensurate with their age. However, because they are deemed to be 'growing up' rather than 'grown up', such responsibilities are often underplayed or undervalued. Taking on responsibility on its own, therefore, is not sufficient for social inclusion, contrary to much government rhetoric on citizenship. What is needed is a reciprocal relationship between adults and young people, where young people's contribution is acknowledged, valued and respected. According to Sennett (2003: 219), 'reciprocity is the foundation of mutual respect', but unless young people are treated on a par with others in society, such mutual respect will not be forthcoming.

Prioritising young people

The majority of the chapter authors and postscript contributors in this volume have noted that young people generally are not a political priority, although they gain a disproportionate amount of political attention. Young people, because of their lack of power and status as voters, taxpayers or citizens, are an ideal scapegoat for governments intent on being seen to implement innovative policies but in reality merely maintaining the status quo of older, more privileged members of society. As is argued in Chapter 4, 'there are no votes in prioritising children or youth', but nevertheless, young people bear the brunt of much of the rhetoric within government initiatives.

It was suggested in the Preface to this book that the situation for young people today within youth policy could be seen as institutionalised 'ageism'. However, ageism is not a term usually applied to people at the younger end of the age spectrum. Thompson (1993) cites two definitions of ageism, both of which apply to older people. One by Fennell *et al* (1988: 97) sees ageism as 'unwarranted application of negative stereotypes to older people' and the other, by Butler (1975: 12), suggests that ageism 'makes it easier to ignore the frequently poor social and economic plight of older people . . . that our productivity-minded society has little use for non-producers . . . those who have reached an arbitrarily defined retirement age'. Without detracting from the justifiable condemnation of ageist policies and practice relating to older people, it could be argued that young people also often share similar experiences of discrimination and prejudice. Scraton (1997: 186) notes, in relation to children, that:

> adult power . . . is a power readily and systematically abused. It is a dangerous and debilitating power, capable of stunting the personal development and potential of even the most resilient children. . . . What is so difficult for adults, as the power-brokers, to accept is that the 'crisis' is not one of 'childhood' but one of 'adultism'.

Social policy has traditionally been seen as 'an ostensibly progressive series of social arrangements concerned with the distribution of resources in order to meet individual and social needs' (Muncie 1999: 207). However, it has increasingly become less concerned with needs and more concerned with control. It could be argued that youth policy has become more reactive than proactive and has increasingly been driven by a concern by better-off adult members of society to maintain the status quo at the expense of giving priority to the development of opportunities for more marginalised younger members of society.

The academic contributions in this book have raised as many questions as they have answered about the issues for young people in relation to social inclusion. Many of these same questions have been critically examined by young people themselves in the postscripts to each chapter. Whilst the book as a whole cannot claim to resolve or alleviate the problems facing young people in our society, it has highlighted their needs and wishes and the barriers they face as they move into adulthood. What is needed in youth policy in the future to ensure young people's social inclusion is a greater emphasis by those in power on acknowledging the needs and priorities of young people, creating a sea change in the ways in which young people's status is viewed by adults and offering young people genuine opportunities for participation more widely within society.

References

Barry, M. (2004) *Understanding Youth Offending: In search of 'social recognition'*, unpublished PhD thesis, Stirling: University of Stirling.

Bates, I. and Riseborough, G. (1993) *Youth and Inequality*, Buckingham: Open University Press.

Bromley, D. (1993) *Reputation, Image and Impression Management*, Chichester: Wiley.

Jeffs, T. and Smith, M. (1996) 'Getting the dirtbags off the streets – curfews and other solutions to juvenile crime' *Youth and Policy*, No. 53: 1–14.

Muncie, J. (1999) *Youth and Crime: A critical introduction*, London: Sage.

Musgrove, F. (1964) *Youth and the Social Order*, London: Routledge and Kegan Paul.

Scraton, P. (1997) 'Whose "childhood"? What "crisis"?', in P. Scraton (ed.), *Childhood in 'Crisis'?*, London: UCL Press.

Sennett, R. (2003) *Respect: The formation of character in a world of inequality*, London: Allen Lane.

Tajfel, H. (1982) *Social Identity and Intergroup Relations*, Cambridge: Cambridge University Press.

Thompson, N. (1993) *Anti-Discriminatory Practice*, Basingstoke: Macmillan.

Wyn, J. and White, R. (1997) *Rethinking Youth*, London: Sage.

Young, J. (1999) *The Exclusive Society*, London: Sage.

Index

abortion 237

abuse *see* domestic violence; emotional abuse; sexual exploitation and abuse; substance abuse

accessibility: leisure activities 134; New Deal for Young People 146; publicity on services 30, 296–7; substance abuse treatment and services 277–9, 282, 290, 291–2, 295

actor network theory (ANT) 73, 76–7, 85, 87

addiction *see* substance abuse

Addiction Severity Index (ASI-X) 277

adoption and teenage mothers 235, 237

Adult Learning Grant 178

adulthood as transitional phase 97, 99–100, 114, 115–16; barriers to reaching 102–8, 109; desire for adult status 2–3, 127; and employment status 100, 105–6, 143, 158; young carers 104–5, 257–9; young mothers 106–7, 238–40, 243, 249

adults as threat to young people 128

Advisory Council on the Misuse of Drugs 276

advocacy: and rights 66; for young homeless 172

age: adverse effects of asylum policy 206–8; *see also* ageism; youth transitions

Age of Legal Capacity Act (1991) 278

ageism 3, 109, 114, 299–300, 301, 302

agency: structure–agency boundary 73, 76; young carers 252

Ainley, P. 99

alcohol abuse 273, 275; drinking culture 119–20; family influences 276; specialist treatment services 277–9, 282

Aldridge, J. 254, 256, 260

All-Wales Youth Offending Strategy 16

Allen, R. 222

amphetamine abuse 273, 280

ANT (actor network theory) 73, 76–7, 85, 87

Anti-Social Behaviour Orders 52, 212, 214

apprenticeships 162–3; modern apprenticeships 178

Aries, P. 98

Asians: British Asian identity 37

ASMA categorisations 275

asylum seekers and refugees 187–201, 300; asylum continuum 188–90; asylum policy 192–3; dispersal policy 191; hostility towards 37, 195, 198–9, 296; policy impacts 192–200, 206–7; right to protection 65; statistics on applications 190–1; use of terms 188; young people's perspective 205–9

attitudes *see* public attitudes

Auld, J. 272

authoritarianism: 'new authoritarianism' 15

autonomy and rights 62–3

'bad' citizenship 39–40, 41–2, 45

Balding, J. 273

Ball, J. 271

Bandman, B. 56–7

Barnard, M. 273

Barry, M. 97

Bates, I. 298

Beattie Report 88

NORTHERN COLLEGE LIBRARY
77076 BARNSLEY S75 3ET